Evolving Psychosis

Evolving Psychosis explores the success of psycho-social treatments for psychosis in helping patients recover more quickly and stay well longer.

Mental health professionals from all over the world share their clinical experience and scientific findings to shed new light on the issues surrounding need-specific treatment. They cover the nature of psychosis, early intervention in psychosis, phase-specific treatment of psychosis and the need for integration. Particular attention is paid to how the treatment can be improved with individually tailored treatment programmes, early intervention, more integration between psychological treatments, and new and better diagnostic concepts.

This book incorporates new and controversial ideas that will stimulate discussion regarding the benefits of early, need-adapted treatment. It will be of interest to psychologists, psychiatrists and other mental health professionals interested in psycho-social approaches to psychosis.

Jan Olav Johannessen is Chief Psychiatrist of the Division of Psychiatry, Stavanger University Hospital in Norway and President of the ISPS.

Brian V. Martindale is on the board of the ISPS, is Chair of the ISPS UK network and Editor of the ISPS books.

Johan Cullberg leads a national multi-centre research project on integrated treatments in first-episode psychosis. He is author of *Psychoses*, also published as part of the ISPS book series.

The International Society for the Psychological Treatments of the Schizophrenias and Other Psychoses Book Series

Series editor: Brian Martindale

The ISPS (The International Society for the Psychological Treatments of the Schizophrenias and Other Psychoses) has a history stretching back some 50 years, during which it has witnessed the relentless pursuit of biological explanations for psychosis. The tide is now turning again. There is a welcome international resurgence in interest in a range of psychological factors in psychosis that have considerable explanatory power and also distinct therapeutic possibilities. Governments, professional groups, users and carers are increasingly expecting interventions that involve talking and listening as well as skilled practitioners in the main psychotherapeutic modalities as important components of the care of the seriously mentally ill.

The ISPS is a global society. It is composed of an increasing number of groups of professionals organized at national, regional and more local levels around the world. The society has started a range of activities intended to support professionals, users and carers. Such persons recognize the humanitarian and therapeutic potential of skilled psychological understanding and therapy in the field of psychosis. Our members cover a wide spectrum of interests from psychodynamic, systemic, cognitive and arts therapies to the need-adaptive approaches and to therapeutic institutions. We are most interested in establishing meaningful dialogue with those practitioners and researchers who are more familiar with biological-based approaches. Our activities include regular international and national conferences, newsletters and email discussion groups in many countries across the world.

One of these activities is to facilitate the publication of quality books that cover the wide terrain that interests ISPS members and a large number of other mental health professionals, policy makers and implementers. We are delighted that Routledge of the Taylor & Francis group has seen the importance and potential of such an endeavour and have agreed to publish an ISPS series of books.

We anticipate that some of the books will be controversial and will challenge certain aspects of current practice in some countries. Other books will promote ideas and authors well known in some countries but not familiar to others. Our overall aim is to encourage the dissemination of existing knowledge and ideas, promote healthy debate and encourage more research in a most important field whose secrets almost certainly do not all reside in the neurosciences.

For more information about the ISPS, email isps@isps.org or visit our website www.isps.org

Evolving Psychosis

Different stages, different treatments

Edited by Jan Olav Johannessen,
Brian V. Martindale and
Johan Cullberg

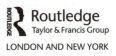

Routledge
Taylor & Francis Group

LONDON AND NEW YORK

First published 2006
by Routledge
27 Church Road, Hove, East Sussex BN3 2FA

Simultaneously published in the USA and Canada
by Routledge
270 Madison Avenue New York, NY 10016

Reprinted 2006

Routledge is an imprint of the Taylor & Francis Group, an informa business

Typeset in Times by RefineCatch Ltd, Bungay, Suffolk
Printed and bound in Great Britain by
TJ International Ltd, Padstow, Cornwall
Paperback cover design by Hybert Design

This publication has been produced with paper manufactured to
strict environmental standards and with pulp derived from
sustainable forests.

British Library Cataloguing in Publication Data
A catalogue record for this book is available from the British Library

Library of Congress Cataloging-in-Publication Data
Evolving psychosis : different stages, different treatments / edited by
Jan Olav Johannessen, Brian V. Martindale, Johan Cullberg.
      p. cm.
   Includes bibliographical references and index.
   ISBN 1-58391-722-5 (hbk.) – ISBN 1-58391-723-3 (pbk.)
   1. Psychoses – Treatment.   2. Psychoses – Prognosis.
      3. Psychoses – Prevention.   I. Johannessen, Jan Olav.
   II. Martindale, Brian.   III. Cullberg, Johan, 1934–
   RC512.E95 2006
   616.89–dc22
                                             2005053669

ISBN13: 978-1-58391-722-0 (hbk)
ISBN13: 978-1-58391-723-7 (pbk)

ISBN10: 1-58391-722-5 (hbk)
ISBN10: 1-58391-723-3 (pbk)

Contents

PART II

Early intervention in psychosis   79

PART III

Phase-specific treatment of psychosis   161

List of tables and figures

Editors' bibliographies

Jan Olav Johannessen has been President of the ISPS since 2000 (www.isps.org) and is a member of the board of the International Early Psychoses Association (iepa@vicnet.net.au). He is Chief Psychiatrist of the Division of Psychiatry, Stavanger University Hospital, Norway. A trained psychotherapist and member of the Norwegian Institute of Psychotherapy, he has a special interest in working psychotherapeutically with young first-episode psychosis patients. He has participated in the development of early intervention strategies nationally and internationally, and is one of the driving forces behind the Scandinavian multi-centre TIPS project (www.tips-info.com). He has published numerous papers on early intervention, epidemiology, quality indicators, antistigma, etc., and has contributed to and edited several scientific and popular books on these and related themes.

Brian V. Martindale is on the board of ISPS, is Chair of the ISPS UK network and Editor of ISPS books. He is currently Western European Zone Representative of Psychiatry for the World Psychiatric Association and on the Board of International Affairs of the Royal College of Psychiatrists. He is Honorary President and former Chair of the European Federation of Psychoanalytic Psychotherapy and is currently head of the Department of Psychotherapy in Ealing, London, and a psychoanalyst. Amongst his publications, he edited the ISPS book *Psychosis: Psychological Approaches and their Effectiveness* (Gaskell 2000).

Johan Cullberg, since his retirement in 2000, has been working as the leader of a national multi-centre research project on integrated treatments in first-episode psychoses. He is also a supervisor of several new clinical psychosis projects and lectures internationally. He was President of ISPS from 1990 to 1996, and his main scientific writing is in social psychiatry, psychoendochrinology, and psychotherapy of psychosis.

Editors and contributors

Donald Addington
Professor and Chair, Department of Psychiatry, University of Calgary, Foothills Medical Centre, 1403 29th Street, NW, Calgary, Alberta, T2N2T9, Canada

Jean Addington
Associate Professor, Department of Psychiatry, University of Calgary, Foothills Medical Centre, 1403 29th Street, NW, Calgary, Alberta, T2N2T9, Canada

Hilary Beard
South London and Maudsley NHS Trust, Department of Psychotherapy, St. Thomas' Hospital, London SE1 7EH, UK

Paul C. Bermanzohn
Psychiatrist, Dutchess County (New York) ACT Team, 4 Jefferson Plaza, Suite 4, Poughkeepsie, NY 12601, USA

Louise Bywood PhD Student
University of Lincoln, Brayford Pool, Lincoln LN6 7TS, UK

Valerie Crowley
Consultant Clinical Psychologist and CAT Therapist, Learning Disability Services Brooklands Hospital, Coleshill Road, Marston Green, Birmingham, West Midlands B37 7HL, UK

Johan Cullberg
Anders Reimers Vag 17, 117 50 S-11750 Stockholm, Sweden

Peter Elwood
Consultant Psychiatrist, The Peter Godgkinson Centre, Lincolnshire Healthcare NHS Trust, Greetwell Road, Lincoln LN2 5UA, UK

David M. Gresswell
Consultant Clinical/Forensic Psychologist, The Francis Willis Unit, The Peter Hodgkinson Centre, Lincolnshire Healthcare NHS Trust, Greetwell Road, Lincoln LN2 5UA, UK

Paul Hammersley MSc, RMN
Department of Psychology, University of Manchester, Oxford Road, Manchester M13 9PL, UK

Susan M. Hingley
Consultant Clinical Psychologist, Clinical Tutor for Psychological Services, St Aidans House, 2a St Aidans Walk, Bishop Auckland, Co. Durham DL14 6SA, UK

Jan Olav Johannessen
Chief Psychiatrist, Stavanger University Hospital, Division of Psychiatry, Postboks 1163 Hillevåg, 4004 Stavanger, Norway

Ian B. Kerr
Consultant Psychiatrist and Psychotherapist, Sheffield Care Trust, Sheffield S10 3TH, and Hon. Sen. Lecturer, School of Health and Associated Research, Sheffield University, UK

Joachim Klosterkötter
Professor and Director, University of Cologne, Department of Psychiatry and Psychotherapy, 50924 Cologne, Germany

Susan E. Mason PhD
Wurzweiler School of Social Work, Yeshiva University, 2495 Amsterdam Avenue, New York, 10033, USA

Patrick D. McGorry MBBS, PhD
Professor and Director, Early Psychosis Prevention and Intervention Centre (EPPIC)/Mental Health Services for Kids and Youth, and Department of Psychiatry, University of Melbourne, 35 Poplar Road, Parkville, Victoria 3052, Australia

Rachel Miller CSW
Hillside Hospital of the North Shore, Long Island Jewish Health System, Glen Oaks, New York, USA

John Read
Director of Clinical Psychology, Senior Lecturer, Department of Psychology, University of Auckland, Private Bag 92019, Auckland, New Zealand

Bjørn Rishovd Rund
Professor of Psychology/Head of Department, Institute of Psychology, University of Oslo, Box 1094 Blindern, 0317 Oslo, Norway

Colin Robertson
Senior Lecturer in Psychology, University of Lincoln, Brayford Pool, Lincoln LN6 7TS, UK

Bent Rosenbaum
Chief Psychiatrist and Consultant Psychotherapist, Unit for Psychotherapy

Education and Research, Department of Psychiatry, Copenhagen County University Hospital, Nedre Ringvej, 2600 Glostrup, Denmark

Colin A. Ross
President, Institute for Psychological Trauma, 1701 Gateway, Suite 349, Richardson, TX 75080, USA

Stephan Ruhrmann
Medical Head of University of Cologne, Department of Psychiatry and Psychotherapy, 50924 Cologne, Germany

Frauke Schultze-Lutter PhD
Scientific-Psychological Head of the Early Recognition and Intervention Centre, FETZ, University of Cologne, Department of Psychiatry and Psychotherapy, 50924 Cologne, Germany

Ann-Louise S. Silver MD
President, USA Chapter of ISPS, 4966 Reedy Brook Lane, Columbia, MD 21044–1514, USA

Erik Simonsen MD
Medical Director, Fjorden County Hospital, Smedegade 10–16, 4000 Roskilde, Denmark

Lars Thorgaard
Consultant Psychiatrist, Psychotherapist and Supervisor, Department of Psychiatry, Herning Hospital, gl. Landevej, 7400 Herning, Denmark

Wilfried Ver Eecke
Professor of Philosophy and Adjunct-Professor of Psychology, Georgetown University, Department of Philosophy, Washington, DC 20057, USA

Foreword

Schizophrenia and related psychotic states have been at the center of interest for much of psychiatry ever since the discipline came into existence. The psychotic states and the schizophrenic syndrome in particular – paradigmatic for severe mental disorder – have been described in great detail, their frequency studied in many countries and their development examined using qualitative and quantitative methods.

The treatment of psychotic states over the past two hundred years is marked by an extraordinary diversity of methods sometimes based on a theory, sometimes on analogies and single observations and sometimes on no more than doctors' and healers' instincts. People with schizophrenia and other psychotic states similar to it have been placed under extreme physical stress, exposed to exclusively psychoanalytic approaches, made comatose, injected with substances that produced fits, given electro-convulsive therapy, forced to take medications, isolated from people and all other stimuli, and given acupuncture and unusual diets.

And there were major areas of neglect, in terms of theoretical development and in terms of treatment practices. Among them were the harmonization of treatment modalities with stages of the illness; the utilization of information about the disease and outcome of treatment obtained from the person who was suffering from it, both in planning treatment and in evaluating it; the need to combine therapeutical approaches (often based on different theories) in treating psychotic states and in preventing psychotic breakdowns or relapses; the imperative need to individualize treatment and tailor it with regard to the patient, the doctor, the environment and the stage of illness; and above all how to ensure that the treatment is based on mutual respect between patient and the person dealing with treatment.

The authors assembled by Drs Johannessen, Martindale and Cullberg address the above areas with competence and vigor. This in itself would be sufficient to recommend the book to psychiatrists and other mental health workers: what is more, the volume is being published at a time when the insights the authors and editors provide are more important than ever before. New treatment modalities, including in particular an ever-increasing number of powerful medications, new theories and practices of rehabilitation, new diagnostic methods and techniques for the examination of the functions of the brain – and also new social and economic pressures on the health system – make it necessary to construct a modern doctrine of dealing with psychotic states. This timely and highly interesting volume makes a valuable contribution to this goal

Professor Norman Sartorius

Preface

There is growing recognition internationally that in the western world the range of treatments offered to people suffering from a psychotic disorder is nowhere near the optimum, which could be provided if sufficient resources were made available.

Evidence exists that comprehensive treatment models which include psychosocial treatment modalities, especially different types of psychotherapeutically-oriented therapies, help patients to recover more quickly and to stay well longer.

It should be every patient's right to be able to narrate his or her unabridged story, and to engage in a therapeutic relationship that is based on both professional skills and a deep respect for the patient as a unique human being, rather than as a biochemical disorder.

The therapy offered should be adapted to each individual's specific needs, with emphasis on adapting to different needs as the therapy progresses.

Nowadays, treatment is often initiated too late in the development of the illness: in most western countries professional help starts two or three years after the psychosis has started. Much of this thinking lay behind the international conference *Schizophrenia and Other Psychoses: Different Stages – Different Treatments?* held in Stavanger, Norway, in 2000.

In this book we present the work of mental health professionals from all over the world who, from different perspectives and different angles, share their clinical experience and scientific findings and shed new light on what we call 'need-specific treatment'. The treatment of first-episode psychosis receives special attention, as it is perhaps the most important phase both in the development of psychotic disorders and in research and further development of clinical methods, especially in psychologically-based treatment possibilities.

In this book we focus on the following:

- The need for individually tailored treatment programmes in psychosis.
- The effectiveness of a broad spectrum of psychological treatments.
- The need for early intervention.

- The need for the development of better integration between some of the most important psychological treatments, such as psychodynamic and cognitive-behaviour therapies.
- The need for new and better diagnostic concepts.

It is also our hope that, after reading this book, the reader will be inspired to make available a broader range of psychologically-based therapeutic tools and strategies that will, in turn, provide a better future for patients suffering from psychotic disorders.

Acknowledgements

First, I would like to express my gratitude to my co-editors Brian Martindale and Johan Cullberg for their valuable help in getting this book together. Without their enthusiasm and experience this book would probably not have surfaced. Brian, being the editor of and driving force behind the ISPS book series, deserves a special thanks for his never-ending optimism and energy.

The members of the board of ISPS also deserve warm thanks for their support.

I would like to thank Catherine Noraas, my secretary, for her help and skill with the practical aspects of bringing into reality a book with more than 20 contributors from all over the world. This is not the easiest of jobs. Not every workplace would allow their chief psychiatrist to be engaged in putting a book together when so many other tasks need to be dealt with. I owe great thanks therefore to my colleagues in the Division of Psychiatry, Stavanger University Hospital, for their inspiration and support, and a special thanks to my boss, Inger Kari Nerheim, for the way she always accepts and supports my work.

Finally, my wife Kristin receives my warmest thanks for the way in which she has supported the work that was involved in this book, as well as all the other tasks her husband inevitably seems to get involved with.

Jan Olav Johannessen
Senior Editor

Introduction

Evolving psychosis: Different stages, different treatments

Jan Olav Johannessen, Brian V. Martindale and Johan Cullberg

This book has come about because it has long been the impression of the editors and many clinicians that there are considerable differences between different stages in the course of psychotic disturbances. Foremost amongst these differences is that it is often easier to understand, reason with, and be with patients with a first-episode psychosis than those with a longer-standing and well established pattern of psychosis.

Psychological treatments are a threatened 'species' in today's health services, which are often dictated by short-term economic considerations and are vulnerable to the marketing strategies of large pharmaceutical companies. A place and space for the more long-lasting psychotherapeutic approaches, such as psychodynamically-oriented psychotherapies, has been hard to defend. Moreover, the statistical measurements used in natural sciences approaches are difficult to apply when demonstrating the effectiveness and cost-effectiveness of such treatments, partly because of difficulties in operationalising the goals.

In addition, most research projects in the field of schizophrenia research has tended to collapse all cases, whether first-episode or multi-episode cases, into a single category. Contemporary research focusing on the first episode is giving us a better basis for understanding the process of becoming psychotic and the ways of relieving it.

In a recent special issue of the *Journal of the American Academy of Psychoanalysis and Dynamic Psychiatry* (2003) focusing on 'The schizophrenic person and the benefits of the psychotherapies', the effectiveness of psychological treatments is clearly demonstrated. Numerous recent projects demonstrate the effectiveness of cognitive-behavioural therapeutic approaches (CBT), in which the procedures are more stringent and the outcomes more clearly defined and measurable than in most psychodynamic approaches.

However, we must not fool ourselves into thinking that we have found *the* psychological treatment for people suffering from psychosis, and fall for the 'zeitgeist' of today. Psychological treatment models draw on rich philosophical, psychological, socio-anthropological and biological traditions from Kant, Nietzsche, Heidegger, Freud, Fromm and Lacan. Indeed it would be easy to fill a book with historical texts, many of which can still contribute richly to the understanding of the human experience of psychosis today.

The idea of phase-specific treatments with its derivative early intervention strategies has its own complex history. The editors of this volume are especially well acquainted with the Scandinavian and Anglo-American traditions which will be explored in some detail. Harry Stack Sullivan pointed out back in 1927 that 'the psychiatrist sees too many end states and deals professionally with too few of the pre-psychotic' (Sullivan 1927: 127). In 1955 Lewis B. Hill stated in his book *Psychotherapeutic Intervention in Schizophrenia* that if 'the crisis is badly treated or is neglected, then the liability to chronic disabling illness is vastly increased. It is quite possible that the thousands of patients in state hospitals diagnosed as chronic undifferentiated schizophrenics are, in fact, the results of inadequately treated acute schizophrenia.' The work of D. E. Cameron (1938), Heinz Häfner (1992) and others has pointed to the possibility of influencing the long-term course through early interventions and thus improving the opportunities for recovery.

Pioneering work developing phase-specific strategies took place in Finland in the 1970s and 1980s. Veikko Tähkä published several books and articles on the theme 'Psychotherapy as a phase-specific interaction: towards a general psychoanalytic theory of psychotherapy'. He suggests that it is legitimate to state that there are therapeutic applications of psychoanalytic theory not only for the treatment of neurosis but also for more severe levels of pathology. However, he clearly indicates that this does not mean widening the scope of application of the classical technique to the treatment of personality disturbances (for which it has not been developed). What it does mean is the application of analytic knowledge to patients who represent earlier and more extensive disturbances of personality development than neurotic patients do, and who therefore also benefit from other aspects of the therapeutic interaction. Tähkä states that there are three levels of pathology: psychoses, borderline states and neuroses. He finds prestructural disturbances in object relations to be treatable, but he thinks it is questionable whether they are analysable. Tähkä further says:

> The analytic as well as any other psychotherapeutic situation tends to become structured so that the patient repeats his/her developmental disturbance in his/her relationship to the therapist, and the therapist on his/her part tries to understand the nature of the patient's phase-specific messages. The immediate goal in working with a psychotic patient must always be to try to restore the patient's sense of reality, and the phase-specific curative factor in the treatment of psychoses seems to be gratification.
>
> (Tähkä 1979: 125)

He sums up by saying that 'for the psychotic patient we have to become an object, for the borderline patient we have to act as an object, and finally, for the neurotic patient we have to liberate the patient from an object which has become superfluous' (131).

J. P. Docherty and colleagues, in their article 'Stages of Onset of Schizophrenic Psychosis' (1978), point to the fact that, almost without exemption, it is possible to describe a process of progressive decline in patients leading up to a psychotic decompensation. This gives us important reasons for wanting to know more about the period of onset of schizophrenic psychoses:

1   For preventive psychiatry – giving us the possibility of reliable early recognition and of staging the degree of psychological and biological decompensation
2   It gives us the possibility of providing stage-appropriate treatment
3   It could give us clues to pathogenesis.

Docherty *et al.* describe the following stages of decompensation (with our elaboration in brackets):

0   Equilibrium (psychological equilibrium)
1   Overextension (becoming psychologically overwhelmed/stressed)
2   Restricted consciousness (referring to attempts to defend against the stress, by psychologically shutting down)
3   Disinhibition (beginnings of a disregard for reality/unmodulated impulse expression begins)
4   Psychotic disorganisation
   a   destructuring of the external world disregarding/distorting painful realities
   b   destructuring of the self disregarding/distorting painful aspects and experiences
   c   total fragmentation
5   Psychological resolution (this period is marked by decreased anxiety and the organisation/consolidation of a psychotic state).

It is important to notice the temporal duration of each of the stages and try to understand the fundamental psychological and biological axes along which decompensation occurs. Docherty *et al.* (1978: 420) state that 'schizophrenic psychosis is one stage in the process of psychological and biological breakdown that has a specific structure and a characteristic unfolding. This structure consists of the sequential appearance of hierarchically ordered distinguishable and recognisable psychological stages.'

Yrjö Alanen, also from Finland, represents the best of the Finnish and Scandinavian tradition in the treatment of psychotic disorders. Alanen (1997) claims that deficient individuation (sense of self) is the most defining psychological feature that characterises schizophrenia-prone individuals, and that disorders of the self/other relationships which contribute to vulnerability to schizophrenia seem to have dissimilar mutual weighting in different cases. He further claims that schizophrenia can be conceived of as the deepest and, hence, the most tragic solution to the problems of human life. Building on Ciompi *et al.* (1982), Alanen underlines the importance of the biological and psychosocial risk factors that contribute to this inadequate psychological individuation. This leads to a tendency to withdrawal and/or excessive dependency, and to failure in the developmental task of becoming an adult. In due course, this results in narcissistic traumata, experiences of loss, in some cases physical stress or the use of drugs, anxiety, panic, resorting to substance abuse, and a loss of grip on the surrounding social reality. Breakdown of the integrity of psychological functions, especially the loss of reality-testing capacities, leads to acutely or gradually developing psychotic states. Alanen thus builds the rationale for a need-adapted treatment of patients with psychoses. He widens the scope from *phase-specific* to *need-specific*, emphasising that there is a manifest heterogeneity within the group of patients called schizophrenic, something that is obvious at the clinical level. Therefore, just as symptoms differ greatly from one patient to another, so also do their therapeutic needs. Alanen underlines that the treatment approach to schizophrenia must be based on case-specific premises, especially with regard to both individual and interactional factors. Alanen's Turku group uses psychoeducational principles in combination with medication and family intervention techniques, as well as individual psychotherapy. According to Alanen, 50% of an unselected group of first admission patients with schizophrenia were without any psychotic symptoms at five-year follow-up when provided with sufficient psychotherapy. The Finnish approach combines different forms of treatment in a flexible way, tailored individually to take into account both the patient's and the family's needs. From the very beginning, the emphasis should be on the establishment of psychological contact with the patient. In the experience of Alanen and his colleagues, many schizophrenic psychotherapy patients manage well without any medication in the later stages of their therapy. Alanen's model is outlined in Figure 1.

One such tool for establishing the treatment of both new and recurrent psychotic patients is to form acute psychosis teams. This is the equivalent of assertive outreach teams or a particular form of community-based mental health team. Alanen (1997: 51) summarises the Finnish tradition as a 'hermeneutic approach, that is, a psychological understanding of problems and the therapeutic situation, and action based on this understanding.' Alanen underlines that the treatment is a process during which the needs may change.

McGlashan and Keats, in their book *Schizophrenia Treatment Process and Outcome* (1989), offer other examples of how the treatment, in this case psychotherapy, should be adapted to each patient's maturational levels and relationship complexity.

From a milieu therapeutic point of view, Gunderson (1978) outlines the

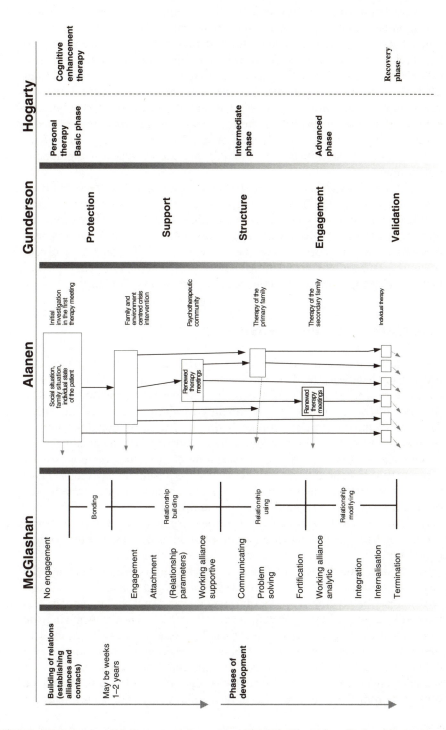

Figure 0.1 Examples of phase-specific approaches.

five most important functions defining the therapeutic processes in psychological milieus as: containment, support, structure, involvement and validation. These functional variables 'reflect operations or processes provided by the staff that are recognisable largely by their effects on the patients' (Gunderson 1978: 327). They exist as un-asked-for potentials or conditions available to be used by patients. As such they have greater relevance to the values and purposes of the therapists than to those likely to be articulated by patients. It should be understood from the start that no single type of therapeutic activity is ideal for all patients or at all times for any given patient. Moreover, no single milieu can optimally provide all types of therapeutic functioning.

Hogarty and his colleagues have developed a model called 'personal therapy' (Hogarty *et al.* 1997). This is a three-stage systematic approach in recognition of the sensitivity of many schizophrenic patients. They stress an important but often neglected fact that it makes no sense to provide advanced psychotherapy for people whose basic needs for food, housing, a decent economy or meaningful occupation are not met. This aspect is often neglected in psychotherapy research, as is the need for long-term follow-up.

THE NATURE OF PSYCHOSIS

We think that the treatment offered to patients suffering from psychotic disorders usually reflects the therapist's underlying assumptions about the basic nature of psychosis. The aim of this book is to expand on the prevalent idea that psychiatric disorders in general and psychosis especially are either dimensional disorders or categorical disorders. The dimensional perspective regards psychosis as a disorder gradually developing from 'normality', with psychological defence mechanisms becoming eroded until there is loss of capacity to withstand internal and external stress, resulting in psychosis. This is also reflected in the so-called 'stress-vulnerability model' which was originally a psychological model (Zubin and Spring 1977).

In Europe today the prevailing view is the German concept of *Einheitspsuchosen* which reflects this dimensional way of looking upon psychotic disorders (Crow 1990).

For a long time, Patrick McGorry of Australia has been advocating the necessity of providing rapid and effective treatment in the very early phases of psychosis, based on just such a dimensional viewpoint. In his chapter 'The Recognition and Optimal Management of Early Psychosis: Applying the Concept of Staging in the Treatment of Psychosis' he argues that even in the very early stages the treatment must be need-adapted, and that it will differ from individual to individual. In particular, he emphasises that the special clinical needs of young people at this phase of illness should be protected from the iatrogenic effects of standard care. The clinical care of first-episode and recent-onset patients must be organised separately from that of chronic patients. A key issue to be addressed is the common prolonged delay in accessing effective treatment (Edwards and McGorry 2002, Johannessen *et al.* 2001). This delay often results in treatment starting in the context of severe behavioural crisis, with crude, typically traumatic and alienating initial treatment strategies and subsequently poor continuity of care and engagement of the patient with the treatment.

The key elements/foci of management in first-episode psychosis are summarised as follows by McGorry:

1   Easy access and early engagement
2   Full assessment
3   Prompt treatment
4   The nature of the attention during the recovery phase.

The term 'the critical period' (Birchwood 1999) refers to the phase of maximum vulnerability to further episodes, and covers the period following recovery from a first episode of psychosis to up to five years subsequently.

In the next chapter, Erik Simonsen from Denmark deals with the very difficult connection between personality and psychosis. Research offers only a limited number of unambiguous answers about its nature. He outlines three different ways in which it could be considered: the disposition or vulnerability model, the pathoplastic model where personality/psychosis is integrated, and the complication model which understands schizophrenia and personality disorders as two different and independent constructs. Simonsen stresses that our understanding of the interface of personality and psychosis is still mainly built upon sophisticated clinical observations and speculations, and that little is based on clinical research. It is also important to remember that many people with schizophrenia have a normal personality. He concludes that the extreme heterogeneity of schizophrenia, its symptoms and its outcome, call for a model that is open to different combinations of factors.

The American Wilfried Ver Eecke provides an in-depth analysis based on the work of Alphonse De Waelhens. De Waelhens understands schizophrenia as the result of a disturbance in a triangular structure in which each of the three angles (maternal figure, paternal figure and child) can play a role. This explanation concentrates upon the desire (as opposed to the behaviour) of the mother, and begins its analysis of the influence of the maternal figure from the period of pregnancy (and not just from the period after birth). After outlining De Waelhens' theoretical contributions, Ver Eecke points to disturbances in very early interpersonal relationships. In his chapter he makes reference to Lacan, Searles, Karon and Van den Bos, Silver, Fromm-Reichmann, Davoine, Gaudrilliere, Pankow, Benedetti and others who have made significant contributions to the field.

In 'Schizophrenia: Pathogenesis and Therapy', Lars Thorgaard and Bent

Rosenbaum from Denmark illustrate the importance of establishing and maintaining an empathic understanding of 'psychic reality' in persons suffering from schizophrenia. The degree of empathy will be crucial to the models we develop about pathogenesis and therapy. They claim that empathy is found to be lacking in many models. They show that established therapeutic practice and diagnostic thinking (according to DSM and ICD) lack this important dimension, and that supplementing this dimension will be of invaluable help in understanding people who suffer from schizophrenia. They 're-classify' schizophrenia as :

1   A separation/attachment disorder
2   A distrust/loss of trust disorder
3   A relation disorder
4   An identity disorder
5   A paroxysmal and relapse disorder
6   A control and loss of control disorder
7   A self-care-failing/care-failing disorder.

EARLY INTERVENTION IN PSYCHOSIS

In the fifth chapter 'A Behavioural Versus a Cognitive Analysis of the Relapse Prodrome in Psychosis', our colleagues from the UK, Louise Bywood, Colin Robertson, David Gresswell and Peter Elwood, challenge Birchwood and Macmillan's (1993) theory of the relapse signature. They provide evidence to illustrate that the same sequential prodromal pattern does not necessarily herald each psychotic breakdown, in contrary to Birchwood and Macmillan's theory that an individual's early/prodromal signs of psychosis are generally stable from relapse to relapse and follow a predictable temporal pattern. Using multiple sequential functional analysis (MSFA), an in-depth qualitative case history methodology, evidence has been found to support the argument that the relapse prodrome is developmental in nature. Bywood and her colleagues present case study extracts to illustrate their findings. MSFA can also be used to design individual treatment packages and create more opportunities for clinicians to implement early intervention strategies to ameliorate a psychotic breakdown.

In the following chapter Frauke Schultze-Lutter, Stephan Ruhrmann and Joachim Klosterkötter from Germany discuss whether schizophrenia can be predicted phenomenologically. Attenuated and transient psychotic symptoms or a combination of risk factor and functional loss are widely used in research for early detection and intervention in psychosis. The authors present an alternative approach: the basic symptom concept. In the Cologne Early Recognition (CER) project, out of two predictive constellations of ten, nine cognitive perceptive basic symptoms per constellation were identified using different methodological procedures and were compared for their prospective accuracy. Both constellations possessed excellent predictive accuracy overall, but Schultze-Lutter *et al.* warn us that their application must be guided by considerations of the potential harm of treatment on one hand and by the apparent imminence of psychosis on the other.

Jean and Donald Addington from Canada describe a phase-specific group treatment for recovery in an early psychosis programme in Chapter 7. They thus illustrate a common feature of early psychosis intervention programmes (phase adapted and structured treatment programmes). This group treatment programme is part of the Calgary Early Psychosis Program (EPP) in western Canada, a well-established comprehensive programme for individuals experiencing a first episode of psychosis. It offers treatment to patients as well as to their families for three years. Treatment includes case management, psychiatric management, cognitive behaviour therapy, group therapy and family interventions. The details of the group therapy component of the programme are described. The Addingtons underline the need to clarify the developmental issues and problems of young patients as these need to be carefully considered when designing relevant groups; group therapy is an excellent modality to address many such issues. They outline groups that have been specifically designed for different phases of illness and recovery following the first episode. One group offers education about the illness and tries to develop an understanding of its impact, how to adjust to it and make future plans. As the individual moves further into recovery, the relevant group moves from educational to cognitive behavioural therapy and eventually to encompassing some aspects of an interpersonal therapy. The chapter offers practical guidance for developing and conducting groups suitable for those recovering from a first episode of psychosis.

Rachel Miller and Susan E. Mason from the USA present a phase-specific psychosocial intervention programme for first-episode schizophrenia with emphasis on the timeliness of interventions and their effects on the patients and their families. The three phases – the acute phase, the healing phase and the maintenance phase – are derived both from the literature and from the clinical experiences of working with 68 first-episode patients. Within each phase, treatment modalities – individual, psychoeducation, group and family interventions – are discussed to explicate the special needs of patients and families as these change over the course of illness. Approaches to psychoeducation are described separately for the patient and for the family within each phase of illness. The goals of treatment are to enhance adherence to treatment, reduce stigma, obtain the co-operation of families, help patients reintegrate into their communities and promote self-esteem and hope. Special attention is given to building a therapeutic alliance and to negative symptoms, cognitive dysfunction, safe sex practices and problems of substance abuse. They conclude that first-episode patients with schizophrenia differ from the chronic population. They and their families have to come to terms with a serious and stigmatising diagnosis for which they have little preparation. Clinical interventions take into consideration the unexpected shock of having to change life expectations. Even where there are no additional resources for treatment of this specialised group, all or part of this treatment plan can be used effectively by focusing on its salient themes: first-episode patients and their families require timely interventions which address their special needs.

PHASE-SPECIFIC TREATMENT OF PSYCHOSIS

The overall approach in Chapter 9 has much in common with the preceding two chapters. Johan Cullberg, from Sweden, looks at the need to identify the different soils within which psychosis takes place in order for optimum treatment to be offered. He demonstrates how psychodynamic thinking is an important tool in this work, depending on what kind of psychosis we are dealing with and in which phase of the disorder we meet the patient. Cullberg's approach is also much in line with the tradition represented by Veikko Tähkä, as outlined earlier. He is pessimistic about the possibilities of the psychoanalytic psychotherapy of chronic schizophrenia, but optimistic about the importance of a dynamic understanding of the psychotic states – not as a means of explaining the ultimate causes, but in the search for a meaning of the psychotic experience in the person's inner world. He points to the new treatment facilities we can find in combined dynamic-cognitive approaches. The primary point he wants us to consider in discussing the appropriateness of dynamic approaches is that the acute psychotic state has a self-healing capacity provided the individual is given an optimal psychological and social milieu. Psychiatry may facilitate the healing process; however, in Cullberg's experience, this capacity is often obstructed by traditional psychiatric care conditions that are counterproductive to these processes. Cullberg outlines how a really effective organisation must put an emphasis on family and network relationships that provide support at times of crisis, on the building of self confidence, on continuity of therapeutic relationships and on skilful psychotherapeutic and pharmacological treatments. If we are to accomplish this, dynamic understandings are pertinent. Therefore, every member of staff working with psychotic patients will have the knowledge, training and supervision to create and maintain therapeutic relationships with their patients.

UK colleagues Ian Kerr, Valerie Crowley and Hilary Beard could be said to have taken up Cullberg's challenge. In their chapter they describe the so-called 'cognitive-analytic therapy' (CAT), an integrative model of psychotherapy developed in the UK by Anthony Ryle. This is a brief, time-limited model of therapy originally designed for a range of 'neurotic' disorders, but its applications have by now extended well beyond this to more 'difficult' groups of patients, such as those with severe personality disorders. It has been applied in a model of how to form group therapy, day hospital or community mental health team work, as well as consultative work not involving patient contact. This has led to a preliminary CAT-based model of psychosis which accounts for many psychotic experiences and symptoms in terms of distorted, amplified or muddled enactment of normal or 'neurotic' reciprocal role procedures and of damage to the self at a meta-procedural level. This CAT-based model may contribute usefully to our understanding of psychotic disorders, as well as complement and extend current models of psychological treatment for this important group of disorders.

Another very important aspect of the treatment of patients with psychosis, especially in the light of phase-specific treatment strategies, is the cognitive functioning of patients with schizophrenia and other psychoses. Bjørn Rishovd Rund from Norway addresses this in his chapter 'Cognitive Remediation of Patients with Schizophrenia: Does it Work?' It has been reliably demonstrated that 60–70% of patients with schizophrenia have persistent abnormalities in various types of cognitive dysfunction. It has also been shown that, to a certain degree, these abnormalities antecede the psychosis – that is, they are present during the prodromal period and are relatively specific for schizophrenia. It is therefore important routinely to recognise those with cognitive deficits, and to find methods of improving cognitive functioning, because these deficits influence patients' ability to function well in the community and are related to their capacity to comprehend social perceptions and to learn social skills. It could be argued that attention should be given to these difficulties from the earliest phase of the illness to maximise rehabilitation potential. Rund presents a programme from his unit in Oslo which includes a controlled treatment study. The primary question asked in the study is whether the cognitive training programme adds anything to the psychosocial (psychoeducative) programme. The conclusion that can be drawn so far from these data is that the treatment (or the natural course of the illness) contributes to an improvement in patients' cognitive functioning. However, it is uncertain whether the cognitive training programme contributes specifically to the improvement.

In her chapter, Susan Hingley from the UK discusses the contribution of psychodynamic theory and practice from the perspective of finding meaning within psychosis. Hearing the patient within can be one of the most important achievements for any therapist hoping to ease some of the suffering and isolation that is inherent to psychosis. She uses the vulnerability-stress model to express an understanding of two of the major contributions of psychodynamic theory – the vulnerability of defence and the vulnerability of the ego – and the part they both play in the development of psychotic experience. If we can understand something of the underlying meaning, importance and purpose of the illusionary or hallucinatory experience, we can begin to build a therapeutic relationship based on common humanity. This provides understanding and empathy alongside caution in avoiding anxiety and confrontation and aims to provide an overall opportunity for the development of a more securely established self with a greater capacity for less distorting defences. This results in a person who is more able to accept and care for themselves and who is more empowered to cope with the world around them.

THE NEED FOR INTEGRATION

As we all know, the concept of schizophrenia is, in many ways, imprecise. Most patients also have some degree of co-morbidity, for example depression or post-traumatic stress disorder (PTSD). Paul C. Bermanzohn from the USA discusses this in his chapter 'Neglected Syndromes of Schizophrenia – Pervasiveness, Profiles and Phenomenology: An Overview of Associated Psychiatric Syndromes'. Bermanzohn discusses the problem of little-examined hierarchical assumptions in DSM-IV causing clinical and epidemiological confusion. In schizophrenia, he writes, this problem has been most evident in the study of concurrent or associated psychiatric syndromes (APS) such as depression, obsessive-compulsive disorder (OCD) and panic disorders. He claims that diagnostic reductionism, the tendency to attribute all of the symptoms and signs shown by those with schizophrenia to the schizophrenia alone, contributes to the widespread tendency to treat schizophrenia as if it were a single, unitary disorder. Bermanzohn's research shows that approximately 50% of patients diagnosed with schizophrenia have one or more APS. This obviously has great importance for our understanding of both the individual's problems and their treatment. Depression, obsessive compulsion and panic/social anxiety should be treated as co-morbid disorders rather than as a part of the schizophrenia syndrome.

In Chapter 14 Colin A. Ross discusses the need for integration of theory and practice in the controversial relationship between dissociation and psychosis. He critiques the rigid conceptual system that dominates North American psychiatry, which maintains that schizophrenia is a valid bio-genetic brain disease treated with medication, while dissociative identity disorder is a neurotic reaction to the environment of questionable validity. He demonstrates that the two categories overlap extensively, and reviews data showing that concordance for schizophrenia in monozygotic twins is around 30%, proving that the environment is the major aetiological factor in schizophrenia. He examines drug trial data which show that anti-psychotic medications are only slightly more effective than placebo. The endogenous biological causation of schizophrenia and the efficacy of anti-psychotic medication have been massively oversold by biological psychiatry. The overlap between dissociation and psychosis occurs at various levels: clinical diagnosis and treatment, structured interviewed diagnosis and measures of psychotic symptoms. He proposes the existence of a dissociative subtype of schizophrenia;

the subtype brings conceptual order and scientific testability to the confusion and overlap between dissociation and psychosis.

Chapter 15 describes 'the stages of treatment of schizophrenia [which] take place within a cultural matrix, in a particular political climate, in treatment settings, whose stability changes, and within evolving family matrices (both our patients' and our own)'. Ann-Louise Silver compares the stages of treatment with the game of chess, and makes reference to Ernest Jones' paper 'The Problem of Paul Morphy' (1931). She also draws a line back to Frieda Fromm-Reichmann's 'principles of intensive psychotherapy' which she characterises as our profession's fundamental text, most of which she believes remains relevant. Her chapter gives us an opportunity to re-examine the roots of our interest in our own psychotherapeutic work with psychotic patients. For example, are we in error when we keep private our personal histories as an extension of analytic anonymity?

Finally, John Read and Paul Hammersley from New Zealand discuss the connection between bad childhoods and later psychiatric illness. Through a review demonstrating a relationship between childhood abuse and schizophrenia in adulthood, they present a preliminary investigation of the relationships between three positive schizophrenic symptoms – hallucinations, delusions and thought disorders – and childhood physical and sexual abuse. Previous findings concerning the high frequency, in abused in-patients, of auditory hallucinations (particularly command hallucinations to kill oneself) and paranoid ideation were confirmed. The hypothesis that auditory hallucinations experienced by abused survivors are 'pseudo-hallucinations' is refuted. Although the connection between abuse and schizophrenia still remains unclear, there should be no doubt that there is a strong connection between abuse, trauma and psychiatric disorders developing in later life. Read and Hammersley end their chapter by illustrating the importance of professionals who, when eliciting the background of the patient, are attuned to the possibility of earlier abuse having contributed to vulnerability to psychosis.

CONCLUSION

Future clinical practice and future research in the area of psychotic disorders require a more refined descriptive methodology, refined diagnostic procedures and refined need-adapted psychosocial methods. Just as it is a sine qua non to look for the person, the human being, behind the diagnosis, it is a sine qua non to offer treatment as early in the illness development as possible. This 'window of opportunity' is probably also a critical period where the psychotherapies are likely to make most impact. Furthermore, it is the relation between therapists and patient which forms the matrix for effective treatment, that is, for change. Although some seminal early analysts were pessimistic about psychoanalytically-orientated therapies being of clinical use in psychosis, much of this book shows how the adaptation of dynamic understandings contributes to the contemporary approaches we should be espousing.

The first step in the psychological treatments of schizophrenia and other psychoses is to establish a relationship to carry the treatment, and this in itself needs to be the foundation of treatment for the years to come in some people. If we manage to establish such a relationship between two human beings, a therapist and a patient, and cement the necessary trust between them, the necessary engagement in each other, then we have accomplished a lot already.

We hope that through this book we have demonstrated that the psychological treatments carry a range of possibilities that must be tailor-made to each patient's individual situation. Where there is no structure, our primary task is to re-establish this structure. When structures begin to be re-established, the first steps towards recovery have been taken.

When we look behind the diagnosis, people with a schizophrenic psychosis can be sad and depressed, obsessed, preoccupied and anxious. They may have panic attacks or be so scared that they have developed PTSD. If we bear these possibilities in mind and meet the patient as early as possible in the illness development, there is a 'window of opportunity' for the patient and the continuing development of better and more need-adapted psychological treatments for this group of patients.

Jan Olav Johannessen
Brian Martindale
Johan Cullberg

REFERENCES

Alanen, Y. O. (1997). *Schizophrenia: Its Origins and Need-Adapted Treatment*. London: Karnac Books.

Birchwood, M. (1999). Early intervention in psychosis: The critical period. In: P. D. McGorry and H. J. Jackson (eds) *Recognition and Management of Early Psychosis: A Preventive Approach*. New York: Cambridge University Press.

Birchwood, M. and Macmillan, F. (1993). Early intervention in schizophrenia. *Australian and New Zealand Journal of Psychiatry* 27: 374–8.

Cameron, D. E. (1938). Early schizophrenia. *American Journal of Psychiatry* 95: 567–78.

Ciompi, L. *et al.* (1992). A new approach to acute schizophrenia. Further results of the pilot project Soteria Bern. In A. Werbart and J. Cullberg (eds) *Psychotherapy of Schizophrenia: Facilitating and Obstructive Factors*. Oslo: Scandinavian University Press.

Crow, T. (1990). The continuum of psychosis and its genetic origins. *British Journal of Psychiatry* 156: 788–97.

Docherty, J. *et al.* (1978). Stages of onset of schizophrenic psychosis. *American Journal of Psychiatry* 135: 420–6.

Edwards J. and McGorry P. D. (2002). *Implementing Early Intervention in Psychosis. A Guide to Establishing Early Psychosis Services.* London: Martin Dunitz Ltd.

Gunderson, J. G. (1978). Defining the therapeutic processes in psychiatric milieus. *Psychiatry* 41: 327–35.

Häfner, H. *et al.* (1992). IRAOS: An instrument for the assessment of onset and early course of schizophrenia. *Schizophrenia Research* 6: 209–23.

Hill, L. B. (1955). *Psychotherapeutic Intervention in Schizophrenia.* Chicago: University of Chicago Press.

Hogarty, G. E. *et al.* (1997). Three-year trials of personal therapy among patients living with or independent of family. I: Description of study and effects on relapse rates. *American Journal of Psychiatry* 154: 1504–13.

Johannessen, J. O., *et al.* (2001). Early detection strategies for untreated first-episode psychosis. *Schizophrenia Research* 51: 39–46.

McGlashan, T. H. and Keats, C. J. (1989). *Schizophrenia: Treatment Process and Outcome.* Washington, DC: American Psychiatric Press.

Sullivan, H. S. (1927/1994). The onset of schizophrenia. *American Journal of Psychiatry* 151 (suppl. 6): 135–9.

Tähkä, V. (1979). Psychotherapy as phase-specific treatment. *Scandinavian Psychoanalytic Review* 2: 113–32.

Zubin, J. and Spring, B. (1977). Vulnerability – a new view of schizophrenia. *Journal of Abnormal Psychology* 86: 103–26.

Part I

The nature of psychosis

Chapter 1

The recognition and optimal management of early psychosis

Applying the concept of staging in the treatment of psychosis

Patrick D. McGorry

EARLY PSYCHOSIS: A NEW REFORM PARADIGM

> The best progressive ideas are those that include a strong enough dose of provocation to make its supporters feel proud of being original, but at the same time attract so many adherents that the risk of being an isolated exception is immediately averted by the noisy approval of a triumphant crowd.
>
> (Kundera 1996: 273)

Over the past decade, there has been a growing sense of optimism about the prospects for better outcomes for schizophrenia and related psychoses, and this has achieved the status of a 'progressive idea'. This has disturbed some (for example, Verdoux 2001) who have urged caution in proceeding with reform. However, while there is a sociopolitical dimension to all successful reform, this one has an increasingly solid basis in evidence. Clinicians and policymakers in particular are enthusiastic about reform based on this idea because of the sound logic behind it and the unacceptably poor access to and quality of care previously available to young people with early psychosis, and are encouraged by the increasing evidence that better outcomes can be achieved. The rationale for, and extent of, this reform is described in Edwards and McGorry (2002) and the latest evidence is reviewed in a balanced manner by Malla and Norman (2002). There has also been considerable resistance and scepticism which helps to keep the reform process 'honest'. In this chapter I will summarise this evidence and provide guidelines for its clinical application.

Key drivers of this paradigm are the special clinical needs of young people at this phase of illness, the iatrogenic effects of standard care and a range of secondary preventive opportunities (Garety and Rigg 2001). This is especially clear when the clinical care of first-episode and recent-onset patients is streamed separately from chronic patients, something which is still difficult to engineer and sustain (McGorry *et al.* 1996). The key failures in care are: prolonged delays in accessing effective treatment, which thus usually occurs in the context of a severe behavioural crisis; crude, typically traumatic and alienating initial treatment strategies; and subsequent poor continuity of care and engagement of the patient with treatment. Young people have to demonstrate a severe risk to themselves or others to gain access and a relapsing and chronically disabling pattern of illness to 'deserve' ongoing care. These features are highly prevalent in most systems of mental health care, even in developed countries with reasonable levels of spending in mental health.

The increasing devolution of mental health care into community settings has provided further momentum, as has a genuine renaissance in biological and psychological treatments for psychosis. Exponential growth in interest in neuroscientific research in schizophrenia has injected further optimism into the field, with a new generation of clinician-researchers coming to the fore. Several countries have developed national mental health strategies or frameworks which catalyse and guide major reform and mandate a preventive mindset and linked reform (WHO 2001). Around the world an increasingly large number of groups have established clinical programmes and research initiatives focusing on early psychosis, and it now constitutes a growth point in clinical care as well as research (Edwards and McGorry 2002). This reform differs fundamentally from previous reforms (such as deinstitutionalisation) in being much more evidence-based, and also in its integration of biological, psychosocial and structural elements of intervention.

Early intervention means early detection of new cases, shortening delays in effective treatment, and providing optimal and sustained treatment in the early 'critical period' of the first few years of illness (Malla and Norman 2002). Even on the basis of our existing knowledge, substantial reductions in prevalence and improved quality of life are possible for patients, provided societies are prepared to pay for it. However, this has not occurred, despite the development of effective treatments (Hegarty *et al.* 1994; Jablensky *et al.* 1999), because we have so far failed to translate these advances to the real world beyond the randomised controlled trial. Early intervention, with its promise of more efficient treatment through an enhanced focus on the early phases of illness, is an additional prevalence and burden reduction strategy, which is now available to be widely tested and, if cost-effective, to be widely implemented. This is hardly a radical goal and would be non-controversial in other areas of healthcare where primary prevention remains out of reach (for example, diabetes and many cancers).

While evidence is a critical element, how much evidence is required before a change in practice is warranted? For asymptomatic patients with increased risk, the onus is clearly on avoiding harm, with attempting to reduce risk as a secondary goal. When patients become symptomatic and impaired, however, the dynamics change. In deciding where the onus of proof should lie here, we should be very clear that the alternative to early and optimal intervention is delayed and substandard treatment with all its human (and inhumane) consequences (Garety and Rigg 2001; Lieberman and Fenton 2000). Even in developed countries, as consumers and carers will readily attest, the timing and quality of standard care is relatively poor, very much a case of 'too little, too late'. In developing countries, a significant proportion of cases never receive treatment (Padmavathi *et al.* 1998). While we do need evidence, there are obvious additional clinical and commonsense drivers for the provision of more timely and widespread treatment of better quality (see Figure 1.1).

EARLY INTERVENTION IN THE REAL WORLD: CONCEPTS, EVIDENCE AND CLINICAL GUIDELINES

Mrazek and Haggerty (1994) have recently developed a more sophisticated framework for conceptualising, implementing and evaluating preventive interventions for mental disorders which supersedes the primary, secondary and tertiary prevention model. This translates into a staged model of intervention for psychotic disorders.

Universal preventive interventions are focused upon the whole population while selective preventive measures are aimed at asymptomatic high-risk subgroups of the population. Indicated prevention is concerned with sub-threshold symptoms which confer enhanced risk of a more severe disorder. Early intervention can be defined as indicated prevention, early case detection and optimal management of the first episode of illness and the subsequent critical period.

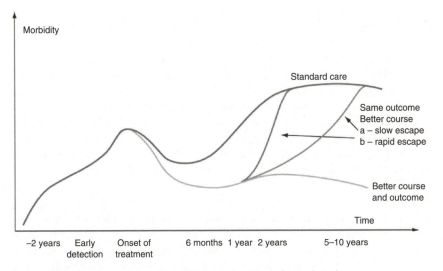

Figure 1.1 Early intervention and possible outcome in psychotic disorders.

Prepsychotic intervention

This is a form of indicated prevention and is currently the earliest possible phase for preventive intervention in psychosis (Mrazek and Haggerty 1994). However, at present it remains a research focus, even though clinical guidelines have been developed to underpin a safe and appropriate clinical response to young people presenting for treatment with potentially subthreshold or prodromal symptoms (Garety and Rigg 2001), since these are distressing and disabling (Häfner *et al.* 1999; Yung *et al.* 1996). Much of the disability and collateral damage associated with psychotic disorders develops during this complex and confusing period and sets a ceiling for recovery, thus influencing the social course of the disorder (Häfner *et al.* 1999). In fact, subthreshold symptoms constitute a risk factor in their own right for more severe disorders (Eaton *et al.* 1995). Since universal and selective prevention remain out of reach at present, indicated prevention marks the current frontier of prevention research in psychotic disorders (Mrazek and Haggerty 1994). Notwithstanding the neurodevelopmental theory of schizophrenia, the illness is relatively quiescent during childhood (Jones *et al.* 1994) with the emergence in adolescence or early adult life of symptoms and disability which can be used to predict full-threshold disorder (Klosterkötter *et al.* 2001; Yung *et al.* 2004). The idea of intervening at this stage of illness raises conflicting concerns. With the passage of time, some of these cases will be seen to have been manifesting an early form of the disorder in question, and the subthreshold clinical features will then turn out to have been prodromal (a retrospective term). On the other hand, others will not undergo transition, and will therefore constitute 'false positives' for the disorder in question. This has caused concerns about the effects of labelling and unnecessary treatment (McGorry *et al.* 2001; Schaffner and McGorry 2001).

Following a series of initial naturalistic studies which created more accurate operational criteria for ultra high risk (UHR; Yung *et al.* 2004), a recent randomised controlled trial in this clinical population has shown a significant reduction in transition rate to psychosis for patients receiving specific treatment comprising very low dose risperidone (1–2mg/day) and cognitive therapy, in comparison to non-specific treatment comprising supportive psychotherapy and symptomatic treatment (McGorry *et al.* 2002). Such patients must be distinguished from a subgroup of the general population who report isolated psychotic symptoms in the apparent absence of distress, disability or progressive change, and who do not desire assistance (McGorry *et al.* 2001; Van Os *et al.* 2001).

Further research is urgently required to clarify the range of treatments which will alleviate distress and disability and reduce the risk of subsequent psychosis in help-seeking UHR patients. While this evidence is being assembled, if people present with a potentially incipient psychosis, there may often be a need for a clinical response. What should the clinician do when approached by a young person, or by the family of a young person, who appears to be at ultra high risk?

For those meeting the criteria for UHR (McGorry *et al.* 2002; Yung *et al.* 2003), the offer, at least, of initial psychosocial treatment, including the emerging range of cognitive therapies, aimed at the relief of such distress and disability in young people, with or without syndrome-based drug treatments such as anti-depressants, seems justifiable. What the patient and family should be told about the level of risk of future psychosis has been debated. However, in our experience, an open approach of disclosure, guided by the curiosity of the patient and family, has worked well, especially since many are well aware of this risk and are already concerned. An optimistic attitude to treatment and recovery in schizophrenia and psychosis generally should be strongly communicated (Harrison *et al.* 2001).

If this offer of intervention is initially refused, as it may well be in this age group, this can usually be accepted, although some kind of assertive monitoring or follow-up may be justifiable, combined with family contact. This is important and necessary because, in addition to the risk of psychosis, there is a higher than expected rate of substance abuse, deliberate self-harm and suicide in this potentially prepsychotic population (McGorry *et al.* 2002).

Not uncommonly, the parents of the young person will be very concerned but unable to persuade them to attend for assessment. Since this is partly due to stigma and self-stigmatisation, the young person should ideally be assessed and offered help in a low stigma setting. This can be accomplished through home visits by the family doctor, the school counsellor or, where these exist, mobile youth mental health teams linked to specialist mental health services. Naturally, a good understanding of the range of normal psychology of adolescents and young adults, and of appropriate interviewing and engagement strategies, is invaluable.

Even if psychosis does emerge and the symptoms cross the threshold for anti-psychotic therapy, a key advantage of this focus on vulnerable, prepsychotic or potentially prodromal young people, in a youth-oriented setting, is that a therapeutic relationship has been securely established. The young person is usually more accessible to therapeutic relationships generally and this means that recommendations re drug therapy are more likely to be accepted when they are made and hospitalisation can be avoided, hence reducing costs and secondary trauma (McGorry *et al.* 1991). Furthermore, the duration of untreated psychosis (DUP) is reduced to an absolute minimum. Even if only a minority of first-episode cases can be engaged prior to psychosis and no transitions to psychosis can be prevented, the advantages are still potentially great. Treatment will be commenced 'on the right foot' in an atmosphere of trust rather than fear and disruption, and with fewer complications.

The final clinical issue in this phase of illness is whether there is a role for anti-psychotic medications prior to patients reaching the threshold for diagnosis of a frank psychotic disorder. Despite the lower risks of disabling side-effects and better efficacy of the novel anti-psychotic drugs (Csernansky *et al.* 2002), and positive early research findings, caution is required here. Novel anti-psychotic medications are clearly not a benign intervention and have increasingly recognised side effects of a different kind. If the indications for broadening the use of anti-psychotic medications beyond frank and persistent psychosis are not very carefully defined and supported by high quality research, then it is likely that much harm could be done. Treatments in the early phase of illness may not only be different but more benign. While anti-psychotics may ultimately not be the appropriate treatment for this phase of illness, at least for some, it is the advent of more benign anti-psychotic medications that has helped to catalyse interest in intervening this early.

In the future a range of other strategies may prove worth trying, such as cognitive remediation, cognitive behaviour therapy and putative neuroprotective agents such as lithium and essential fatty acids (Berger *et al.* 2002). The safety, acceptability and efficacy of all interventions need to be thoroughly tested through further clinical research. The value of such research cannot be overestimated given the critical nature of this phase of illness in relation to outcomes for patients. However in most clinical settings, because of the lack of streamed first-episode psychosis programmes, very few of these patients get anywhere near mental health services. Hence this focus is still a long way off in terms of reform priorities.

Early case detection in first-episode psychosis

Once the currently accepted threshold for treatment with anti-psychotic medication – the first clear and sustained emergence of psychotic features – is reached, there is a firm foundation for early intervention. Despite this, and the severity of these disorders, for a substantial proportion of people such treatment is surprisingly delayed, often for prolonged periods (McGlashan 1999; Norman and Malla 2001). Indeed for some, especially in the developing world (Padmavathi *et al.* 1998), treatment is never accessed. This focus is concerned, however, with the timing of intervention.

The duration of untreated psychosis (DUP), as a marker of delay in delivering effective specific treatment, is a potentially important variable in relation to efforts to improve outcome in first-episode schizophrenia, and more widely in first-episode psychosis (McGlashan 1999; Norman and Malla 2001).

DUP is important because, unlike other prognostic variables such as genetic vulnerability, gender and age of onset, it is a potentially malleable variable which can become the focus of intervention strategies. Psychosis may be an easier and less conflicted target to detect than schizophrenia (Driessen *et al.* 1998). Schizophrenia, which requires a period of frank psychotic features for diagnosis, may take time to emerge as a stable diagnosis, and our primary treatment target is positive psychotic symptoms for which we prescribe anti-psychotic medications (notwithstanding their effects on other symptom domains). A strong and extensive literature supports a correlational link, albeit moderate, between DUP and both short- and long-term outcome (McGlashan 1999; Norman and Malla 2001), although two recent studies have cast doubt on the link (Craig *et al.* 2000; Ho *et al.* 2000).

Assuming the link is as robust as it seems, there is a further question. Is the association causal? That is, is delay in treatment (prolonged DUP) a risk factor for worse outcome? Or is the link due to a common underlying factor, namely a more severe form of illness, which has a more insidious onset with more negative symptoms, more paranoid ideation, less salience and awareness of change and less willingness to seek and accept treatment? Even if this is so, DUP may still be a key intervening variable through which these clinical features influence outcome, and hence reducing it may mitigate their effect (McGorry 2000).

In addition to the evidence-based argument (Norman and Malla 2001) there is a strong clinical appreciation, derived from patients and families directly, of the destructive effects of delay and the range of negative psychosocial outcomes which accumulate during the period of untreated psychosis. These include vocational failure, self-harm, offending behaviour, family distress and dysfunction, aggression, substance abuse and victimisation by others (Garety and Rigg 2001). Even those who have questioned the relationship between DUP and outcome are either extremely vague about how long one should wait to intervene in cases of clearcut psychotic disorder (Verdoux 2001) or strongly support the idea of intervening as soon as a diagnosable psychotic disorder emerges which is impacting on functioning or quality of life (Ho *et al.* 2000). Since we do have effective treatments available, therapeutic nihilism, the underlying premise of a 'wait and see' attitude, is not justified.

Mental health services, in partnership with local communities, primary care and individual clinicians, should therefore embark upon a range of strategies to reduce delays in treatment onset (Larsen *et al.* 2001). This is not a process which has been seen as part of the mandate of clinicians or clinical services, where resources are scarce. It is more common, understandable and possibly even necessary for the latter to regulate their workload by restricting access to new patients. There may be a natural reluctance to widen access because of a lack of resources, due to inadequate funding, to cope with a feared influx of referrals.

The effect of early detection strategies in community psychiatry settings (such as community education and mobile detection teams) will probably be twofold, as witnessed in recent studies (Malla *et al.* 2003; McGorry 2000).

First, if intensive efforts are made to improve mental health literacy in the general community, improve recognition skills among general practitioners through training and consultation-liaison, and improve access to, and engagement with, specialist mental health services, then the duration of untreated psychosis for the average case should be substantially reduced, especially the relatively small subgroup with a very long DUP. This should make the work of the service easier and result in a reduced need for inpatient care and involuntary treatment (Larsen *et al.* 2001).

Second, there will be an increase in treated incidence of psychosis and hence workload, and a corresponding reduction in the prevalence of hidden psychiatric morbidity in the community (McGorry 2000). More resources will be required for services to become proactive in this way, to undertake the detection role and cope with the additional caseloads. Such a role should be built into the mandate of modern community-based mental health services and hence adequately funded.

Optimal and intensive phase-specific intervention in first-episode psychosis and the critical period

The third and most robustly evidence-based preventive focus is enhancing the quality of treatment. As Malla and Norman (2002) put it, there is a lot more to early intervention than intervening early. The notion that optimal treatment of the early phase of a disorder could shorten the duration of illness and thus reduce the prevalence of the disorder, and further have a positive medium- to long-term effect on the course and outcome, is an attractive idea. However, the treatment should be phase-specific. This introduces the idea of 'staging' into psychiatric treatment, an idea which has been rarely applied. Staging means that the treatment in earlier phases of illness should be different, more benign and potentially more effective than in later phases. The best examples of this lie in the cancer field (Moody-Ayers *et al.* 2000).

The idea of a critical period during which the disorder is more responsive to intervention has recently been developed for psychotic disorders and fits with the patterns of illness severity found in recent follow-up studies as well as the developmental stage of life in which these illnesses emerge (Birchwood *et al.* 1998; Harrison *et al.* 2001; McGorry and Jackson 1999).

Since it does not require as much of a change in role as the previous two preventive foci (prepsychotic intervention and early case detection), more intensive phase-specific treatment during the first episode of psychosis, and beyond into the critical period, is the most feasible proposition for most clinicians and researchers interested in secondary prevention.

In general, there is some evidence that such intensive treatment of young people at this phase of illness is effective (McGorry *et al.* 1996; Nordentoft *et al.* 2002) and cost-effective (Mihalopoulos *et al.* 1999) in real-world settings at least in the short term, although more research is certainly required to examine the longer-term impact and to determine the most appropriate service models.

Whether it is possible to reduce the intensity of treatment over a longer timeframe or not is an important secondary research question. Recent studies suggest that treatment intensity should not be reduced within the first five years for the majority of patients (Gitlin *et al.* 2001; Linszen *et al.* 2001; Robinson *et al.* 1999).

First-episode psychosis

The key elements of management in first-episode psychosis are summarised as follows.

1. Access and engagement

Most people, though not all, who develop psychotic disorders are young people with little or no experience of mental health services. They lack knowledge, carry the same fears and prejudices as the rest of the community regarding mental illness and will generally be reluctant to seek or accept help. This is exaggerated by the sense of invulnerability which is part of normal adolescence and the presence of psychotic symptoms. Access to and engagement with services are processes that can be markedly enhanced by the way services are designed and operated. Mobile assessment available around the clock in a setting that suits the individual patient and family is a key advance in improving access to care. This should ideally be offered even prior to a crisis or high risk situation having developed, so that a calm and careful process of assessment and initial management can be undertaken.

Engagement with services is made more difficult if a traumatic crisis and involuntary treatment is the initial experience of the young patient and family. While inadequate resources are typically a structural obstacle, many services still shield themselves behind convenient interpretations of local mental health legislation requiring patients who are not actively seeking help on their own behalf or who reject it, especially first-episode cases, to develop suicidal or violent behaviour before even direct assessment is offered. Although crises cannot always be avoided, their frequency can be reduced substantially if resources are devoted to a mobile early detection and assessment service (McGorry and Jackson 1999).

2. Assessment

The initial assessment should focus on the major diagnostic issues and levels of risk of harm to self or others. The rest can be pieced together over time. A key issue is to determine whether the patient is clearly psychotic and, if so, whether there is also a major mood syndrome present. This can be difficult. Substance abuse and dependence are frequently comorbid with positive psychotic symptoms, and should not lead to exclusion of the patient from treatment.

As early detection strategies begin to bite, it is also likely that more subthreshold cases, including those with isolated psychotic symptoms (Van Os *et al.* 2001), will be assessed. Some of these patients have psychotic symptoms that are not typical in the textbook or diagnostic manual and may confuse clinicians. Many of these patients do request and require treatment, and further research is required to define carefully the range of appropriate treatment for such patients, though the onset of clearcut and sustained positive psychotic symptoms represents a watershed for any given patient.

Although the novel anti-psychotics have broader effects than on positive symptoms alone, the clear emergence of frank and sustained positive symptoms is currently a necessary step to considering their use in clinical settings. Hence in first-episode detection and diagnosis psychosis is an appropriate target which is a necessary way-station en route to schizophrenia as currently defined. Secondary targets within the psychosis spectrum include mania, depression, PTSD and a range of other comorbid syndromes, rather than DSM or ICD diagnoses per se, because they constitute a better guide to drug therapy.

3. Acute treatment

The initial decision is whether inpatient care is required. This will be influenced by patient factors, the degree of family and social support, the range of services available and local policies. Where it is possible, home-based acute care is preferred for a range of reasons and can be achieved in over 50% of cases with a highly structured and intensive approach (McGorry and Jackson 1999). An anti-psychotic-free period of at least 48 hours is usually advisable, during which benzodiazepines only are prescribed to alleviate the distressing symptoms of agitation, anxiety and insomnia. If sustained psychosis is confirmed, then anti-psychotic medication may be commenced. Reversible medical illnesses and drug intoxications should also be identified during this period.

Second-generation or novel anti-psychotics are indicated where possible as first, second and even third line therapy because of their better tolerability and greater efficacy. The starting dose should be very low and be increased to an initial 'step' or target dose and held there for the effect to be evaluated. Further increases should only occur in the setting of poor response and only then at intervals of approximately three weeks to allow the effect of the change in dose to become clear. More rapid increases in dose in first-episode psychosis lead to greater risk of side effects, especially extrapyramidal features, with no clear benefit. We now know that these dosages are sufficient to produce sufficient levels of D2 blockade in the CNS to bring about a clinical response and that the threshold for clinical response is lower, albeit narrowly, than the threshold at which neurological and other side effects begin to manifest (Kapur *et al.* 2000; Nyberg *et al.* 1995).

These low doses of anti-psychotics are not intended or expected to deal immediately with the behavioural disturbances and associated symptoms frequently seen in this acute phase. The latter should be managed if at all possible with benzodiazepines and psychosocial strategies during this period, since the use of parenteral or sedating oral typical neuroleptics will inevitably produce aversive side effects and undermine, perhaps terminally, an already fragile process of engagement and adherence to treatment.

Emergency situations requiring urgent sedation can be managed with intramuscular benzodiazepines such as midazolam or lorazepam in most cases. In occasional cases this will be ineffective and a short-acting sedating neuroleptic is the next best option. Repeated injections are rarely required with good nursing care, a supportive milieu and liberal use of benzodiazepines in the acute phase.

Naturally intensive psychosocial support is essential for the patient and family during this highly stressful period, though services are often unable to provide this due to inadequate funding, low morale and poor skills, combined with an unfortunate lack of awareness or acknowledgement of its critical role. This is a deficiency in urgent need of reform.

Home-based care is less stressful for the patient, in particular, and usually results in a reduced need for acute medication. It is more likely to be feasible with earlier intervention; however, the presence of manic features makes it more difficult to carry out home-based intervention. Indeed, the identification and treatment of the major affective syndromes, especially mania, is a key issue in the treatment of first-episode psychosis. A manic syndrome is present in up to 20% of cases of first-episode psychosis and should be rapidly treated with a mood stabiliser, ideally lithium carbonate or alternatively sodium valproate, to promote full recovery while minimising anti-psychotic dosages. Subsyndromal manic features are even more frequent. Depression, unless clearly dominating the clinical picture, commonly resolves in parallel with the positive psychotic symptoms; however, if it persists or worsens during the post-psychotic period, it should be actively treated with a combination of anti-depressants and psychological intervention. More detailed descriptions of the principles and practice of acute care can be found elsewhere (Edwards and McGorry 2002; McGorry and Jackson 1999).

4. The recovery phase

Up to 85–90% of first-episode patients will achieve a remission or partial remission of their positive psychotic symptoms within the 12 months following entry to treatment, though some potentially responsive patients will fail to engage with treatment or rapidly cease adherence to medication. This is balanced by the persistence of vulnerability in most patients and the tendency to recurrence, which may be subtle (Gitlin *et al.* 2001). A range of psychosocial strategies can augment and broaden the scope and depth of the recovery process; these include psychological interventions, family interventions and group-based recovery programmes (Malla and Norman 2002). Some of these will increase the remission rate for positive symptoms and they all aim to improve negative symptoms, functioning and quality of life. Rapid discharge of responding patients following an acute first episode of psychosis to unsupported general practitioners is poor practice. It represents a missed opportunity for maximising and consolidating recovery and for secondary prevention. An integrated shared care model with the GP and other agencies is likely to prove more beneficial in minimising relapse and promoting more complete recovery.

The critical period

This term can be regarded as covering the period immediately following recovery from a first episode of psychosis and extending for up to five years subsequently, and is based on the notion that this is the phase of maximum vulnerability (Birchwood *et al.* 1998). A number of recent research studies have focused on the treated course of early psychosis (Gitlin *et al.* 2001; Linszen *et al.* 2001; Malla and Norman 2002). These have shown that the early course of illness for both schizophrenia and affective psychosis is turbulent and relapse-prone, with up to 80% of patients relapsing within a five-year period and between acute relapses there may be additional persistence of subclinical yet disabling clinical features. These findings suggest that, if possible, drug therapy should be continued for most if not all patients for longer than 12 months after recovery from a first psychotic episode.

However, it should be remembered that a subsample, at least 20%, never relapse, that some will not relapse for a prolonged period and that relapse prevention is not the sole consideration in treatment but rather a means to an end. Adaptation to illness is a challenging and often overwhelming task for these young people, and they usually need to be given time and special help to come to an acceptance of their need for maintenance treatment (Carpenter 2001; Jackson *et al.* 1998). A concerted effort should be made to maintain the engagement of most patients with clinical care during the early years after onset and to have in place a written relapse plan so that action can be taken if symptoms re-emerge, whether on or off medication. A good therapeutic and personal relationship with the patient and family is the key to success and should be nurtured, though continuity of care is at a premium in public psychiatry in developed countries. This deficiency is the Achilles heel of the system, leaving patients, who often have significant problems with trust and in forming social relationships, with no safety net. Even with standard care, however, it has been shown that outcome at 13 years is much more positive than expected, supporting the notion of an early critical period, which may be turbulent, but this turbulence seems to abate after two to five years (Harrison *et al.* 2001). With optimal care such outcomes could be substantially improved (Falloon 1999).

CONCLUSION

Despite and partly because of the poor quality of standard treatment for schizophrenia and other psychoses in real-world settings in both developed and developing countries (WHO 2001), there is growing support for a more preventive stance towards treatment, one which translates into a staged model of intervention according to duration and severity of illness. Primary prevention, specifically universal and selective preventive intervention, is beyond our capacities at the present stage of knowledge. However, indicated prevention for subthreshold symptoms has been endorsed as the frontier of prevention research in schizophrenia (McGorry and Jackson 1999), while early detection and optimal early treatment are clearly within the mandate of clinicians and services, and can be justified despite predictable academic scepticism. This scepticism must be appropriately addressed through rigorous clinical research, but it may prove difficult to dissipate fully, and should not be allowed to snuff out precious therapeutic optimism, which can improve morale within services as well as patient outcomes. Realistic optimism has been in short supply in the treatment of schizophrenia and this deficiency has contributed to the serious gap between efficacy and effectiveness in treatment, as well as suicide rates (McGorry *et al.* 1998; Power and McGorry 1999; Power *et al.* 2003). Evidence will be a vital guide, because new clinical and ethical issues are being brought to light as the frontier advances (though they are essentially the same as in the rest of medicine), and it is important that changes in mental health care are based on solid foundations, not shifting sands, as so often in the past. Nevertheless, dispersing the mists of pessimism, which have shrouded the clinical care of people with schizophrenia, fuelled suicide and enhanced stigma, is an overdue and worthwhile endeavour. The treatment objectives and approaches reviewed here characterise recent steps in this direction, in the confident belief that further progress will occur.

ACKNOWLEDGEMENT

Kundera extract reproduced from Milan Kundera (1996). *The Book of Laughter and Forgetting*. London: Faber and Faber, with permission.

REFERENCES

Berger, G. E. *et al.* (2002). Implications of lipid biology for the pathogenesis of schizophrenia. *Australian and New Zealand Journal of Psychiatry* 36: 355–66.

Birchwood, M. *et al.* (1998). Early intervention in psychosis: The critical period hypothesis. *British Journal of Psychiatry* 172 (supplement 33): 53–9.

Carpenter, W. T. (2001). Evidence-based treatment for first-episode schizophrenia? *American Journal of Psychiatry* 158: 1771–3.

Craig, T. J. *et al.* (2000). Is there an association between duration of untreated psychosis and 24-month clinical outcome in a first-admission series? *American Journal of Psychiatry* 157: 60–6.

Csernansky, J. G. *et al.* (2002). A comparison of risperidone and haloperidol for the prevention of relapse in patients with schizophrenia. *New England Journal of Medicine* 346: 16–22.

Driessen, G. *et al.* (1998). Characteristics of early- and late-diagnosed schizophrenia: Implications for first-episode studies. *Schizophrenia Research*: 33: 27–34.

Eaton, W. W. *et al.* (1995). Prodromes and precursors: Epidemiological data for primary prevention of disorders with slow onset. *American Journal of Psychiatry* 152: 967–72.

Edwards, J. and McGorry, P. D. (2002). *Implementing Early Intervention in Psychosis: A Guide to Establishing Early Psychosis Services*. London: Dunitz.

Falloon, I. R. H. (1999). Optimal treatment for psychosis in an international multisite demonstration project. *Psychiatric Services* 50: 615–8.

Garety, P. A. and Rigg, A. (2001). Early psychosis in the inner city: A survey to inform service planning. *Social Psychiatry Psychiatric Epidemiology* 36: 537–44.

Gitlin, M. *et al.* (2001). Clinical outcome following neuroleptic discontinuation in patients with remitted recent-onset schizophrenia. *American Journal of Psychiatry* 158: 1835–42.

Häfner, H. *et al.* (1999). Depression, negative symptoms, social stagnation and social decline in the early course of schizophrenia. *Acta Psychiatrica Scandinavica* 100: 105–18.

Harrison, G. *et al.* (2001). Recovery from psychotic illness: A 15- and 25-year international follow-up study. *British Journal of Psychiatry* 178: 506–17.

Hegarty, J. *et al.* (1994). One hundred years of schizophrenia: A meta-analysis of the outcome literature. *American Journal of Psychiatry* 151: 1409–16.

Ho, B. C. *et al.* (2000). Untreated initial psychosis: Its relation to quality of life and symptom remission in first-episode schizophrenia. *American Journal of Psychiatry* 157: 808–15.

Jablensky, A. *et al.* (1999). *People Living with Psychotic Illness: An Australian Study 1997–98*. Overview of the method and results of low prevalence (psychotic) disorders as part of the National Survey of Mental Health and Wellbeing. Report published on behalf of Low Prevalence Disorders Study Group, Commonwealth Department of Health and Age Care, Canberra, Australia, 1999.

Jackson, H. *et al.* (1998). Cognitively-oriented psychotherapy for early psychosis (COPE). Preliminary results. *British Journal of Psychiatry* 172 (supplement 33): 93–100.

Jones, P. *et al.* (1994). Child developmental risk factors for adult schizophrenia in the British 1946 birth cohort. *The Lancet* 344: 1398–402.

Kapur, S. *et al.* (2000). Relationship between dopamine D_2 occupancy, clinical response, and side effects: a double-blind PET study of first-episode schizophrenia. *American Journal of Psychiatry* 157: 514–20.

Klosterkötter, J. *et al.* (2001). Diagnosing schizophrenia in the initial prodromal phase. *Archives of General Psychiatry* 58: 158–64.

Kundera, M. (1996). *The Book of Laughter and Forgetting*. London: Faber and Faber.

Larsen, T. K. *et al.* (2001). Early detection and intervention in first-episode schizophrenia: A critical review. *Acta Psychiatrica Scandinavica* 103: 323–34.

Lieberman, J. A. and Fenton, W. S. (2000). Delayed detection of psychosis: Causes, consequences, and effect on public health. *American Journal of Psychiatry* 157: 1727–30.

Linszen, D. *et al.* (2001). Early intervention and a five year follow up in young adults with a short duration of untreated psychosis: Ethical implications. *Schizophrenia Research* 51: 55–61.

Malla, A. K. *et al.* (2003). A Canadian perspective programme for early intervention in non-affective psychotic disorder. *Australian and New Zealand Journal of Psychiatry* 37: 407–13.

Malla, A. K. and Norman, R. M. G. (2002). Early intervention in schizophrenia and related disorders: Advantages and pitfalls. *Current Opinion in Psychiatry* 15: 17–23.

McGlashan, T. (1999). Duration of untreated psychosis in first-episode schizophrenia: Marker or determinant of course? *Biological Psychiatry* 46: 899–907.

McGorry, P. D. (2000). Evaluating the importance of reducing the duration of untreated psychosis. *Australian and New Zealand Journal of Psychiatry* 34: 145–9.

McGorry, P. D. and Jackson, H. J. (eds) (1999). *The Recognition and Management of Early Psychosis: A Preventive Approach.* Cambridge, UK: Cambridge University Press.

McGorry, P. D. *et al.* (1991). Post-traumatic stress disorder following recent-onset psychosis: An unrecognised post-psychotic syndrome. *Journal of Nervous and Mental Disorders* 179: 253–8.

McGorry, P. D. *et al.* (1996). The Early Psychosis Prevention and Intervention Centre (EPPIC): An evolving system of early detection and optimal management. *Schizophrenia Bulletin* 22: 305–26.

McGorry, P. D. *et al.* (1998) Suicide in early psychosis: Could early intervention work? In R. J. Kosky *et al.* (eds) *Suicide Prevention: The Global Context.* New York: Plenum.

McGorry, P. D. *et al.* (2001). Ethics and early intervention in psychosis: Keeping up the pace and staying in step. *Schizophrenia Research* 51: 17–29.

McGorry, P. D. *et al.* (2002). Randomized controlled trial of interventions designed to reduce the risk of progression to first episode psychosis in a clinical sample with subthreshold symptoms. *Archives of General Psychiatry* 59: 921–8.

Mihalopoulos, C. *et al.* (1999). Is phase-specific, community-oriented treatment of early psychosis an economically viable method of improving outcome? *Acta Psychiatrica Scandinavica* 100: 47–55.

Moody-Ayers, S. Y. *et al.* (2000). 'Benign' tumors and 'early detection' in mammography-screened patients of a natural cohort with breast cancer. *Archives of Internal Medicine* 160: 1109–15.

Mrazek, P. J. and Haggerty, R. J. (eds) (1994). *Reducing Risks for Mental Disorders: Frontiers for Preventive Intervention Research.* Washington, DC: National Academy Press.

Nordentoft, M. *et al.* (2002). OPUS-study: Suicidal behaviour, suicidal ideation and hopelessness among first-episode psychotic patients. A one-year follow-up of a randomised controlled trial. *British Journal of Psychiatry*, 43: s98–106.

Norman, R. M. G. and Malla, A. K. (2001). Duration of untreated psychosis:

A critical examination of the concept and its importance. *Psychological Medicine* 31: 381–400.

Nyberg, S. *et al.* (1995). D$_2$ dopamine receptor occupancy during low-dose treatment with haloperidol decanoate. *American Journal of Psychiatry* 152: 173–8.

Padmavathi, R. *et al.* (1998). Schizophrenic patients who were never treated – a study in an Indian urban community. *Psychological Medicine* 28(5): 1113–7.

Power, P. and McGorry, P. D. (1999). Initial assessment of first-episode psychosis. In P. D. McGorry and H. J. Jackson (eds) *The Recognition and Management of Early Psychosis: A Preventive Approach*. New York: Cambridge University Press.

Power, P. *et al.* (2003). Suicide prevention in first episode psychosis: the development of a randomised controlled trial of cognitive therapy for acutely suicidal patients with acute psychosis. *Australian and New Zealand Journal of Psychiatry* 37: 414–20.

Robinson, D. G. *et al.* (1999). Predictors of relapse following response from a first episode of schizophrenia or schizoaffective disorder. *Archives of General Psychiatry* 56: 241–7.

Schaffner, K. F. and McGorry, P. D. (2001). Preventing severe mental illnesses – new prospects and ethical challenges. *Schizophrenia Research* 51: 3–15.

Van Os, J. *et al.* (2001). Prevalence of psychotic disorder and community level of psychotic symptoms. *Archives of General Psychiatry* 58: 663–8.

Verdoux, H. (2001). Have the times come for early intervention in psychosis? *Acta Psychiatrica Scandinavica* 103: 321–2.

World Health Organisation (2001). *Mental Health: New Understanding, New Hope*. Switzerland: World Health Organisation.

Yung, A. R. *et al.* (1996). Monitoring and care of young people at incipient risk of psychosis. *Schizophrenia Bulletin* 22: 283–303.

Yung, A. R. *et al.* (2003). Psychosis prediction: 12-month follow up of a high-risk ('prodromal') group. *Schizophrenia Research* 60: 21–32.

Yung A. R. *et al.* (2004). Risk factors for psychosis in an ultra high-risk group. Psychopathology and clinical features. *Schizophrenia Research* 67: 131–42.

Chapter 2

Personality and psychosis*

Erik Simonsen

INTRODUCTION

> Clinicians are sometimes prone to forget that every schizophrenic patient also has a personality. These characterological problems may therefore result in noncompliance with medication, alienation of the family members and other supportive persons in the environment, denial of illness, and inability to function in vocational setting.
>
> (Gabbard 1994: 207)

In psychotherapy with schizophrenic patients, the therapist must make an effort to build an alliance with the person behind the illness. The therapeutic process will progress if the patient and the therapist are able to create a meaningful mutual dialogue. However, the person behind the illness in schizophrenia is often deeply disturbed and part of the illness itself. Our assumptions and understanding of how this link takes shape are limited. We do not know how and when the personality structure becomes inflicted and what kind of impact this impairment has on the therapeutic development and outcome. Therefore, this relationship between personality and schizophrenia is difficult to investigate.

Historically, premorbid personality has always been considered a risk factor for the development of psychosis. However, there is controversy over whether there is a continuum from personality deviance to psychosis, or if they are two separate categories of disorder; it is hard to conceptualise this kind of link precisely. Early personality characteristics may simply reflect an underlying common core defect. In other words, it is likely that certain premorbid personality traits precede the first psychotic breakdown and that the psychotic episode itself can damage the personality structure, both during the course of psychosis and in the aftermath. It is, therefore, impossible to separate this relationship from a discussion of the models of schizophrenia itself.

---

* This chapter originally appeared in Martindale, B. and Johannessen, J. O. (2004). *Different Stages – Different Treatments*. London: Brunner-Routledge.

The DSM classification system has separate axes for personality disorders (such as schizoid personality disorder) and syndromes (such as schizophrenia). This separation is meant to facilitate both progress and a better understanding of the relationship between the disorders. However, most clinicians exclude an evaluation of the patient's personality and his or her disorders when the patient has met the criteria for schizophrenia. This attitude reflects the clinical ambiguity regarding a closer evaluation of personality and psychosis. It also reflects the powerful conceptual issues in diagnostic strategies and our current classification systems.

Due to methodological difficulties, researchers are often cautious about studying personality in schizophrenia. However, innovative theories about the development of schizophrenia have placed a focus on the need for new strategies in early detection and intervention. It is likely that the earlier we intervene and treat in schizophrenia, the less damaged the personality will be; a less damaged personality might be an indicator of a good outcome and it might favour psychotherapy instead of medication in early stages of schizophrenia. It is important to try to identify those at special risk and treat them as early as possible. From this perspective, it is important to take a look at the personality structure as an important part of the stress-vulnerability model of schizophrenia. Are there specific personality features which are forerunners of psychosis?

The methodological problems are numerous and, for the most part, remain unsolved. They range from insufficient personality assessment instruments, skewed and biased samples, lack of control groups and biased retrospective studies to changes in definition of those variables under investigation (diagnostic criteria for the personality disorders and schizophrenia).

Our current knowledge of this relationship stems mainly from the following different research strategies:

- Retrospective studies of schizophrenic patients
- Cohort studies
- Follow-up studies of child clinical populations
- Prospective studies of high-risk populations for schizophrenia
- Comorbidity of personality disorders and schizophrenia
- Outcome studies of schizophrenia.

Before summarizing important findings from these different research strategies, I will highlight the current conceptualisations of schizophrenia and personality, and models of their relationship.

THE CONCEPTS OF SCHIZOPHRENIA AND PERSONALITY

Schizophrenia is a heterogeneous group of morbid conditions and multiple manifestations. The term covers diverse clinical pictures and processes. It is a 'catch-all' diagnosis. Therefore, it is not surprising that research only offers a limited number of unambiguous answers to the question of the relationship between personality and early psychosis. It is likely that the three different psychopathological processes (positive psychotic, negative and cognitive disorganised) are of importance to the overall symptomatology of the disorder.

The current neo-Kraepelin era, for reliability reasons, strictly focuses on a descriptive approach to the definition of schizophrenia. This is most notably illustrated by the use of diagnostic criteria in the *DSM-III* (and later *DSM-IV*) and *ICD–10* classification systems. On the contrary, in *ICD-8*, the self and personality of the schizophrenic patient was still in focus: '[T]he disturbance of personality involves its most basic functions, which give the normal person his feeling of individuality, uniqueness and self-direction.' This prototypical approach, in which patients are compared to 'ideal types', has been overtaken by the polythetical approach whereby patients are defined by overt signs and sets of criteria.

These set criteria-based definitions of schizophrenia are arbitrary and pseudo-scientific. They may impair a holistic view of the patient's psychopathology. Consequently, they may cut the treatment planning and the approach to the patient into pieces. Both Bleuler and Jaspers suggested a much broader, dynamic, phenomenological-oriented approach to describing the schizophrenic patient. By doing so, they offered clinicians a better sense of what it is to be a schizophrenic patient. These kinds of description paved the way for our understanding of how to build a mutual therapeutic alliance with the schizophrenic patient.

Likewise, the boundaries of a definition of personality are difficult to draw. As with schizophrenia, the definition of personality reflects the kind of problem scientists decide to study and the empirical procedures used to investigate their questions. One issue is how to select and organise the pervasive, multiple-function patterns of personality functioning; that is, to what extent should the definition be governed solely by theory, vulnerability and dispositional factors, or overt behavioural, symptomatic manifestations? Another controversy is whether to follow a categorical or a dimensional approach. Most recently there has been a movement to study dimensions of personality instead of categories. Additionally, there have been great advances in the methodology of personality disorder assessment, both from a categorical and a dimensional approach. But, so far, very few studies have been carried out using the new instruments covering these general personality dimensions – the Revised NEO Personality Inventory (NEO-PI R), the Temperament and

Character Inventory (TCI) and the Millon Clinical Multiaxial Inventory (MCMI) – and, frequently, the findings are nonspecific.

The most notable instruments for measuring or assessing schizotypy, available for several years, are: the Structured Interview of Schizotypy (SIS), the Structured Interview for Schizotypy–Revised (SIS-R) and the Schizotypal Personality Questionnaire (SPQ).

MODELS OF THE RELATIONSHIP BETWEEN PERSONALITY AND PSYCHOSIS

There are three different ways to look at the relation of personality and psychosis: the disposition or vulnerability model, the personality/psychosis integrated model and the complication model.

Historically, the disposition or vulnerability model (Figure 2.1) regards premorbid personality as part of a continuum of mental illness and/or as a disposition to psychosis. This model is supported by the clinical observations of Kraepelin, Kretschmer and Bleuler (Bleuler 1911/1950; Kraepelin 1919; Kretschmer 1970), as will be described later.

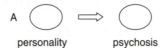

personality   psychosis

Figure 2.1 The disposition or vulnerability model.

Moving on to the integrated model (Figure 2.2): in the psychotic phase of schizophrenia there is a pervasive intrusion in nearly all aspects of the psychic life, including personality. Eugen Bleuler was one of the first to describe how 'single emotionally charged ideas or drives attain a certain degree of autonomy so that personality falls to pieces. These fragments can then exist side by side and alternately dominate the main part of the personality, the conscious part of the patient' (Bleuler 1911/1950).

personality/psychosis

Figure 2.2 Personality/psychosis integrated model.

From a phenomenological point of view, Jaspers describes how the patient's awareness of his/her own personality changes under the psychotic process. Unlike in the normal experience, particularly at the time of puberty, a profound transformation has taken place (Jaspers 1968). The patient has the feeling of being another person; that his or her own personality has disappeared or different personalities are present at different times. Jaspers uses the term 'perplexity' to describe the unpleasant feeling of confusion the patient experiences from not being in control of self and personality.

This integrated model corresponds to a biological approach to the understanding of schizophrenia, where many different neurobiological domains such as perception, thought processing, emotionality, affect, personality and so on are involved.

Historically, the complication model (Figure 2.3) corresponds best to Jasper's idea that mental illness as a biological process deteriorates the person and his personality. According to Jaspers (1968), the personality and its deviances are regarded as part of the illness. The positive, negative and cognitive disorganised symptoms in schizophrenia will tend to develop and enhance disordered personal relationships for the schizophrenic patient. A countless number of characterological problems will occur, such as an inability to make meaningful contact, inappropriate reaction to minor events, excessive aggression, withdrawal and isolation, selfishness, unpredictable behaviour, loneliness, hypersensitivity and so on.

In summary, personality disorders may act as a forerunner and/or a risk factor (A); be a representation of (including early signs of) the illness itself (B); or may become a deteriorating effect of the psychosis (C). However, it may not be possible in clinical practice to separate the models from each other.

These three different approaches to our current understanding will be elaborated further, from both a clinical and an empirical point of view.

DESCRIPTIVE CLINICAL PSYCHOPATHOLOGY

Kraepelin tried to trace the early courses of 'dementia praecox' and from his clinical observations he coined the term 'autistic temperament'. Kraepelin's portrait of the preschizophrenic personality is close to what we now term the 'schizoid personality'. He regarded the person to be reclusive and disinclined to be open or to become involved with others; they withdrew from games and other pleasures, and were impassive and resistant to influence.

It was Bleuler, however, who coined the term 'schizoid', which he found to be represented in all cases to a varying degree. It achieves its full level of morbidity in schizophrenia, and is found to a moderate degree in the schizoid personality: 'people who are withdrawn, suspicious, incapable of

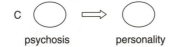

Figure 2.3 The complication model.

discussion, people who are comfortable dull' (Bleuler 1924: 441). On the basis of case studies, Bleuler found that only one quarter had a pathological schizoid personality disorder and one third had emotional and behavioural problems to a lesser degree. Jung, an erstwhile pupil of Bleuler, likewise saw the schizoid position as a general personality dimension and coined the term 'introversion':

> They are mostly silent, inaccessible, hard to understand ... with no desire to affect others, to impress, influence, or change them in any way ... which may actually turn into a disregard for the comfort and well-being of others. One is distinctly aware then of the movement of feeling away from the object.
>
> (Jung 1921: 247)

The schizoid personality has been portrayed by other psychoanalysts such as Fairbain, Deutsch, Guntrip, Klein, Kernberg and Akhtar. They took an overall nosological, developmental or meta-psychological approach, and were not interested in the schizoid personality as a forerunner of schizophrenia.

Kretschmer had the same idea as Kraepelin: that psychotic symptoms were a reaction to stress in a particularly vulnerable personality. He describes two variants of the schizoid type: the anaesthetic-schizoid and the hypersensitive-avoidant, the hypersensitive being 'timid, shy, with fine feelings, sensitive, nervous, excitable' and the anaesthetic as 'a nothing, a dark hollow-eyed nothing – affective anaemia. Behind the ever-silent façade, which twitches uncertainly with every expiring whim – nothing but broken pieces, black rubbish heaps, yawning emotional emptiness, or the cold breath of an artic soullessness' (Kretschmer 1970: 155).

Arieti's clinical observations are interesting because they correspond well with the two different personality types that were later supported by empirical data. He describes a schizoid and a 'stormy' personality as 'prepsychotic personalities'. The schizoid persons 'appear markedly detached, as if something unnatural and strange divided them from the world', while the stormy personality is more outgoing in his attempts to find 'a reliable meaning for his existence' (Arieti 1974: 105).

It is only within the last 30 years that clinical portrayals of the premorbid personality were linked to more well-defined research strategies.

RETROSPECTIVE STUDIES ON PERSONALITY AND PSYCHOSIS

Retrospective studies in which schizophrenic patients, or their informants, recall premorbid features is an unreliable research method as it is skewed by recall bias.

Eugen Bleuler's son, Manfred Bleuler, investigated records from 351 hospitalised schizophrenic patients and found that 34% had a schizoid constitution (Bleuler 1970). Their personality traits varied: suspicious-oversensitive pedant, reckless and callous, paranoid, shy and delicate, fanatic, bigotedly pious and eccentric. Furthermore, he found that 29% had a less marked single schizoid feature.

In the Bonn study of 477 schizophrenic patients, one third were more or less schizoid, nearly half of these with depressive traits (Gross and Huber 1993); one seventh had a sensitive-inhibited personality disorder (or 'hypersensitive' according to Kretschmer).

LONGITUDINAL AND HIGH-RISK STUDIES OF PERSONALITY AND PSYCHOSIS

Prospective longitudinal studies compare the premorbid characteristics of those who go on to develop schizophrenia with those who do not. Useful information from these studies is limited as schizophrenia is a relatively rare illness, and one needs a huge number of representative individuals to get the necessary statistical power for prediction. The observations and measurement of the children in these studies are often vaguely defined. Nevertheless, these studies confirm clinical observations that preschizophrenic children are often more introverted, shy and weak in contact in early childhood (Ellison *et al.* 1998).

High-risk and adoption studies, most often studies of children of schizophrenic mothers, are less time-consuming and costly to carry out. In a Danish-American high-risk study of children of schizophrenic mothers, school-teacher ratings of behaviour were used (Olin and Mednick 1996). Of the children, 31% went on to develop schizophrenia in their forties. They were rated in school as more passive and unengaged, hypersensitive to criticism and, for the males, also more disruptive and hyperexcitable. However, the Danish psychiatrists reported the schizophrenic group in the premorbid phase to be eccentric, peculiar and cognitively impaired, but they found no signs of schizoid behaviour!

FOLLOW-UP STUDIES OF PERSONALITY DISORDER

McGlashan (1991) investigated a group of patients with severe personality disorders, and found that, of 105 patients with borderline and/or schizotypal personality disorders, at a mean of 15 years' follow-up 17 patients had become schizophrenic. Only the schizotypal personality disorder was a predictor for schizophrenia (not borderline!). Additionally, symptoms of magical thinking, suspiciousness, social isolation, transient delusional experiences, poor premorbid quality of work and low IQ showed predictive power (McGlashan 1991).

PROSPECTIVE STUDIES ON FIRST-EPISODE PSYCHOSIS

In a prospective study, with a well-defined sample of 69 first-episode psychotic patients, Dalkin and his colleagues found a positive association between schizoid, paranoid and explosive personality traits and later schizophrenia (Dalkin *et al.* 1994).

Three-dimensional premorbid personality structures were found in analyses of a sample of 112 patients with relatively recent-onset psychosis (Cuesta *et al.* 1999). Schizoid premorbid traits were associated with the negative dimension, schizotypal traits with the positive dimension and sociopathic traits with the disorganised dimension.

Sociopathic dimension $\rightarrow$ disorganisation
Schizotypal dimension $\rightarrow$ positive psychotic symptoms
Schizoid dimension $\rightarrow$ negative symptoms

Other studies support the validity of these findings (Berenbaum and Fujita 1994; Dalkin *et al.* 1994; Jackson *et al.* 1991; Parnas and Joergensen 1989).

GENETICS AND THE SCHIZOPHRENIA SPECTRUM PERSONALITY DISORDERS

Most genetic studies confirm a link between premorbid personality in schizophrenia and the schizophrenia spectrum personality disorders (i.e. schizotypal, schizoid and paranoid). To a much lesser extent, there is evidence of a link to anti-social, explosive personality traits. There seems to be a common inheritance of these cluster A personality disorders and schizophrenia. Torgersen reviewed twin, adoption and family studies of the common genetic disposition to some personality disorders and schizophrenia (Torgersen 1994). Not all studies pointed in the same direction; some studies showed different associations. The schizotypal personality disorder has the strongest association to schizophrenia (twin, adoption, family), followed by paranoid (family, adoption?), schizoid (family?, adoption?) then avoidant (twin) (question marks suggest an unclear association). Among the schizotypal criteria, social anxiety, constricted affect and odd speech are most clearly genetically related to schizophrenia.

However, one might question whether these personality traits are specific to schizophrenia and not mental illnesses in general. In a meta-analysis of studies, Berenbaum and Fujita (1994) found no differences in premorbid introversion between schizophrenics and neurotics, but they did find that schizophrenics are more peculiar. Both groups are more introverted and peculiar than normal controls.

COMORBIDITY OF PERSONALITY DISORDERS AND SCHIZOPHRENIA

The comorbidity of a personality disorder and schizophrenia may reflect different situations:

- The disorders have causal factors in common with an increased risk of having both disorders.
- There may be insufficient delineation between the disorders on the level of criteria.
- Personality pathology precedes schizophrenia and/or schizophrenia deteriorates personality.

The prevalence of personality disorders in schizophrenia varies greatly between studies, ranging from 7% to 57%. These findings are, of course, highly dependent on sample and research methods. In a study of 112 in-patients, of which one third had schizophrenia, Jackson and colleagues found that schizophrenia was associated with anti-social and schizotypal personality disorders (Jackson *et al.* 1991). It is likely that more severe forms of schizophrenia – those which need hospitalisation – also have the most severe personality traits such as schizotypal and anti-social behaviour. These findings are in accordance with the already mentioned studies on premorbid personalities in schizophrenia.

PERSONALITY, SCHIZOPHRENIA AND OUTCOME

To what extent, if any at all, is outcome related to personality traits?

Torgalsboen (1999) found that schizoid features and conduct disorders were more often present in childhood among non-recovered schizophrenic patients. Furthermore, these traits were related to the presence of a personality disorder at first admission. In the Bonn study, schizophrenic patients with an additional personality disorder had a highly significantly unfavourable outcome, which was more prominent than that of those who had a schizoid constitution (Gross and Huber 1993).

In a Swedish, 14–17-year follow-up study of 110 first-time-admitted schizophrenic patients, the personality pathology for negative outcome was: personality deviation in adolescence, disturbed contact ability, avoidance behaviour, social isolation, introversion and low self-esteem (Jonsson and Nymann 1991).

Personality disorders, particularly anti-social personality disorder, predicted relapses of psychosis in schizophrenia according to a Dutch study (Dingemanns *et al.* 1998).

DIATHESIS-PERSONALITY-STRESS MODEL

How can we summarise these data regarding personality and schizophenia in a more comprehensive model? Zuckermann (1999) has suggested a diathesis-personality-stress model for the etiology of schizophrenia (see Figure 2.4). He defines it as a modified Meehl model in which stress (biological in this case) acts on genetically vulnerable brain systems, while familial-interpersonal stress is involved in shaping the vulnerable personality (Meehl 1990). Genetic dispositions, and prenatal and perinatal factors, constitute the brain of a person at risk. The brain pathologies may produce abnormal personality traits and disorders and, in this model, three main personality dimensions. Neglect, family pathology and other environmental factors enhance the risk for inappropriate social behaviour, and cognitive disturbances create communication and learning difficulties. Negative feedback facilitates further social isolation, social anxiety, and peculiar behaviour and speech. The personality is now very vulnerable to even minor stressors; psychosis might be the consequence.

This useful model includes neurobiological vulnerability, the dimensional thinking of forerunners in the symptom complex, the most robust findings of preceding schizotypal traits and the importance of emotional stress in the family prior to the breakdown in psychosis.

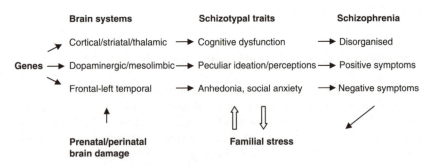

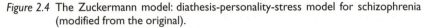

Figure 2.4 The Zuckermann model: diathesis-personality-stress model for schizophrenia (modified from the original).

PSYCHOTHERAPY OF SCHIZOPHRENIA

What has this discussion of the links between personality and schizophrenia to do with the aim of this book, which is to underline the importance of delivering different treatment at different stages? Is it possible to intervene and treat personality deviances in psychotic-prone patients and, by so doing, prevent the patient from becoming psychotic?

Psychotherapy is about how to assess and understand the dynamics of personality traits and symptoms and to teach patients to cope with or modify symptoms.

Most clinicians do not regard psychotherapy as prevention for psychotic-prone patients. Why is this so? Basically, I think it is a question of the relationship between therapist and patient. Is it more important to get in touch with the person behind the illness and address therapeutic interventions from there? Or is it better for the patient if the treatment focuses on how to control symptoms? Clinicians interested in the psychotherapy of schizophrenic patients will argue that it is important to obtain a dynamic concept of schizophrenia, which also keeps a language for the self and for the changes of personality. Symptoms can be conceptualised and understood in relation to the self, interpersonal relatedness and personality structure in a developmental theory. This will create a framework for the psychotherapy of schizophrenic patients.

Manfred Bleuler's opinion about schizophrenia was that behind or beside psychotic phenomena, signs of a normal intellectual and emotional life can be discovered. He argued that research into the clinical course of the illness confirmed what clinicians had realised: in the schizophrenic, the healthy human is hidden and remains hidden, even if psychosis is long lasting. He thought that the healthy life of the schizophrenic would never be extinguished (Bleuler 1970).

This is an important assumption when establishing a therapeutic alliance with a psychotic patient. But it is equally important that therapy addresses characterological problems, if present. All interventions should be tailored to the person behind the illness, his or her unique needs and individuality. These efforts to build a therapeutic alliance are crucial to impede a poor outcome.

In cognitive-behavioural therapy, problem-solving, control of psychotic symptoms and relapse prevention are the centre of focus. This method has influenced traditional psychodynamic-oriented, supportive psychotherapy and provided important knowledge regarding how to engage the person behind the illness. In this way, cognitive therapy tailors the therapeutic strategy, leading to a close agreement with the patient of what he or she needs to do and how to do it.

Hogarthy (2002) has formulated a personal psychotherapy of schizophrenia. The therapeutic set-up is very flexible and need-adapted in its approach. Different needs in different phases of illness require different treatment strategies. Even at long-term follow-up, patients who have been treated in this way achieved better role performance and social adjustment, but not fewer symptoms.

McGlashan (1989) identified, in a 15-year follow-up study, a group of schizophrenic patients who were able to integrate their psychotic experiences into their psychic life. These patients had gained from their acceptance and knowledge of their psychotic episode. A 'sealing over' group, who remained negative towards their psychotic experiences, had a less favourable outcome. The rate of drop-out from psychotherapy in schizophrenia is an immense problem and is closely linked to this 'sealing over'. As with borderline patients, a longer-term hospitalisation, prior to or concomitant with psychotherapy, may tailor the treatment to the patient (Gunderson 1987).

Psychotherapy may not change symptoms to a great extent or promote full recovery, but it may improve quality of life and overall adaptation to the environment (Rund 1990). However, many patients fear improvement and choose to stay in their psychotic world with devils, hallucinations and autistic fantasies. They would rather be an eccentric personality than face the anxiety and stress of reaching back to the real world.

CONCLUSION

The premorbid personality of patients with psychiatric disorders, especially in schizophrenia, is of longstanding theoretical, nosological and therapeutic interest. The nature of the link between abnormal personality and schizophrenia remains unclear.

Recent research into early intervention strategies has highlighted the need for a better understanding of prepsychotic personality. Several important questions have been raised. Are premorbid peculiarities early, subclinical, phenotypic variations and mild forms of the disorders itself, or do they represent a coexisting genetic or developmental disposition? Do they represent independent, potentially protective or vulnerable variables? How specific and sensitive are these traits if they represent an early stage of schizophrenia? To what extent should the alteration and deterioration of the personality be part of the diagnostic criteria in schizophrenia, or should they be rated as separate features on a separate axis? Consequently, which therapeutic intervention, psychosocial and/or pharmaceutical, should be prescribed to prevent the odd personality from drifting into psychosis?

Due to heavy methodological difficulties and the burden of large-scale studies, very little empirical research has been carried out to answer these challenging questions. To further our understanding of the interface between personality and psychosis, we are compelled mainly to seek the clinical observations and speculations made by psychopathologists like Kraepelin, Bleuler and Jaspers.

Unlike bipolar illness, where the patient's personality can be assessed while s/he is euthymic, schizophrenia, to some extent, is nearly always there and the effect of psychosis on the personality is persistent, not intermittent.

Schizophrenia seems to be closely related to the so-called schizophrenia personality disorders (*DSM-IV* cluster A), either because they have a genetic disposition in common or because the spectrum personality disorders are precursors of or dispositions to schizophrenia. To a much lesser extent, anti-social personality disorder seems linked to schizophrenia.

Many schizophrenic patients have a normal personality. It might be useful to take a dimensional approach to understanding the illness in patients for whom there seems to be a linear progress in psychopathology towards a sudden qualitative different breakdown under stress. The schizoid, schizo-typal and anti-social features seem to be important personality dimensions and precursors in schizophrenia linked respectively to negative, positive and disorganised symptoms.

Another important finding is that if personality disorders are still present after recovery from psychosis, it is likely that they are predictors of an unfavourable outcome.

The extreme heterogeneity of schizophrenia, its symptoms and outcome, calls for an open model of schizophrenia. Schizophrenia is a brain disease, and genetic and environmental factors play a particular role in its etiology and symptom formation. The symptoms seem to cluster in three ways: deficits, positive psychotic and disorganised symptoms. Personality dimensions seem to play a role in each of these clusters, either as pathways to a full-blown syndrome or as independent risk factors.

A shift from a categorical to a dimensional way of conceptualising schizophrenia and personality disorder will enhance our understanding and pave the way for more fruitful validation of prevention strategies and predictors of outcome. Personality and its disorders will be elucidated as risk factors and pathways to psychosis. Psychotherapy deals with personality problems and how to cope with symptoms. Research has shown that the schizophrenic patient does benefit from a psychotherapeutic experience. This new focus on personality dimensions and their treatability through psychotherapy has important implications for treatment approaches following the early detection of schizophrenia.

REFERENCES

Arieti, S. (1974). *Interpretation of Schizophrenia*. Northvale, NJ: Jason Aronson.
Berenbaum, H. and Fujita, F. (1994). Schizophrenia and personality: Exploring boundaries and connections between vulnerability and outcome. *Journal of Abnormal Psychology* 103: 148–8.
Bleuler, E. (1911/1950). *Dementia Praecox or the Group of Schizophrenias* (translated by J. Zinkin). New York: International Universities Press.

Bleuler, E. (1924). *Textbook of Psychiatry*. New York: Macmillan.

Bleuler, M. (1970). Some results of research in schizophrenia. *Behavioral Science* 15: 211–8.

Cuesta, M. J. *et al.* (1999). Premorbid personality in psychoses. *Schizophrenia Bulletin* 25: 801–11.

Dalkin, T. *et al.* (1994). Premorbid personality in first-onset psychosis. *British Journal of Psychiatry* 164: 202–7.

Dingemans, P. M. *et al.* (1998). Personality and schizophrenic relapse. *International Clinical Psychopharmacology* 13 (supplement 1): 89–95.

Ellison, Z. *et al.* (1998). Childhood personality characteristics of schizophrenia: Manifestations of, or risk factors for the disorder? *Journal of Personality Disorder* 12: 247–61.

Gabbard, G. O. (1994). *Psychodynamic Therapy in Clinical Practice*. Washington: American Psychiatric Press.

Gross, G. and Huber, G. (1993). Premorbid personality in schizophrenia: The contribution of European long-term studies. *Neurology, Psychiatry and Brain Research* 2: 14–20.

Gunderson, J. G. (1987). Engagement of schizophrenic patients in psychotherapy. In J. L. Sacksteder (ed), *Attachment and Therapeutic Process: Essays in Honor of Otto Allen Will, Jr.* Madison, CT: International Universities Press.

Hogarthy, G. E. (2002). *Personal Therapy: A Guide to Individualized Treatment*. New York: Guilford Press.

Jackson, H. J. *et al.* (1991). Diagnosing personality disorders in psychiatric inpatients. *Acta Psychiatrica Scandinavica* 83: 206–13.

Jaspers, K. (1968). *General Psychopathology* (translated by J. Hoenig and M. W. Hamilton). Chicago: University of Chicago Press.

Jonssen, H. and Nymann, A. K. (1991). 14–17 years outcome of 110 first-time admitted schizophrenic patients. *Acta Psychiatrica Scandinavica* 83: 342–6.

Jung, C. G. (1921). *The Psychological Types*. Zurich: Rascher Verlag.

Kraepelin, E. (1919). *Dementia Praecox and Paraphrenia*. Edinburgh: Livingstone.

Kretschmer, E. (1970). *Physique and Character, and Investigation of the Nature of Constitution and Theory of Temperament*. New York: Cooper Square Publishers.

McGlashan, T. H. (1991). The schizophrenia spectrum concept: The Chestnut Lodge follow-up study. *Schizophrenia Research* 1: 193–200.

Meehl, P. E. (1990). Toward an integrated theory of schizotaxia, schizotypy and schizophrenia. *Journal of Personality Disorders* 4: 1–99.

Olin, S. S. and Mednick, S. A. (1996). Risk factors of psychosis: Identifying vulnerable populations premorbidly. *Schrizophrenia Bulletin* 22: 223–40.

Parnas, J. and Joergensen, A. (1989). Premorbid psychopathology in schizophrenia spectrum. *British Journal of Psychiatry* 155: 623–7.

Rund, B. R. (1990). Fully recovered schizophrenics: A retrospective study of some premorbid and treatment factors. *Psychiatry* 53: 127–39.

Torgalsboen, A. K. (1999). Comorbidity in schizophrenia. A prognostic study of personality disorders in recovered and non-recovered schizophrenic patients. *Scandinavian Journal of Psychology* 40: 147–52.

Torgersen, S. (1994). Personality deviations within the schizophrenia spectrum. *Acta Psychiatrica Scandinavica* 90 (supplement 34): 40–4.

Zuckermann, M. (1999). *Vulnerability to Psychopathology – A Biopsychosocial Model*. Washington: American Psychological Association.

Chapter 3

A post-Lacanian view of schizophrenia*

Wilfried Ver Eecke

INTRODUCTION

In this chapter I will propose that the theory of Jacques Lacan as presented by Alphonse De Waelhens is close to the empirical phenomena of schizophrenia, and can serve as a theory by which to understand different successful approaches to the treatment of schizophrenics. I will do so by first underlining a possible paradox in De Waelhens' presentation (1978), and will then use that paradox to move to a better post-Lacanian theory.

APPARENT INCONSISTENCY IN DE WAELHENS' PRESENTATION OF THE CAUSE OF SCHIZOPHRENIA

One can find in De Waelhens (1978) two versions of a psychological causal explanation of schizophrenia. The first causal explanation is derived from a student of Lacan: Piera Aulagnier. De Waelhens presents his explanation as a variant of the theory of the schizophrenogenic mother, even though he adds that schizophrenia must be understood as the result of a failure in a triangular structure in which each of the three angles (maternal figure, paternal figure and child) can play a role. Compared with some Anglo-American variants, this causal explanation has two unique features: it concentrates upon the desire (as opposed to the behaviour) of the mother and it begins its analysis of the influence of the maternal figure from the period of pregnancy (and not just from the period after birth).

De Waelhens, making use of a study by Aulagnier (1964), points to a number of observations about mothers of normal children: the narcissistic investment of the pregnant woman in her pregnancy; the transformation of

* I wish to thank Mark Nowacki for the stylistic improvements he suggested.

The ideas of the paper delivered at the ISPS conference at Stavanger, June 2000, have been incorporated, with modifications, in: De Waelhens, A. and Ver Eecke, W. (2001). *Phenomenology and Lacan on Schizophrenia, after the Decade of the Brain* (pp. 70–82). Leuven: University of Leuven Press.

that narcissistic involvement into expectation of a future child by the work of the imagination; the unconscious acceptance of the sexual origin of the child; the rather quick overcoming of post-partum depression; the delicate balance of feeling of oneness-in-otherness with the baby; and the support provided by the mother for the child as it learns to live with its body, even its paining body.

Mothers of schizophrenic children tend, according to Aulagnier's report, to lack the work of imagination that transforms narcissistic involvement into expectation of the future child; they tend to repress unconsciously the idea of the sexual origin of the child; and they tend to imagine themselves as the creator of the child. They also have a harder time overcoming post-partum depression and show a disturbance in the delicate balance of the feeling of oneness-in-otherness with their children. (For a confirmation of many elements of this report see two case studies in Karon and VandenBos 1981: 329–353.) This latter disturbance is conceptualized as leading to difficulties for the child in inhabiting its own body since the child needs to deal with the paradox of experiencing its own body as other from but still desirable by the mother.

One strain of thought in this explanation – which De Waelhens will be able to use legitimately to diminish the apparent contradiction of having two different causal explanations – is the claim that the mother represses the sexual origin of the child which in turn leads to difficulties in recognizing the otherness of the child. As a consequence, the mother does not do the necessary work of imagination to provide the desirable balance in the feeling of oneness-in-otherness with the baby. Using Lacanian language, De Waelhens summarizes this situation as pointing to 'the mother's incapacity to construct a corporeal signifier' which 'must result in a "massive castration" of the future subject. . . . The foreclosure of the name-of-the-father has here its point of origin' (De Waelhens 1978: 64).

Thus one strain of thought in the causal explanation of schizophrenia tied to the function of the maternal figure leads to the claim that the maternal figure helps to lay the groundwork for a failure in the paternal function. This explanation thus has a connection with the second explanation, which claims that schizophrenia results from a failure in the paternal function. That second causal explanation presented by De Waelhens is derived directly from Lacan; more specifically it is derived from Lacan's interpretation of Judge Schreber. The explanation starts by accepting that the child has a symbiotic relation with its mother. In that relation the child creates an imaginary solution to its problem of dependence upon others for survival. That illusion can be conceptualized as the child's attempt to situate itself in a maternal space characterized by the possibility of fusion with the mother. If the fusion is not total, the child still imagines itself to be the sole object of the desires of a mother considered omnipotent.

Lacanian theory argues that the normal way for a child to correct its illusionary vision of others and itself is for the mother to show respect for a third, normally the father. That third – the father – need not be physically present; he need not even be alive. Therefore, Lacan summarizes his views using the formula that the mother must show respect for the name-of-the-father. Such respect by the mother gives a double message to the child. On the one hand, it shows the child that the mother is not omnipotent, and, on the other hand, it shows the child that it is not the only object of the mother's desires. After first trying to destroy the message by either interrupting communication between mother and father or by wishing the father to be gone (or dead), the child moves towards a more constructive solution. The child borrows the insignia of the father and carries them as regalia (glasses, hat, shoes) before selecting unconsciously a mark in the father with which to identify in the hope of thereby re-appropriating some of the esteem of the mother. That mark is the signifier which, from then on, will unconsciously organize the desire of the child.

Of the many consequences created by that move, it is important to mention two explicitly. First, by that move – which corresponds to the Freudian Oedipus complex – the child substitutes mediation for immediacy. Indeed, the child in the post-Oedipal period unconsciously aims to maintain the esteem of the mother not by being directly present to the mother but by incorporating in itself something for which the child guesses the mother has great affection: some mark in the father. Second, the child has made a move in which similarity and difference are united. Indeed, whereas previously the child situated itself as the object of the mother's desire, now the child situates itself differently: it positions itself as wanting to be like the father who is respected by the mother. Still, the child feels itself to be the same child in both positions. Lacan called that move – which synthesizes similarity and difference – the paternal metaphor. The absence of such a move is considered the structural cause of schizophrenia, which is expected to erupt if the proper occasion presents itself. Lacan conceptualizes that occasion as the appearance of an 'A-Father' figure in the emotional life of the patient (De Waelhens 1978; Lacan 1977; Laplanche 1969).

ADDRESSING THE APPARENT INCONSISTENCY

De Waelhens senses the problem lurking within his dual causal explanation of schizophrenia when he asks, in a special section on 'The Relative Role of the Mother and Father in Psychosis', the following: 'Could we not be reproached for having located the origin of psychosis both in the child's relationship to the mother, and in his relationship to the father?' (De Waelhens 1978: 137). De Waelhens answers his own rhetorical question by arguing that the two causes are in effect not two separate causes but rather two causes that reinforce each other and thus become part of a single more general cause. Thus, the schizophrenogenic mother who during pregnancy omits the work of the imagination does not create a chain of signifiers into which the child will be introduced. If the child has not been introduced to the world of signifiers then it cannot effectively internalize a paternal signifier, for the child has remained alien to the world of signifiers. On the other hand, if the father is 'a caricatural personage' (ibid.: 138) how can the mother show respect for him and introduce him to the child?

Thus De Waelhens presents the overall cause as both a defective maternal and a defective paternal role. As the maternal role consists of, among other things, creating (by fusion, by mirroring) the basis of self-esteem, and as the paternal role consists of, among other things, introducing a sense of finitude, of limit, of separateness and of law – connected by Lacan with the introduction of language (Fink 1996; Muller and Richardson 1982) and conceptualized by Freudians as the imposition of castration – the schizophrenic seems to be in need of help from two contradictory directions. But how can one claim that a patient needs at the same time fusion and separation, for instance? This claim is a paradox only if one has a static view of human development in which one sees one or the other element missing. It is not a paradox if one has a dynamic view of human development in which one postulates the need for the simultaneous healthy presence of both. This is similar to the view developed by Blatt when he argues that human beings need both 'the development of satisfying interpersonal relationships and a well-differentiated sense of self' and that 'these two developmental processes evolve in an interactive, reciprocally balanced, mutually facilitating fashion from birth through senescence' (Blatt 1995: 1012).

The view that both the maternal and the paternal function have been defective in the schizophrenic goes a long way towards explaining the advice of experienced and successful therapists of schizophrenics.[1] Harold Searles, for example, advises that first, it is mandatory to:

> foster the necessary emotional atmosphere in the sessions for the development of the contented, unthreatened emotional oneness to which I refer by the term 'therapeutic symbiosis' – a form of relatedness of the same quality as that which imbues the mother–infant relatedness in normal infancy and very early childhood.
>
> (Searles 1986: 598)

He advises, second, that 'limit-setting is one of the major dimensions of therapeutic technique in this work' (ibid.). Furthermore, Searles points to a dialectical connection between the two above requirements. In a passage which De Waelhens or Lacan could have written, Searles writes:

> The analyst is able firmly to set and maintain limits to the extent that he is aware of, and accepting of, his own individual limitations. But the very nature of the work with schizophrenic patients, who themselves have so

much unresolved infantile omnipotent striving, is such as powerfully to evoke the analyst's unconscious fantasies of omnipotence.

(Searles 1986: 601)

And, 'An analyst who, for whatever unconscious reasons, cannot become able to live comfortably with the possibility that his patient may never become free from psychosis cannot, by the same token, foster the necessary ... "therapeutic symbiosis" '(ibid.: 598). Thus the therapist who cannot control his own sense of omnipotence in healing schizophrenics will not only be incapable of setting the necessary limits for his patients (he will be defective in his paternal function) but he will also not be able to create the necessary therapeutic symbiosis (he will be defective in his maternal function). In summary, a successful maternal function (e.g., therapeutic symbiosis) requires the incorporation of a paternal function (acceptance of finitude, limit-setting).

The above reading of Searles allows me to make two points. The first point is a practical one. If effective therapy requires such contradictory capabilities, it is no wonder that Blatt can conclude: 'Significant differences exist in therapeutic efficacy among therapists, even the experienced and well-trained therapists in the TDCRP [Treatment of Depression Collaborative Research Program]' (Blatt *et al.* 1996: 1281–2). All indications are that a similar statement can be made for therapists of schizophrenia. Searles gives us a test, a criterion for effectiveness in psychotherapy. De Waelhens' theory, as it is informed by Lacan, can provide a reason why the criterion given by Searles is necessary. My second point is theoretical. For the maternal function and the paternal function to be effective, feelings of grandiose omnipotence must be checked. When De Waelhens wrote his book, Lacan had articulated that requirement explicitly for the maternal function by insisting that a mother needs to acknowledge her own lack by showing respect for the name-of-the-father. Lacan had not yet articulated the requirement so well for the paternal function. He does so later (Evans 1996), when he writes that the father should be a symbolic father: a subject himself submitted to the law and thus subject to finitude (death) and limitation, rather than an imaginary omnipotent father (Evans 1996; Lacan 1993).

BROADENING THE SEARCH FOR A SOLUTION TO THE DUAL CAUSAL THEORY

Since the publication of De Waelhens' book several of Lacan's seminars have become available, and Lacan scholarship has also developed. Scholars and therapists using the ideas of Lacan have pointed out that while Lacan's use of the name-of-the-father as the crucial element in the definition of psychosis and of schizophrenia is a very important conceptual achievement, Lacan's account is still a negative definition (Calligaris 1991; Vergote 1998).[2] One can find in Lacan's work elements that go beyond his own negative definition when he points to schizophrenia as the failure of the symbolic system to get hold of the imaginary (Fink 1997), because both the symbolic and the imaginary are deficient. As a result of these deficiencies the stitching of the symbolic to the imaginary, the creation of anchoring of meaning is defective. In Lacan's technical language, the schizophrenic lacks 'button ties' – also called 'anchoring points' or 'quilting points' (Fink 1997; Moyaert 1993). Consequently, the patient is confronted with the horror of the Real that can neither be imagined nor symbolized (Evans 1996).[3] This line of thinking explicitly takes the road suggested by De Waelhens; that is, the failure of the symbolic is also a failure of the imaginary. However, the solution suggested by De Waelhens can now be better articulated because recent theoretical developments have made us aware of the multiple failures that are possible in both the imaginary and the symbolic.

The possibility that the imaginary system may fail in many ways becomes obvious if one recalls that Lacan twice revised his mirror stage theory. In his original presentation Lacan located the achievement of the child and the reason for its jubilation in the fact that it had now created a unified total body image instead of experiencing itself as body parts. In his first revision, Lacan located the reason for the jubilation of the child in the child's discovery of the mother's narcissistic involvement with the child. The mother's involvement is noticeable in the child's search for the mother's eye when it sees itself in the mirror. According to this reading, it is the mother's emotional involvement with the child that allows the child to invest emotionally in its own body (Fink 1997; Simiu 1986; Ver Eecke 1984). In his second revision, Lacan accepts the idea from one of his students, Rosaline Lefort, that the child not only needs to create a unified body image but that it also has to create a body image that performs the role of container to some contained (Lacan 1988). Lacan explicitly connects the idea of the body as container to a contained with his theory of the mirror stage by means of his famous flower vase, in which a concave mirror allows a person to see flowers separated from a vase as being within the vase (Lacan 1977). For a human being, the body image as container needs to have a place for needs, feelings, faeces, urine, food and even pain. The baby's task of creating a body image as container requires the skilled help of a maternal figure.

Similarly, the multiple ways in which the symbolic system may fail can also be better understood in the light of later developments in Lacan's thought. Indeed, De Waelhens reconstructs Lacan's thesis on the basis of his article summarizing the seminar on psychosis. In that summary the major reason for the failure of the symbolic is because the mother shows no respect for the word (name) of the father (Lacan 1977). It is true that Lacan adds one paragraph at this point about the deficiencies of the father himself, but it is almost presented as an afterthought. However, in the full seminar, Lacan stresses at length that the paternal function requires a symbolic father not an imaginary father (Lacan 1993). He defines an imaginary father as someone who 'manifests himself simply in the order of strength and not in that of the pact' (ibid.: 205). He describes the consequences of such a paternal figure as follows: 'We are all familiar with cases of these delinquent or psychotic sons who proliferate in the shadow of a paternal personality of exceptional character, one of these social monsters referred to as venerable' (ibid.: 204). Later, Lacan conceptualizes this notion of the symbolic father as the 'barred Other' (Evans 1996). Thus, in light of the full development of Lacan's thought we can argue that the father, too, can contribute to the failure of the symbolic order in a child. He can do so because he presents himself more as an imaginary rather than as a symbolic father.

Finally, the failure of the symbolic may not just be the result of a deficiency in the symbolic or in the imaginary; it may also be attributed, in some cases, to the horror of the Real itself. This possibility arises because Lacan seems to accept two moments in the development of the child where language emerges. On the one hand, Lacan describes the result of the Oedipal complex as the establishment of the symbolic order and thus the creation of an effective signifier. On the other hand, he also comments on Freud's analysis of his grandchild who, as an infant, did not cry when his mother left him because he had, first, created a transitional object (the spool) and then, second, replaced the spool with the words 'fort-da' (away-here) (Lacan 1977). Thus, in his dual theory of the origin of language, Lacan allows for the possibility that something might go wrong in the use of language (the symbolic) before the Oedipal period, at a time when the imaginary seems to dominate. Indeed, children may not succeed in using either transitional objects or words to deal with a departing mother, or they may do so in a radically defective way.

There may be multiple reasons for failures of the symbolic. Furthermore, these multiple reasons may exert their influence independent of or in addition to maternal and paternal influences. Two cases might illustrate my claim.

VandenBos presents a case of a child whose parents were going through a divorce, but where the family doctor played the major role in creating the symptom. The boy was sent to the doctor because he was quite 'nervous' and was placed on mild tranquilizers. The boy asked for an explanation from his doctor, who told him that he had bad nerves. To the boy's further questions the doctor answered that nerves were like worms under the skin. The boy was sent to VandenBos because he 'was compulsively splashing water on his face and soaking his hands . . . as many as 20 to 30 times a day. He would wake up in the middle of the night to do the same thing' (Karon and VandenBos 1981: 159). VandenBos discovered that the boy knew about worms from fishing. He knew that if they dried, they burst open. He was therefore afraid that his bad nerves were going to burst open and hence he tried to keep them wet. The nervousness changed into compulsive behaviour because of the explanation given by an outsider (the family doctor) about the child's nervousness.

Lefort presents another case, that of Robert, who was grossly neglected by his mother (he was twice brought to hospital in a state of acute wasting before he was one year old). However, a surgical team greatly contributed to the child's difficulties with developmental tasks, because they administered an antrotomy at the age of five months without anaesthetics while simultaneously forcing a bottle of sweetened water in the boy's mouth in order to prevent him from crying. Lefort writes that she had the impression that the boy's horror 'fantasies had become reality' (Lacan 1988: 100).

In the case presented by VandenBos, the family doctor unwittingly helped create the horror of the Real by making a connection between the boy's nervousness and worms. In the case presented by Lefort, the encounter with life itself created too much of a horror (not being fed, and being operated on without anaesthetics).

As I mentioned before, the later Lacan argues that psychosis is the reaction to the Real which cannot be signified by the imaginary or by the symbolic. As the Real is horrifying, the lack of its mastery by signifying leads to very defensive strategies. In presenting psychosis as a reaction to a developmental failure at two levels, an opening is created for a more complex definition of schizophrenia. Indeed, a psychotic reaction is not a reaction to the failure of the symbolic alone (i.e. a failure of the paternal metaphor). It is a reaction to the joint failure of the imaginary and the symbolic. I will therefore articulate the connection and the difference between the functions of the imaginary and the symbolic.

Let me start by clarifying the imaginary as it is created in the mother–child relationship. The challenge in the mother–child relation is for the mother to introduce distance between herself and the child while creating a deep form of caring unity with her child. The child's challenge is to use the gift of caring unity with the mother as the basis for accepting itself as embodied and to use the gift of distance offered by the mother as a method to separate itself from its mother.

The challenge of the symbolic is for both the mother and the father to introduce and make acceptable to the child the idea of finitude, which implies for the child the acceptance of its place in the legitimate order of human beings. The painful dimension in this challenge is that the symbolic dislodges the child from its imagined privileged place with its mother. This involves the experiencing of a narcissistic wound. However, it also results in the child discovering its own identity and a direction for its own desire. Both result from the child borrowing, through identification, a basic mark from the father. That identity is signalled by the name given to the child, but is only significant if the child accepts that identity, which in turn means that the child in its unconscious has been marked and grounded in a central meaning-giving signifier. The early Lacan called this meaning-giving signifier the name-of-the-father. The later Lacan splits the two moments involved in his original concept of the name-of-the-father. He differentiates the fact of receiving a name from the phenomenon of accepting the meaning associated with it (my name is John Smith and I have the choice of honoring or dishonoring that name). Lacan continues to call the first moment the fundamental signifier, now also referred to as S1, and he calls the second moment S2. The first moment is associated with the negative experience of alienation (my name is something different to the inner feeling of my selfhood and is imposed on me without my consent). The second moment is associated with separation (how I choose to individuate myself – as honoring or dishonoring my given name) (Fink 1996). Through this move Lacan connects his original idea of the name-of-the-father as the fundamental signifier with his other idea of meaning consisting in a chain of signifiers. S1 and S2 are seen to be the beginning of an infinite series of signifiers: S1, S2, S3, S4 . . .

The case of Robert presented by Rosaline Lefort in a seminar given by Lacan illustrates the claim that psychosis is not just the failure of the symbolic but rather the failure of the symbolic because of an already failed imaginary. We do not hear about Robert's father. At the time of Robert's treatment the mother was diagnosed as a paranoiac and confined (Lacan 1988). His mother kept him with her, moving from house to house. She neglected his essential needs so much that at five months old he arrived in a hospital with acute 'hypertrophy and wasting'. After an infection which necessitated an operation he was isolated and 'fed on a drip'. At nine months he was returned to his mother, only to come back to the hospital two months later, 'again in a state of acute wasting' (ibid.: 91). Five months later the mother legally abandoned the child. As a foster child, Robert changed residence twenty-five times before he was four years old (ibid.). As indicated before, the therapist discovered that Robert had undergone an antrotomy at the age of five months without anaesthetics: 'Throughout the painful operation a bottle of sweetened water had been kept forced in his mouth' (ibid.: 100).

Some of Robert's symptoms were: his extreme lack of coordination in movement; his hyperagitation; his lack of coordinated speech (he would frequently utter screams and guttural, discordant laughter, and he yelled two words: Miss and Wolf); his prehensive activity was uncoordinated – 'he would throw his arm out to take hold of an object and if he didn't reach it, he couldn't correct it, and had to start the movement all over again from the beginning' (ibid.: 92); and he had convulsive fits of agitation without real convulsions, 'during each of the routine moments of his daily life – the pot, and above all the emptying of the pot, undressing, feeding' (ibid.: 92). 'One evening, after going to bed, he tried to cut off his penis with a pair of plastic scissors, while standing on his bed in front of the other terrified children' (ibid.: 93).

> The business of undressing was for him the occasion for genuine crises
> . . . one having lasted three hours, during which the staff described him as
> possessed. He howled – Wolf!, running from one bedroom to the next,
> smearing the other children with faeces that he found in the pots. It was
> only once he was tied up that he calmed down.
>
> (ibid.: 96)

Using the three categories of Lacan, the therapist Lefort writes about
Robert:

> I had the impression [that] it was Robert's tragedy that all his oral-
> sadistic fantasies had been realised in the actual events of his life. His
> [horror] fantasies had become reality . . . the image that Robert had
> constructed of a starving, paranoiac, dangerous mother, who certainly
> attacked him. Then the separation, a bottle held by force, making him
> swallow his cries. The force-feedings with the tube, twenty-five moves in
> succession.
>
> (ibid.: 100)

Lefort continues: 'I had the impression that this child had sunk under the
real, that at the beginning of the treatment there was no symbolic function
in him, still less an imaginary function' (ibid.). Lacan corrects Lefort by
adding: 'But he did have two words' (ibid.). The treatment consisted of
restoring the imaginary and the symbolic so that the horror of the Real
diminished, if it did not disappear.

   Lefort's effort to restore the imaginary could be described almost completely in object-relations terminology. The body had to be accepted as a
container-contained with reference to milk, faeces and urine. Lefort remained
present to Robert as a stable object even though he was aggressive or peed
on her. This, writes Lefort, helped Robert; but it only allowed him to create a
bad self-image, as is evident from the following:

> [W]hen I had to frustrate him – he ran to the window, opened it and cried
> out – Wolf! Wolf!, and seeing his own image in the glass, he hit it, crying
> out – Wolf! Wolf! That is the way Robert represented himself, he was the
> Wolf!
>
> (ibid.: 95)

Then, in two phases, Robert reconstructed a good self-image using two forms
of mirroring separated by a symbolic act. Robert first projected his bad
image onto the therapist and separated himself from her. Lefort was:

> made to swallow the bottle of dirty water and was on the receiving end of
> the aggressive pee. So I was the Wolf! Robert separated himself from it
> during one session, by shutting me in the toilets, then returned to the

room where we had the sessions, all alone, climbed into the empty bed, and started to moan. He could not call me, yet I did have to come back, since I was the permanent person. I came back. Robert was stretched out, pathetic, his thumb now within an inch of his mouth. And, for the first time in a session, he held out his arms to me and let himself be consoled.

(ibid.: 97)

Robert then used a symbolic act in which he renamed himself. Lefort describes it this way:

Robert, completely naked and facing me, collected up the water in his cupped hands, raised it to the level of his shoulders and let it run the length of his body. He started afresh several times, and then he said to me, softly – Robert, Robert.

(ibid.: 98)

He then repeated the scene with milk. The separation of the good boy (Robert not Wolf!) from the therapist was performed in another form of mirroring:

He first tried to differentiate himself from me by sharing with me. He gave me everything to eat, saying, while touching himself – Robert, then touching me – Not Robert. I made great use of this in my interpretations to help him and me.

(ibid.: 99)

CONCLUSION

Robert is a case where there is not just a failure of the symbolic. It is a case where there is abuse of the symbolic – the patient calls himself Wolf instead of Robert – in order to structure an already deficient imaginary. Let us start with the deficient imaginary. Robert had not only failed at separating himself as a good object from a maternal figure. He had not yet established himself as a good object. Robert beat his own image and called it Wolf. He had created a bad self-image. But the creation of the bad self-image was an achievement of the therapy. Robert's self-image had no place for the things that go in and out of the body: milk, urine, faeces. The milk and the bottle had been so much connected with deprivation and pain that the imaginary assumption of his body must have become unacceptable. The digestive body is for Robert one horror story. As reported by Lefort, all digestive functions are used aggressively (the milk, the urine and the faeces). The symbolic order is then used by Robert to create distance between himself and his digestive body that is unacceptable. He gives up his Christian name Robert and calls himself Wolf, signifying his radical badness. Thus the obvious failure in the symbolic order in which Robert does not call himself Robert but Wolf is more than a failure of the symbolic. It is, first of all, failure to imaginarily inhabit his body because that body was made the source of pain by others. And Robert needed to be a loved body for those others who had hurt him in order to be able to accept himself as embodied (Moyaert 1993).

Lacanian theory does not require that physical pain be inflicted on a child in order for that child to fail in its imaginary effort to inhabit its body. Crucial is that the child experiences itself as lovable by others but in its own right. In a case presented by Karon, there is no indication that physical pain was inflicted upon the child, with one possible exception: the toilet training was completed early. There was evidence that the child was not treated as lovable in his own right. Indeed, while trying to praise the child the mother proudly showed trivial achievements and did not show real achievements. Karon writes: 'Consciously, she was attempting to impress people with the accomplishments of her son; unconsciously, she was convincing them of his worthlessness by presenting the worthless productions first and the worthwhile productions later or not at all' (Karon and VandenBos 1981: 340). Even though physically-inflicted pain is not a necessary condition, in the case of Robert it was occurring within a context in which Robert experienced himself as worthless and unlovable. So let us be clear: Lacanian theory does not make pain as such the cause of failure in the imaginary. It is the dialectic between the experience of pain and the experience that one is not lovable which creates a difficulty for the child in properly constructing a body image it can inhabit. A body which has been constructed as an unlovable and paining body requires distortions in the symbolic world. Sometimes these symbolic distortions are as visible as the imaginary distortions.

What a Lacanian theory is better able to point to than object relations theory, in the case of Robert, is the crucial usage made by Robert of one of the two words he knew: Wolf! Robert lets go of his bad self by abandoning his self-given name Wolf! He creates a good self-identity by publicly accepting his Christian name. Words and the symbolic organize the progress in the imaginary.

NOTES

1 Successful interventions with schizophrenics can therefore be assumed to be complex interventions which address both the imaginary and symbolic deficiencies of the schizophrenic. The imaginary develops in relation to a maternal figure. The symbolic develops through the introduction of a third, normally the father. In my article, 'Lacan's theory and Karon's Psychoanalytic Treatment of Schizophrenics (Ver Eecke 2001), I try to explain the success of Karon's interventions with schizophrenics by pointing to the double dimension of his interventions. His interventions

first repair an imaginary defect (e.g., by justifying a terrible feeling), and second, introduce a symbolic distinction and prohibition (your murderous feeling is justified, but it is stupid to act upon it). In the first chapter of the book *Phenomenology and Lacan on Schizophrenia, after the Decade of the Brain* (De Waelhens and Ver Eecke, 2001), I demonstrate that other therapists who report successes in treating schizophrenics, such as Frieda Fromm-Reichman, Harry Stack Sullivan, Harold Searles, Bertram Karon, Ann-Louise Singer, Y. Alanen, Gisela Pankow, Françoise Davoine, Jean-Max Gaudillièrere, Piera Aulagnier, Gaetano Benedetti, Isidro Vegh, Contardo Calligaris, and Willy Apollon, use similarly complex interventions.

2 Vergote and several of his students at the University of Leuven have not only pointed out that Lacan's definition of schizophrenia as foreclosure of the name-of-the-father is a negative definition, they have also provided a positive definition. Thus, in a review of De Waelhens' book *La Psychose*, Vergote argues that De Waelhens, like Lacan, over-emphasizes the ruptures that are necessary in the development of the child (including the rupture imposed by the paternal metaphor) and neglects to analyze the 'necessary presence which precedes, supports and maybe even helps to achieve the ruptures and upheavals in the constitution of the subject' (Vergote 1973: 781). Vergote then identifies that which has to be present as the drives, as they find or do not find representation. Vergote thus points to the Freudian economic point of view as the place where a more positive definition of schizophrenia should be sought (Vergote 1973). Ten years later, Vergote formulates his objection to De Waelhens' and Lacan's views by his claim that understanding schizophrenia by means of a genetic constitution – including the idea of a paternal metaphor – is inadequate. Such a point of view, according to Vergote, does not permit one to understand why it is that the predominant experience of the schizophrenic is not an anxiety-provoking experience of the body broken into parts but rather an experience of the body which is in the process of breaking up under the influence of imaginary aggression that devours from the inside, that corrupts and turns pleasure into pain, and that tears a human being apart (Vergote 1984). Another ten years later, Vergote reminds us that Freud made the distinction between the physiological body and the psychic body (Vergote 1994). Vergote then points out that the skin as physiological separation of the body is insufficient to protect the psychic self from invasion. That protection is provided by the creation of a psychic body image (ibid.). The body image is created through the interaction of parents and child in dealing with bodily needs, in the way the parents respond to, satisfy or reject these needs (ibid.). Rudolf Bernet makes use of Schopenhauer to clarify the great challenge of human beings to deal as conscious beings with the demands of the body. In order to be effective, the energy of the body needs to find some representation so as to guide its attempt at satisfaction. But no representation is a satisfactory translation of the demand for fulfillment of the original need. When the child does not succeed in connecting its bodily energy and needs to some form of representation then the energy races unbound and blindly and creates in the schizophrenic the experience of a body falling apart (Bernet 1996). Paul Moyaert in turn points out that the Lacanian definition of schizophrenia as foreclosure of the name-of-the-father can only point to deficiencies. Such an understanding of schizophrenia does not allow us to understand what the schizophrenic is trying to do. Such a definition thus eliminates the dynamic point of view which is essential in a psychoanalytic approach. Moyaert then points out that the drives without representation are experienced as a danger. Moyeart is thereby able to explain the self-mutilation of the schizophrenic as an attempt to deal with the badness of the body because its drives are experienced as the source of displeasure (Moyaert 1998). In order to provide a positive definition for schizophrenia so as to

complement Lacan's negative definition, Vergote and his students concentrate upon the problem for the human being of finding representations for the demands of the body. If that search fails then the body and its demands are experienced as dangerous. The human being will then be forced to fight its own embodiment. Thus, the dynamic point of view is reintroduced in the theory of schizophrenia. In Lacanian terms one can say that Vergote and his students point to a deficiency other than the failure of the symbolic by the foreclosure of the name-of-the-father. That other deficiency is one connected to the construction of a body image by creating representations for the drives. Lacan uses the concept of the imaginary to cover that domain. Schizophrenia can therefore be defined as a failure of both the symbolic and the imaginary.

3 Michael Robbins, a non-Lacanian, shows nicely that the language of the schizo-phrenic – schizophrenese – is such that it sometimes intends to be a substitute for reality, not a way to signify that reality (Robbins 2002).

REFERENCES

Aulagnier-Spairani, P. (1964). Remarques sur la structure psychotique. *La Pschanalyse* 8: 47–67.

Bernet, R. (1996). Over de premissen van Lacan: Manifestatie en terugtrekking van het onbewuste in de drift, de voorstelling and het affect. In N. Kok and K. Nuijten (eds) *In Dialoog met Lacan*. Amsterdam: Boom.

Blatt, S. J. (1995). The destructiveness of perfectionism: Implications for the treatment of depression. *American Psychologist* 50: 1003–20.

Blatt, S. J. *et al.* (1996). Characteristics of effective therapists: Further analyses of data from the National Institute of Mental Health Treatment of Depression Collaborative Research Program. *Journal of Consulting and Clinical Psychology* 64: 1276–84.

Calligaris, C. (1991). *Pour une Clinique Différentielle des Psychoses*. Paris: Point hors Ligne.

De Waelhens, A. (1978). *Schizophrenia. A Philosophical Reflection on the Structuralist Interpretation of J. Lacan* (translated by W. Ver Eecke). Pittsburgh: Duquesne University Press.

De Waelhens, A. and Ver Eecke, W. (2001). *Phenomenology and Lacan on Schizophrenia, after the Decade of the Brain*. Leuven: University of Leuven Press.

Evans, D. (1996). *An Introductory Dictionary of Lacanian Psychoanalysis*. London and New York: Routledge.

Fink, B. (1996). The subject and the other's desire. In R. Feldstein *et al.* (eds) *Reading Seminars I and II. Lacan's Return to Freud*. New York: State University of New York Press.

Fink, B. (1997). *A Clinical Introduction to Lacanian Psychoanalysis. Theory and Technique*. Cambridge, MA: Harvard University Press.

Karon, B. P. and VandenBos, G. R. (1981). *Psychotherapy of Schizophrenia. The Treatment of Choice*. New York: Jason Aronson.

Lacan, J. (1977). *Écrits. A Selection* (translated by A. Sheridan). New York: W. W. Norton and Company.

Lacan, J. (1988). *The Seminars of Jacques Lacan. Book I. Freud's Papers on Technique 1953–1954* (edited by J. Miller, translated by J. Forrester). New York: W. W. Norton.

Lacan, J. (1993). *The Seminars of Jacques Lacan. Book III. The Psychoses 1955–1956* (edited by J. Miller, translated by R. Grigg). New York: W. W. Norton.

Laplanche, J. (1969). *Hölderlin et la Question du Père*. Paris: Presses Universitaires de France.

Moyaert, P. (1993). Schizophrénie et paranoïa. *Psychanalyse. L'homme et Ses destins* 255–81.

Moyaert, P. (1998). Schizofrenie vanuit psychoanalytisch perspectief. *Tijdschrift voor Psychoanalyse* 4: 132–49.

Muller, J. P. and Richardson, W. J. (1982). *Lacan and Language. A Reader's Guide to Écrits*. New York: International Universities Press.

Robbins, M. (2002). The language of schizophrenia and the world of delusion. *International Journal of Psychoanalysis* 83: 383–405.

Searles, H. F. (1986). *My Work with Borderline Patients*. Northvale, NJ: Jason Aronson Inc.

Simiu, D. (1986). *Disorder and Early Alienation: Lacan's Original Theory of the Mirror Stage*. Doctoral dissertation. Washington, DC: Georgetown University.

Ver Eecke, W. (1984). *Saying 'No'*. Pittsburgh: Duquesne University Press.

Ver Eecke, W. (2001). Lacan's theory, Karon's psychoanalytic treatment of schizophrenics. *Psychoanalysis and Contemporary Thought* 24: 79–105.

Vergote A. (1973). Raisons de la déraison. *Revue Philosophique de Louvain* 71: 772–85.

Vergote, A. (1984). La psychose. In G. Florival (ed.) *Études d'Anthropologie Philosophique* Louvain-La-Neuve: Éditions de l'Institut Supérieur de Philosophie.

Vergote, A. (1994). La constitution de l'ego dans le corps pulsionnel. In G. Florival (ed.) *Dimensions de l'Exister*. Louvain: Editions Peeters.

Vergote, A. (1998). Le plaisir destructeur transfiguré en hiérogamie. In D. Devreese *et al.* (eds), *Schreber Revisité*. Louvain: Presses Universitaires de Louvain.

Chapter 4

Schizophrenia
Pathogenesis and therapy

Lars Thorgaard and Bent Rosenbaum

INTRODUCTION

The overall aim of this chapter is to illustrate the importance of establishing and maintaining an empathic understanding of the reality of suffering from schizophrenia. Our degree of empathy is crucial to the models we develop about pathogenesis and therapy. More often than not, however, it is precisely empathy that is found to be lacking in many models.

It is our conviction that it can be invaluable to supplement established therapeutic practice and diagnostic thinking (according to DSM and ICD) with systems of classification based on an empathic understanding of how it really must be for any given person to suffer from schizophrenia. This addition may be of great importance to the therapeutic process which, to a large extent, is dependent on how the patient is met and received by the professionals working in psychiatry.

MODEL FOR PATHOGENESIS

Eugen Bleuler (1983) devised the classifications 'diagnostic' and 'pathogenetic' to distinguish between basic and accessory symptoms and primary and secondary symptoms respectively (Bleuler 1908). In making his pathogenetic classification, Bleuler was inspired by Freud and the early psychoanalysts. The secondary symptoms were viewed as reactive to the primary ones, and could be understood psychologically as expressions of the patient's efforts to adapt to, and work with, their inner and outer predicaments. However, there continues to be confusion of Bleuler's diagnostic and pathogenetic classifications, although this clear distinction between symptoms is largely ignored and unrecognised today. Many have mixed the two (Cullberg 1984; Kringlen 1990; Strömgren 1969; WHO 1973), illustrating the great difficulties that have always been present in understanding some of the psychodynamic and dynamic pathogenetic processes in schizophrenia. The pathogenetic classification implied that the so-called secondary symptoms of schizophrenia are reactive to, and can be understood and looked upon as psychopathological understandable reactions to the consequences of, the very basic disorder.

In this model of pathogenesis many symptoms in schizophrenia are secondary to others, and reflect the efforts made by the sufferer in trying to come to terms with primary basic problems or fundamental deficits. They become distorted due to either a primary deficit or indispensable instinctive or unconscious defences implying distortions in themselves. Equal consideration should be given to each, as these distortions will deteriorate and aggravate further.

Although there is still no final or reliable clarification of the primary symptoms in schizophrenia, recent research seems to indicate they are to be found among the expressions of the so-called 'Ich-Störungen'. However, the point that will be made here is that it is not essential for a pathogenetic understanding and explanatory view of schizophrenia to concern itself with primary aetiology; rather, it is important to try to illustrate and produce a thesis about elements of the pathological process and its interactions (Thorgaard and Rosenbaum 1996).

Our view concurs with Bleuler's with respect to the idea that the primary deficits must have been present earlier in life (pre-morbidly) without developing into a manifest disorder. If this is true, it follows that ways of adapting to these deficits must have been possible. Furthermore, we should assume that this capability can be repeated. If this is not possible, by implication schizophrenia would be an inevitable process leading to unavoidable dementia, and we know this to be untrue. A proportionally large number of spontaneous remissions do occur. According to this theory, schizophrenia develops as a 'process disorder'. In our view, schizophrenia involves a process that develops from a special personality complex or frame ever-increasingly towards autism, depending on the survival instincts. Such an additional emotional withdrawal takes place according to both external and internal reality and, therefore, is not solely a withdrawal into the internal as is often mistakenly thought. According to Manfred Bleuler (1972), Minkowski has distinguished between 'rich' and 'poor' autism. The internal life of the rich form is compared with lively dreams; in the poor form it dries out and becomes a rigid system which may be cold, impersonal, timeless and impossible to influence. In the poor form, you will presumably find the above-mentioned negative spiral of withdrawal from autism to more severe autism.

Contemporarily, there is a tendency to ignore the concept of ambivalence, which was considered important by earlier researchers and teachers. Ambivalence is often defined in terms of opposing feelings that the person suffering from schizophrenia simultaneously and very painfully experiences. This may be true in many cases but, in other instances, the person experiences not only two opposing feelings but also many other feelings and thoughts which are painfully felt to be incompatible with each other. It is important to supplement this further with phenomenological descriptions. The person may be characterised by having an insufficiently developed capacity to bear, contain and integrate feelings of ambivalence. He or she must constantly suffer the pain of containing opposing feelings and must protect him/herself against that pain by unconscious splitting of feelings and by withdrawal from both the inner and outer worlds: namely, by increasing autism. Thus, the idea of ambivalence is dynamically closely connected with the idea of autism. Dynamically the autism could be assumed to be secondary to the undeveloped capacity to bear feelings of ambivalence. The formal thought disorders must also be viewed, to some extent, as reactive to the inability to bear ambivalence (Thorgaard and Rosenbaum 1996).

WORKING WITH LOSS AND CONTAINMENT OF GRIEF

The aetiology of this process disorder of schizophrenia is very complex, and the pathogenetic and psychodynamic complexities are not particularly clear. According to Zubin and colleagues (1977), multiple aetiological factors and pathogenetic chains create an extremely vulnerable state of mind. One can say that schizophrenia is a disorder characterised by vulnerability.

We have devised a dynamic model for this (Thorgaard and Rosenbaum 1996), which includes the following characteristics:

- Aetiology is multi-factorial.
- Both protective and predisposed conditions exist, internal and external, as well as environmental and genetic.
- Some genes are seen as protective, while others predispose individuals to the disorder. The interaction is surely dynamic, so that, in this instance also, schizophrenia is a 'disease of balance'. External conditions might be used as protection against shifts in such genetic balances, as well as to prohibit/inhibit shifts in genetic balances.
- Prenatal infections and/or birth trauma, with subclinical brain damage for example, can be part of a pathogenetic chain. Both internal and external environmental factors and genetic conditions can be protective or can predispose pathogenetic results from such aetiological factors. The significance of factors that affect the quality and solidity of personality structure would, presumably, compensate for such predisposed elements, according to the total vulnerability (Tienary's 1990 adoption studies indicate this). When these factors have negative influences they can provoke pathogenetic effects.
- Before vulnerability is expressed as manifest illness, there are likely to have been several preceding attempts at complex internal and external self-healing. The person will have tried, either instinctively, consciously or unconsciously, to protect him/herself against the consequences of

vulnerabilities by means of psychological adaptive defences. Bleuler's secondary symptoms are supposed to be the crudest way of expressing such adaptive defences. It is probable that many of what have hitherto been known as primary symptoms could also be seen as psychological, understandable adaptive defences.

The following statement, while generalising, nonetheless poses a most fundamental view: the vulnerability in schizophrenia expresses itself most critically in an inadequately developed capacity to bear, to endure, to contain and to work through mourning processes.

Working through mourning – or grief work – does not only refer to the predicament of bearing, accepting and working upon losses. A developed capacity to endure, contain and work through mourning means that an individual is able to endure and bear the frustrations, loss and dissatisfactions as well as the pleasures of ordinary life. One might justly propose that such a lack of capacity to deal with losses and grief is fundamental to many psychopathological conditions of a widely differing nature. Pathological mourning processes are often seen in connection with disease and disease processes. However, whatever the aetiology, we assume that this capacity for the prospective sufferer from schizophrenia is reduced and thus creates vulnerability from the outset. The Kleinian dynamic psychopathology understanding (Klein 1946) is therefore valid. The prospective schizophrenic, owing to his/her vulnerability, from the outset must begin a process of excessive and defensive fragmentation of what, in fact, should be linked or gathered. The mental foundation of life – self-agency, self-coherence, self-affectivity and self-history (Stern 1985) – is, from its beginning, vulnerable, and this vulnerability is essentially expressed as a basic lack of capacity to mourn. In this way the pre-psychotic person differs markedly from other persons who suffer from different kinds of psychopathological processes, since pathological mourning processes, while important, are not that fundamental.

A FUNDAMENTAL DYNAMIC UNDERSTANDING OF SCHIZOPHRENIA

The following statement illustrates a fundamental psychodynamic thesis: *every psychopathological symptom protects against something even worse, an even worse alternative* (Thorgaard 1995). This thesis is especially valid in psychotic conditions.

This thesis implies that symptoms are viewed as creative expressions from the mind. Symptoms are internally created adaptations, expressed both inwardly (body–mind) and outwardly (motor acts, behaviour and speech). Such creations or strategies in psychosis, however insufficient, inadequately compensating or painful they might be, enable the individual to cope in the best possible manner with what might otherwise be unbearable and/or extremely threatening. In schizophrenia, it is the existence and the preservation of the personality which is at risk: threats against self-agency, self-coherence, self-affectivity and self-history. What we consequently witness is a life-and-death struggle in which the processes of symptom formation are intended to protect against the disastrous experience of disintegration. The process of symptom formation is an attempted defence against the wordless experiences of an imminent disaster underlying the so-called 'Ich-Störungen'.

This is where nature intervenes. When faced with the worst situation thinkable, namely the disintegration of mental life, it seems that humans instinctively try to find an effective counter-move. When anticipating catastrophe this is achieved by killing the body–mind in an effort to terminate the present condition of the mind and its associated sufferings.

We now understand that suicide, along with suicidal impulses and fantasies, is a reactive measure employed to combat the experience of disintegration and the ensuing catastrophic consequences. The fundamental psychodynamic thesis can now be supplemented thus: *every psychopathological symptom in psychosis protects against that which is even worse – i.e. suicide or the threatening impulse to kill oneself – in order not to experience the disintegration* (Thorgaard 1995).

This thesis is useful in that it ensures that the risk of suicide is always in focus. More fundamentally, it reminds us of the deepest roots of man's wish, will and capacity to survive. This wish and will is illustrated by the processes of symptom formation: a wish to survive in spite of the ongoing existential sufferings arising from the experience of disintegration and its consequences. We have, therefore, a deep understanding of and respect for the vital aspects of this compulsive repetition, although in this context in a more differential basic and radical way than that of classical psychoanalysis.

THE SELF-DESTRUCTIVE AND 'SELF-DE-STRUCTURALISING' PROCESSES IN SCHIZOPHRENIA

One theme of this chapter is to emphasise suicide and suicidal thoughts as a means of opposing the worst thinkable human experience: the catastrophic experience of mental disintegration. We especially emphasise the parallel ongoing exceptional wish to survive and to live. This wish is also contained in, and is the matrix behind, most of the psychopathological symptoms in schizophrenia. The creation of symptoms, which imply further disintegration, can be seen and understood as attempts to grieve (but grieving on a false trail seen from a more healthy perspective), and attempts to preserve – in an existential borderland – at least an illusion of unity through surviving by 'help' from the processes in and behind the symptom formations.

Paradoxically, however, this implies an even greater splitting of the mind (Thorgaard and Rosenbaum 1996).

The symptom formations express what we might call the secondary disintegrations and their manifestations. The symptom formations tell us the narrative of the patient's attempts to bear the unbearable: his or her attempts to mourn. However, the grieving is on false trails. The attempts at self-healing can perhaps be expressed in proverbs or formulae: 'With evil shall evil be banished' (that is to say, disintegration is met with disintegration) or 'Desperate ills need desperate remedies'.

This 'secondary evil' is the secondary splitting processes giving birth to the symptom formations, especially the positive symptoms of hallucinatory thinking and delusions. It all happens in the cause of survival, albeit at enormous cost: schizophrenia is characterised by 'grief on false trail'.

TO REALISE AN ORDINARY LIFE . . . OR NOT! (OR: TO BE OR NOT TO BE)

An ordinary life has to be realised, brought into being. It comprises what is common and inevitable to mankind: all that is given and conquered, taken and lost throughout an ordinary life. This is founded upon a complex bio-psychological basis.

An ordinary life is started by a conception without complications. Conception has its own physiological substratum and its own emotional environment. It is significant whether a child is conceived predominantly in love and concern, and whether the pregnancy develops in a conducive psychological milieu as a supplement to a healthy physiological milieu. The absence of damaging influences on the mother and foetus, which could damage the developments of mental life and arrest the developmental processes in the brain, is crucial. All of the above are part of the process to a delivery ideally free from complications. These occurrences are the conquests of an ordinary life. The newborn has a brain and nervous system with the potential to develop further in interplay with others, and by means of that interplay starts the creation of a new unique mind. This happens in a conducive ('good-enough': Winnicott 1965) environment. Within the right timings, such a child will be able to conquer the processes of individuation. They will experience a mixture of joy and anxiety, when hindrances or obstacles in life have to be overcome. They will gradually develop a capacity to bear and endure absence and loss. They can go to school without too much separation anxiety, and later move away from home and establish a relatively attained independent life (while maintaining the capacity for dependence). They will attain knowledge about sex differences. Their earliest loves, other than with parents and siblings, will have been experienced. Furthermore, the potential to become involved, both emotionally and physically, with members of the opposite – or the same – sex will be developed, along with enjoying the delights of and procuring the capability for love. They will be able to appreciate the indispensability of friendship, but also from time to time do without it. It will be possible to get an education, training and a job. The ordinary life consists of pursuing life's goals. There is a sense of eternity in having children and grandchildren. The ordinary life, in old age, ends with a relative reconciliation with loss, illness and, finally, death. An ordinary life also consists of dealing with loss when life's goals and expectations are not met. An ordinary life is based on a fundamental capacity and capability for living and on a predominance of non-vulnerability. An ordinary life is also based on the capability to manage vulnerability in order that the vulnerable moments in life may be managed, overcome and adapted to. In other words, one can grieve!

The predicament of the situation in schizophrenia is that the life of the individual is deprived of many of the givens and conquests found in the ordinary life of most people. The predicament for many of our patients is a life full of renunciations of the ordinary life so desperately longed for. To make matters worse: the predicament in schizophrenia is often inundated with unfortunate, extremely distressing and miserable life conditions.

Ordinary life and living makes increasing demands on the pre-psychotic individual, but there are also enormous demands related to bearing, tolerating, containing and working upon frequently distressing and unfortunate life experiences. At a certain point it just won't do any longer to try to adapt and to carry on with oneself 'in spite of': schizophrenia is a disorder characterised by living much of a life 'in spite of'.

This tragic failing to adapt will usually occur in early youth and adult life, when demands for independence and separation are at their highest. Here the desperate, prolonged attempts to balance life – to adapt to life – often fail. It happens most often with a 'straw that broke the camel's back', related to the so-called stressors which we often lose sight of with our non-empathic eye. Thus, schizophrenia is a disorder characterised by the constant necessity of having to balance life, and by 'the final straw that broke the camel's back'.

Paradoxically, what is needed is a capacity to cope with unbearable grieving processes but the capacity is basically insufficient. This wounded bedrock gives sequelae in relation to all the grieving processes and demands for grief work found in all lives, demands which are also inevitable in the psychotic and pre-psychotic life. The future sufferer from schizophrenia experiences increasing, distinct, pronounced and painful difficulties in bearing and containing the ordinary life.

In order to try to master living, they will develop subtly pathological grief processes which exceed the normal ones. These pathological grief or mourning processes unfold before us through the evolution of symptom formations. More healthy grief processes, however, are also available. In spite of these, the predicament of schizophrenia is to live in, and make a life from, the split world of these falsely-based grieving processes – 'on false trails'. This must be done because of the extremely painful experience of feeling both different and incapable which is enforced by confrontations with reality.

The person suffering from schizophrenia faces a future having accumulated a mountain of grief and mourning, a rock which is instinctively pushed to the fore, where attempts are made to get rid of it by comminuting, dividing and making distortions from it. It is a mountain of grief derived from loss and renunciation in the ordinary life. This mountain also includes missed opportunities to work through loss and failure to deal with new beginnings in the usual life-conquests from which the individual is more and more isolated. The person suffering from schizophrenia perceives this ability to be possessed by the majority of others. A defence against isolation is to isolate oneself further: schizophrenia is a disorder characterised by isolation and isolating oneself.

When the evolution described is at its highest, a manifest psychotic breakdown seems inevitable. The breakdown sets in with double intent: as a defence against the mountain of grieving and, simultaneously, as an instinctively desperate, despairing, abortive and unsuccessful attempt to break through: schizophrenia is characterised by attempts to break through. Depressive phenomena, still present at this stage, mirror the more healthy grief work attempted by a still existing, relatively healthy and reality-based, reality-testing part of the personality. The patient with still-existing depressive symptomatology is more healthy than when his affective symptoms and signs have disappeared. The patient then falls into a more disintegrated state. Both states of mentality can be, and often are, present simultaneously. The 'balance of power' – so to speak – between the more healthy part of the mentality and the psychotic parts (Bion 1957/1987) is decisive. Consider the most disorganised state in schizophrenia as the condition with predominant negative symptoms; a state dominated by depressive symptoms and positive symptoms reflects a still-fighting, reality-oriented part of the mentality.

At a decisive point in this process the observer will recognise a crucial change in reality testing. The patient is now fighting against reality with the aid of multiple internal splittings. This becomes the process based on the formula 'With evil shall evil be banished' or 'Desperate ills need desperate remedies'. The healthier parts of the mentality, which are able to experience reality as it is, are combated by means of splitting. Comminution, however, can never annihilate the mind. In other words, we are witnessing an extremely active and malignant self-destructive process – a 'self-de-structuralising' process – in which reality is attacked actively from inside in a desperate attempt to at least survive and to avoid or postpone suicidal processes and suicide. The price for survival, however, is extremely high. We really should consider it a miracle that the suicide rate among sufferers of schizophrenia is not even greater. When the patients are most suicidal, they are also in the most intensive and painful emotional contact with their tragic predicament. One could say that they are in a more healthy, but also a life-threatening, contact with reality! They are in emotional contact with the past, with the here and now and with the prospect of living with an ailment felt to be endless: schizophrenia is felt and experienced as 'a never-ending disorder'.

In other words, reality is de-structuralised, is 'de-structed' from within through an instinctive destruction of the mind, which is the 'apparatus' used to measure, weigh and estimate reality.

The knowledge we have gained thus far is summarised and contained in the subcategories presented in the following classification. This is not an ordinary psychiatric classification, but a classification intended as an aid to enable professionals to attain empathy as to what it is really like to suffer from schizophrenia.

A GENERAL DYNAMIC CLASSIFICATION OF SCHIZOPHRENIA BASED ON EMPATHY

To summarize, schizophrenia is always:

- felt as a 'process disorder'
- felt as a 'vulnerability disorder'
- characterised by efforts to grieve, but the grieving is 'on false trails'
- experienced as a 'self-destructive and self-de-structuralising disorder'
- experienced as living most of one's life 'in spite of'
- felt as a constant necessity of having to 'balance one's life'
- experienced as a disorder about 'the final straw that breaks the camel's back'
- felt as a disorder characterised by 'isolation and isolating oneself'
- felt and experienced as an 'attempt to break through'
- felt and experienced as a 'never-ending story disorder'.

If these subcategories can be integrated into the very bones of professionals (and into society), we will be better equipped to acquire and preserve some empathic understanding of the predicament in schizophrenia. The therapist will then have an opportunity to feel the burdens of the accumulated mountain of grief and to feel the attempts at trying to balance the ongoing processes of the disorder. It will enable therapists to gain respect for the 'in spite of' battle for a life and living, and to be able to look for the last straw that breaks the camel's back. It will enable them to keep a keen eye on all risks of self-destruction and suicide and to experience the horror of the predicament in the feeling contained in: 'this is a never-ending story'.

Most importantly, some parts of our loss of empathy come from the patient, who is unable to contain empathy with him/herself, if we can literally discuss such a concept. Empathy with oneself means being in emotional contact with the full horror of the schizophrenic predicament, which in turn implies that the patient will be closer to suicide. The therapist must know about these matters and must use emotional knowledge to meet the patient, where the patient really is, in order to establish a relationship. Søren Kierkegaard's (1848) statement about meeting the ones who suffer and seek help by meeting them where they are is meaningful here, because a way of understanding Kierkegaard is to accept that the sufferers do not know where they are: knowing that would imply the deepest suffering!

The patient and therapist must jointly try to find ways of creatively utilising the emotional knowledge of the therapist and seek its transformations. The therapist must lead by showing that it is possible for them to bear and contain this empathy.

A DYNAMIC SUBCLASSIFICATION OF SCHIZOPHRENIA BASED ON EMPATHY

Sufferers from schizophrenia are all unique. Their differences vary from time to time and according to circumstances. It is valuable to perform an additional diagnostic exercise with each individual patient. The aim is to help the therapist to have or regain even more specific empathy, in addition to the empathy gained from already having integrated the general dynamic classification presented above. The objective is to try to differentiate between the divisions used in the following dynamic subclassification and to rank them in relation to each individual patient at any particular moment and in the particular circumstances of life and of the therapeutic process.

The question is: what primarily and secondarily characterises empathic understanding? The ranking of psychodynamic themes to identify which is primary and which secondary does not exclude the others, because all the characteristics are contained in all patients – and especially in all therapist–patient relations. It is usual to find all the elements, although some will be in the foreground and others more in the background in the experience of the patient. The following dynamic subclassification acts as an aid to where to look and focus.

For the sake of convenience, we have presented this subclassification under brief headings: for example, schizophrenia is a 'separation/attachment disorder'. By this, we mean that a person suffering from schizophrenia is unable to form attachments and/or cope with separation in the usual way, and it is experienced by the person as a disordering of attachment and separation; and so on throughout the list.

Schizophrenia is:

- a separation/attachment disorder
- distrust/loss of trust disorder
- a relation disorder
- an identity disorder
- a paroxysmal and relapse disorder
- a control and loss of control disorder
- a selfcare-failing/care-failing disorder

Schizophrenia is a separation/attachment disorder

Enormous problems and sufferings arise from the incapacity to separate and to attach, which exists in the predicament of schizophrenia. This seems to be one of the most fundamental deficits in schizophrenia (Bion 1962; Thorgaard and Rosenbaum 1996). Being unable to bear, endure and contain separation will result in an inability to attach oneself, and not being able to attach oneself will result in an inability to separate. This double incapacity can be uncovered in the life history and its consequences, and it is especially recommended that it be sought within the therapeutic relationship. This ranking involves an incapacity to be alone and to be together, to attach oneself and to be close.

Schizophrenia is a distrust/loss of trust disorder

The patient has serious problems and conflicts in taking the risks of having confidence in, believing in and trusting reality. There will be a tendency to misunderstand facts of life – as opposed to the general shared understanding. It should preferably be sought and investigated in the patient's relations to significant others and especially in the therapeutic relationship, where the therapist will feel him/herself kept at a distance or excluded. There will be a constant discreet and/or extreme (paranoid) distrust, to test whether the therapist is trustworthy or not. The relation is often dominated by paranoid rejections, behind which deep attachment wishes are hidden.

Schizophrenia is a relation disorder

Being in a relationship with others is experienced as painfully impossible and is associated with overwhelming feelings of impotence and helplessness. The patient withdraws from contact in order to keep at a distance the feelings of impotence, the missing vitality and incapability of living in relation with others. He/she desperately tries to keep intense longings for relationships (e.g. friendships and love relations) at bay. More often than not, there is a hidden and painful vulnerability to narcissistic injuries. This results in withdrawal from relations, and the withdrawal reveals a grandiose paranoid autistic world, which is often inhabited by persecuting revenge fantasies, often acted out as suicide attempts. The patient withdraws from the therapist too, because of fear of losing control over their inner world and the risk of insulting and damaging the other. The fear of losing is painfully present in every relationship.

Schizophrenia is an identity disorder

This is a predicament dominated by constant feelings of disintegration (whether primary or secondary disintegration). Answers to inner painful questions such as, 'Who am I?', 'Who is who?' or 'Who is doing what and with whom?' can never be taken for granted. This is also true of feelings of owning a secure sexual identity. The incoherence and instability of identity is also reflected in shifting feelings of inferiority and grandiosity – and, quite often and at worst, feelings of non-existence! In the therapeutic relationship, the patient will identify him/herself with the therapist – for better or for worse.

Schizophrenia is a paroxysmal and relapse disorder

This implies having some empathy with the horrific experience of suffering from a disorder with the prospect that one never knows when it will break out or return. How can the patient cope with such uncertainty? The patient can be literally afraid of moving, or can create hypotheses – seldom told to us, and most often false solutions – about what provokes and what prevents a breakdown. In this way, life is even more restricted, thus making things even worse, to the point of not doing anything at all in order to try to prevent a feared catastrophe.

Schizophrenia is a control and loss of control disorder

Imagine trying to have empathy with the existence of an ailment constantly dominated by the attempt to maintain a vulnerable control of one's feelings of, and demands for expressing and getting satisfaction from, love, hate, anger, sexuality and so on. Or try to imagine the task of always struggling to control the urge to commit suicide, and of being continuously and painfully aware of the expressions from your body and trying to control the body. Imagine the feeling of being controlled by something or somebody when, mostly, you fear not having any control at all. Think about a predicament where you can never be at peace from fears of, and anxieties about, losing control. When loss of control has occurred once, when will it happen again? How can one live and cope with this uncertainty?

Schizophrenia is a selfcare-failing/care-failing disorder

Failing to take care of oneself is expressed in a good deal of the symptom-atology – especially in the negative symptoms but also in elements of self-destructive behaviour. One can reflect upon possible defensive aspects to this: not to feel, not to expect anything at all, not to feel one's needs and so on. The most important and painful observation is, however, that this selfcare-failing disorder is all too often responded to by care-failing from the community, from the professional community and from therapists. Care-failing is a common response to schizophrenia, partly – but only partly – due to the patient's selfcare-failing.

CONCLUSIONS

The general classification system, based on attempts to empathise with the predicament of schizophrenia, will give us some subheadings for the work to be done with every patient suffering from schizophrenia:

- Affirming and reassuring the patient with the aid of our improved knowl-edge: this is made possible with the help of our regained and improved empathic understanding. This is the foundation for all therapeutic efforts.
- Help and support to grieve: this can only be provided in intensive psychotherapy. It demands a therapist who is sensitive to the many meanings of trauma and loss.
- Self-construction as a creative counter-move against self-destruction: this demanding process is best served by early and continuing intervention and intensive psychotherapy. It demands a therapist with intuition and creative thinking.
- Help and support to live 'in spite of' and hopefully later 'by virtue of': this demands the therapist's integrity.
- Help to believe and trust that improvement is possible and that some or all of these sufferings can be transformed and terminated as a result of 'good-enough' treatment (Winnicott 1965): the therapist's stability, patience and sense of non-intrusion is critical here.

Finally, the subcategories of the dynamic subclassification must be given priority. Depending on which subcategories are given priority in the sug-gested exercise, the therapist, together with the patient, can also name the work which shall be given first and second priority in the therapeutic process. To decide and to name the work to be done means to name a disorder in a new way; and which, in contrast to other diagnostic namings (DSM or ICD), is understandable and meaningful to both patient and therapist.

The therapeutic work to be undertaken is to help and support the patient:

- to endure the consequences of his/her incapacity to separate and attach, and to help improve the remaining capacity
- to dare to trust
- to be and to stay in a relationship
- to develop a more secure feeling of identity
- to endure and to develop more creative coping strategies towards having a paroxysmal and relapse disorder
- to work with the loss of control disorder or the fear of losing control, and gradually develop more creative and realistic adaptations to these fears and/or
- to work with selfcare-failing and with the complex interaction between selfcare-failing and care-failing.

This classification and naming of the therapeutic work to be undertaken with every individual suffering from schizophrenia is not an alternative to the diagnostic namings in the DSM and the ICD, but it can be used as an important supplement to the psychiatry of today.

REFERENCES

Bion, W. R. (1957/1987). Differentiation of the psychotic from the non-psychotic personalities. In W. R. Bion *Second Thoughts. Selected Papers on Psycho-Analysis*. London: Maresfield Library.

Bion, W. R. (1962). The psycho-analytic study of thinking. *International Journal of Psycho-Analysis* 43: 306–10.

Bleuler, E. (1908). Die Prognose der Dementia Præcox (Schizophreniegruppe). *Allgemeine Zeitschrift für Psychiatrie und Psychisch Gerictliche Medizin* 65: 436–64.

Bleuler, E. (1983). *Lehrbuch der Psychiatrie* (15th edn), Berlin, Heidelberg, New York: Springer Verlag.

Bleuler, M. (1972). *Die Schizophrenen Geistesstörungen im Lichte Langjähriger Kranken- und Familiegeschichten [The Schizophrenic Disorders: Long-term Patient and Family Studies]*. Stuttgart: Georg Thieme Verlag.

Cullberg, J. (1984). *Dynamisk Psykiatri [Dynamic Psychiatry]*. København: Hans Reitzel.

Kierkegaard, S. (1848/1964). Synspunktet for min forfatter-virksomhed [The view of my work]. In S. Kierkegaard *Samlede værker [Collected works]*, Vol. 18. København: Gyldendal.

Klein, M. (1946). Notes on some schizoid mechanisms. *International Journal of Psychoanalysis* 27: 99–100.

Kringlen, E. (1990). *Psykiatri [Psychiatry]*. Oslo: Universitetsforlaget.

Stern. D. (1985). *The Interpersonal World of the Infant*. New York. Basic Books.

Strömgren, E. (1969). *Lærebog i Psykiatri [Handbook of Psychiatry]*. København: Munksgaard.

Thorgaard, L. (1995). Hvad er god supervision? [What is good supervision?]. In L. Thorgaard and K. Valbak (eds) *Kontaktpersonen – Relationsbehandling i Psykiatrien* [*The Primary Care-Person: Relation-Treatment in Psychiatry*]. Århus: Psykoterapeutisk Forlag.

Thorgaard, L. and Rosenbaum, B. (1996). Tidlig og vedholdende intervention ved schizofreni. Bind I. En forsknings-behandlingsmanual til Det Danske Nationale Schizofreniprojekt – DNS [Early and enduring intervention in schizophrenia. A research manual in relation to the Danish National Schizophrenia Project – DNS]. (Only published for use by research teams in Denmark).

Tienary, P. (1990). Genes–environment interaction in adoptive families. In H. Häfner and W. F. Gattaz (eds) *Search for the Causes of Schizophrenia. II*. Berlin: Springer Verlag.

Winnicott, D. W. (1960). The theory of the parent–infant relationship. In M. R. Khan and J. Coles (eds) *Maturational Processes and the Facilitating Environment: Studies in the Theory of Emotional Development*. London: Hogarth.

World Health Organisation (1973). *Report of the International Pilot Study of Schizophrenia*. Geneva: Author.

Zubin, J. *et al.* (1977). Vulnerability – a new view of schizophrenia. *Journal of Abnormal Psychology* 86: 103–26.

Part II

Early intervention in psychosis

Chapter 5

A behavioural versus a cognitive analysis of the relapse prodrome in psychosis

Louise Bywood, David M. Gresswell, Colin Robertson and Peter Elwood

Max Birchwood's (1995) theory of the relapse signature suggests that an individual's early/prodromal signs of psychosis are generally stable from relapse to relapse and follow a predictable temporal pattern. Such symptoms usually occur over a period of less than four weeks, with non-psychotic phenomena occurring early in the illness, followed by the development of frankly psychotic symptoms. This chapter challenges Birchwood's theory and provides evidence to illustrate that the same sequential prodromal pattern does not necessarily herald each psychotic breakdown. By using multiple sequential functional analysis (MSFA; Gresswell and Hollin 1992), an in-depth qualitative case history methodology, evidence has been found to support the argument that the relapse prodrome is developmental in nature. Furthermore, Bandura's (1977) social learning model of human behaviour is used to explain how the prodrome is influenced in its development by the continuous reciprocal interaction between personal, behavioural and environmental factors over the course of the illness. Case study extracts are presented to illustrate this finding. A forensic case study is also presented to show how MSFA can be used to explore and predict the developmental nature of the prodrome and create greater understanding of an individual's early signs of psychosis. This clinical assessment tool can also be used to design individual treatment packages and create more opportunities for clinicians to implement early intervention strategies to ameliorate a psychotic breakdown.

INTRODUCTION

Schizophrenia for the majority of its sufferers is considered to be an episodic condition. Each psychotic episode brings with it an increased probability of future relapse and residual symptoms (McGlashan 1988), as well as accelerating social disablement (Hogarty *et al.* 1991). In a prospective study by Shepherd *et al.* (1989) which looked at five-year outcome following a first presentation of psychosis, 16% of patients experienced only one psychotic episode, 32% experienced several episodes with no or minimal impairment between breakdowns, 9% suffered impairment after the first episode with subsequent exacerbation and no return to normality and 43% experienced increasing impairment with each episode and no return to normality. Thus, as each psychotic breakdown may result in the growth of residual symptoms, the prevention or amelioration of relapse is of huge importance. Indeed, people diagnosed with schizophrenia are able to recognise and respond to reduced wellbeing (McCandless-Glimcher *et al.* 1986).

The concept of prodromal symptoms in schizophrenia has traditionally referred to the subtle pathological deviations in thought, affect and behaviour that precede the initial onset of psychosis (Bustillo *et al.* 1995). However in more recent years prodromal symptoms have also referred to the early warning signs (EWS) of impending relapse in individuals already diagnosed as having schizophrenia (e.g. Herz and Melville 1980). Bustillo *et al.* argued that to restrict the definition of EWS to non-psychotic phenomena related to a conceptual distinction that was irrelevant to clinical action. Attempts to predict the onset of psychosis from non-specific or dysphoric prodromal symptoms alone have yielded poor sensitivities, but results have been more promising when low-level psychotic symptoms are included in the predictor variables (Birchwood *et al.* 2000). Thus the effective clinical use of the relapse prodrome/EWS depends on including both psychotic and non-psychotic symptoms as EWS.

Birchwood's theory of the relapse signature

Birchwood *et al.* (1989) developed the Early Signs Scale (ESS) to detect prodromal signs of relapse. The scale was designed in accordance with information obtained from an extensive interview administered to 42 individuals with schizophrenia and their carers. The interviews elicited precise details of changes in behaviour observed prior to the most recent hospitalisation and the interval between onset of symptoms and re-admission. The ESS contains 34 items which measure an increase in early signs on a four-point scale, ranging from 0 (not a problem/zero times a week) to 3 (marked problem/at least once a day). The scale is divided into four subsections: anxiety/agitation, depression/withdrawal, disinhibition and incipient psychosis.

Birchwood *et al.*'s (1989) prospective study using the ESS found that psychotic relapse was preceded by non-psychotic dysphoric symptoms including anxiety, dysphoria, interpersonal sensitivity/withdrawal and low-level psychotic thinking, including ideas of reference and paranoid thoughts. This study also suggested that there were differences in the amplitude and timing of symptoms and that the pattern of prodromal symptoms showed subject variability: some may 'peak' on anxiety symptoms, others on disinhibition and so forth. Thus Birchwood (1992) proposed that it may be more appropriate to think of each individual's prodrome as a personalised relapse signature which includes core or common symptoms, together with features unique to each patient. Such symptoms generally occur in a predictable order over a period of less than four weeks, with non-psychotic phenomena occurring early in the illness, followed by the development of frankly psychotic symptoms. The same sequential pattern of symptoms identified in patients each time they relapse is termed the relapse signature (Birchwood 1992).

CHALLENGES TO THE THEORY OF THE RELAPSE SIGNATURE

The evidence presented by Birchwood (1996) in support of his relapse signature theory is scant. A single case example is presented where the prodromes of four episodes (the total EWS score, as measured by the ESS, at two weekly intervals over an eight-week period) are juxtaposed into one figure. When the total EWS scores for each of the four prodromes are separated out, it becomes evident that each prodrome does not follow the same sequential pattern. For example, in Relapse 1 there was a decrease in EWS scores for the first six/seven weeks, whereas in Relapse 4 there was a very gentle increase in EWS scores over the same time period. In Relapse 2 there was a steady increase in EWS scores from weeks four to eight, whereas in Relapses 1, 3 and 4, the increases in scores are more pronounced in weeks six to eight. Furthermore, Birchwood does not present information on each of the subsections of the ESS (anxiety/agitation, depression/withdrawal, disinhibition and incipient psychosis), only the total EWS scores: thus it is not possible to tease out more specific differences. It is arguable that increases in one subsection of the scale (e.g. anxiety/agitation) could cancel out decreases in other subsections (e.g. disinhibition) and so forth. Thus, by reporting only the total EWS scores, the detail of the sequential development of the prodrome is masked. A quantitative change in symptomology, as measured by the ESS, fails to expose the developmental nature of the relapse prodrome.

Based on the above critique of Birchwood's work with the ESS, it is proposed that the prodrome is not as static a phenomenon as Birchwood's theory of the relapse signature suggests – but rather that it is developmental in nature and can change in content and pattern from relapse to relapse. By taking an idiographic, behavioural approach and analysing the functions of prodromal behaviour, rather than examining an increase in symptomology, the progressive nature of the prodrome can be explored. It is proposed that multiple sequential functional analysis (MSFA; Gresswell and Hollin 1992), an in-depth, qualitative case study methodology designed to capture the changing functions of behaviour as they develop over time, can be applied to understand further the developmental nature of an individual's prodrome.

Taking a social learning theory approach (Bandura 1977) to the functions of behaviour, it is hypothesised that the development of the prodrome will be influenced by continuous reciprocal interaction between personal, behavioural and environmental factors over the course of the illness. In each functional analysis paradigm, an A:B:C sequence is applied to understand the function of prodromal behaviours: A refers to environmental and behavioural antecedents to B the behaviour, which produce C the environmental and behavioural consequences. In MSFA, one A:B:C sequence becomes part of an individual's learning history and hence antecedent to the next A:B:C stage and so on. An A:B:C analysis was conducted for each relapse so that the differences between an individual's prodromes could be easily discerned.

CASE STUDY SUMMARIES

The main differences between the relapse prodromes of two individuals are summarised in Tables 5.1 and 5.2. The names and personal details of the individuals and their families have been changed to preserve anonymity. The

Table 5.1 Summary of main differences between relapse prodromes – Sue

Behaviours	Second prodrome	Third prodrome
Incipient psychosis	Auditory and tactile hallucinatory experiences: hears motorbikes; feels heart taken out of body. Preoccupied with belief boyfriend/ex-boss/Prince Charming are going to save her. Believes black and white cars have special meaning and that TV is sending messages. Feels physically sick: believes pregnant with ex-boss's child. Headache and belief she is going to die. Development of paranoid, sexual and religious delusions: believes Jack/father were sexually abusing her and her children; believed Jesus was a homosexual.	Daydreaming about running a business. Escalating paranoid delusions: Miles, new boyfriend, is involved in drugs, is a paedophile, believes she is a sex object for his pleasure. Believes army spying on her. Believes someone is being punished for her being attractive.
Depression/ withdrawal	Slept less as felt less tired. Optimistic in mood. Increasingly motivated to look after and clean home. Highly concerned with appearance and self-care. Some socialisation with friends. Felt increasingly isolated living alone.	Much more sociable and confident: develops a sexual relationship with Miles. Stable levels of good motivation. Scared to sleep at night.

Disinhibition	Laughing inappropriately. More freedom as living alone therefore increasingly bizarre behaviour: bathing fully dressed; dancing around house. Increasingly assertive/rude to parents.	Slightly elevated mood. Spends large sums of Miles' money on unwanted items. Increasingly assertive with Miles, Jack and children. Gets rid of TV and radio. Outrageous dress, very short haircut, acting/feeling drunk.
Anxiety/ agitation	Low levels of anxiety – feels less stressed as living on her own.	Stressed re custody battle for children. Initially less anxious/more stable, then increasingly anxious and fearful for her safety, becoming less anxious when the children go to stay with their father.
Others	Highly dependent on and feels like controlled by parents. Obsessive writing to boyfriend. More stable ability to function as living alone. Loses weight after ceasing medication; appetite remains normal.	Ceases medication. Increasingly independent. Sexual intercourse enjoyable. Comfort eating followed by deterioration in appetite after children leave home. Fluctuating ability to function while living with children/being responsible for them.
Length of prodrome	Two months approx. from ceasing medication to re-admission to hospital.	17 months approx. from ceasing medication to re-admission to hospital.

summary tables have been designed so that they are easily comparable with the categorisation of early signs in the ESS. Thus the tables have been divided into the four sections of symptomology used in the ESS: anxiety/agitation, depression/withdrawal, disinhibition and incipient psychosis. In addition, a section for 'others' has been included in order to account for prodromal behaviours that cannot be easily categorised in the four main sections. The concept of the prodrome used equated with Birchwood's theory of the relapse signature, which defined the onset of the prodrome as a quantitative change on the ESS and/or the appearance of individualised prodromal signs. The offset of the prodrome was defined as either re-admission into hospital or an increase or change in medication (Birchwood 1995). The duration of the relapse prodrome has also been included in the summary tables to illustrate differences in the length of the relapse prodromes.

Case Study 1: The development of Sue's relapse prodrome

Case Study 1, summarised in Table 5.1, illustrates the main differences between Sue's second and third relapse prodromes. In her second prodrome, Sue was living alone in a large house and was being financially and emotionally supported by her parents. She had separated from her husband who had custody of their children. The content of Sue's relapse prodrome was coloured by her environment. For example, her incipient psychosis focused on the development of her paranoid, sexual and religious delusions involving her father and her ex-husband Jack. She had limited opportunities to socialise as she was living alone and was therefore generally more withdrawn and socially isolated. Her disinhibited behaviour was confined to within the home. In comparison, in her third prodrome, the content of her irrational beliefs was influenced by her new relationship with Miles. Her anxiety levels fluctuated with the responsibility of looking after her children and, because she was more motivated and sociable, her disinhibited behaviour was much more public.

Sue's experience of her two prodromes was very different. Furthermore, such differences in the content of her early signs automatically affected the sequential, temporal pattern of development of the prodromes. The duration of each prodrome was also very different: the second prodrome was two months in length whereas the third prodrome was approximately 17 months in duration. Thus this case study also provides evidence that the prodrome differs in length from relapse to relapse and that such deterioration does not necessarily fit into a four-week time window as Birchwood's theory of the relapse signature suggests.

Case Study 2: Subtle changes in Max's prodromal behaviour

The case study of Max, summarised in Table 5.2, illustrates some more subtle changes in prodromal behaviours, which developed over eight psychotic breakdowns. For example, the levels of depression experienced by Max differed between breakdowns: in his third prodrome Max was extremely depressed whereas in his eighth prodrome he experienced only occasional periods of low mood. Following his arson offence in his third prodrome, Max's paranoia in the fourth prodrome focused on his irrational belief that everyone thought he was a criminal. The content of his paranoid beliefs, however, had significantly changed by his fifth prodrome: Max, who was living in a caravan at the time, believed his neighbours could read his thoughts and stayed up all night to talk to him through the caravan walls. Other behaviour which reflected Max's attempt at coping with his illness also affected the development of his prodrome. In his second prodrome he became highly concerned with his appearance and subsequently developed a new interest in weight training. In his fourth prodrome, however, Max was living in a caravan, where he became very lonely, bored and depressed. He started to gamble in order to pass the time of day. As Max became addicted to gambling he resorted to borrowing money from his parents. His relationship with his parents subsequently deteriorated and Max's ensuing financial problems made him feel highly anxious and physically sick.

The lengths of Max's prodromes varied from relapse to relapse. In the earlier years of his illness his prodromes were much greater in length (ranging from two years two months in his second prodrome to 58 months in his fourth prodrome), whereas in the later stages of his illness they were shorter in duration (from one month in his fifth prodrome to one year in his eighth prodrome). Thus this case study provides evidence that not only does the relapse prodrome change in content, but also in duration. Factors such as Max's greater understanding of his illness, the development of different coping strategies, his manipulation of medication and his build-up of trust and contact with psychiatric services all interactively contributed to changes in the duration of his relapse prodromes.

A BEHAVIOURIST VERSUS A COGNITIVE ANALYSIS OF THE RELAPSE PRODROME

Birchwood proposes that an individual's relapse signature represents a juxtaposition of early symptoms intrinsic to the illness and a psychological response that centres on the individual's search for meaning and control (Birchwood and Macmillan 1993). Thus Birchwood (1995) accounts for variation in the nature and timing of an individual's early signs (i.e. relapse signature) by integrating an individual's own idiosyncratic response to emerging relapse. This cognitive explanation examines individuals' attributional processes during the prodromal stage and attempts to distinguish between primary prodromal changes and secondary attributions (i.e. patients' ideas of causality). Birchwood's cognitive explanation for the variation in early signs suggests that such symptoms arise from the way in which individuals explain and interpret internal and external events (Gumley et al. 1999). This cognitive analysis of early relapse draws upon Maher's (1988) model of delusional formation and Weiner's (1985, 1986) attribution theory (as cited in Birchwood 1995). Birchwood suggests that ambiguous and novel perceptual-cognitive changes are provided with a construction which is likely to be abnormal in view of the initial experience, but which nevertheless offers the individual some relief, thus reinforcing the tenacity with which it is held. Such delusions are regarded as an adaptive response to preserve order, integrity and meaning (Roberts 1991; Strauss 1991; as cited in Birchwood 1995).

However, Birchwood refers to Weiner's attribution theory to explain why,

Table 5.2 Summary of main differences between relapse prodromes – Max

Behaviours	Second prodrome	Third prodrome	Fourth prodrome	Fifth prodrome	Sixth prodrome	Seventh prodrome	Eighth prodrome
Incipient psychosis	Escalating paranoia. Hears voices and believes people talking about him.	High paranoia, low paranoia, increasing paranoia. Fluctuating paranoia, hears voices talking about him. Believes people can read his thoughts. Olfactory hallucinations.	Believes everyone knows he is a criminal. Paranoia stabilises. Believes ducks laughing at him. Spasmodically hears voices. Believes neighbour is a drug dealer.	Believes that neighbours can read his thoughts and that they stay up all night to talk to him through the caravan walls. Hears voices calling him a 'nonce' and telling him to commit suicide.	Believes neighbours shouting sexual insults at him through caravan walls.	Low-level paranoia: believes people talking to him through caravan walls.	Preoccupied with death. Low-level paranoia: believes people in upstairs flat are talking about him.
Depression/withdrawal	Feels very lethargic. Increasingly depressed.	Extremely depressed. Increasingly withdrawn.	Increasingly lonely, bored and depressed. Disrupted sleep.	Depressed. Disrupted sleep.	Miserable, cold, demoralised, depressed.	Extremely isolated and depressed. Lethargic, sleeping 12 hours a day. Barely eating.	Occasional periods of low mood. Increasingly demotivated, bored and withdrawn.
Disinhibition	None.	Aggressive outburst: hits brother.	Unruly and disruptive behaviour.	Assaults old man. Damages flat doors.	None.	Two overdoses of medication.	None.

					Assaults neighbour. Steals books.	Arson: sets fire to his room in a residential home.	
Anxiety/agitation	Mildly distressed at feeling emotionally flat.		Scared he may be assaulted by neighbours. Moderately anxious.	Highly anxious and distressed.	Financial problems make him highly anxious and physically sick.	Feels physically weak. Highly concerned about appearance and physique (has lost weight).	Highly concerned about appearance/neglected appearance. Increasingly uncomfortable in shared house.
Others	Stops medication. Deterioration in concentration and ability to carry out daily living skills. Rationalises paranoia. Requests re-admission.	Threatens to take another overdose in order to be re-admitted to hospital.	Purposefully ceases medication.	Ceases medication. Turns up at friends' houses, uninvited, with overnight bag. Contacts CPN for support.	Abusing alcohol. Becomes addicted to gambling. Discontinues medication 'on advice' of a psychiatrist.	Increasingly difficult to function; leaves work. Loses track of time. Loses weight.	Regularly drinking and smoking. Starts weight training. Increasing communication problems. Contacts mother for help.
Length of prodrome	One year.	Four months.	Two to three months.	One month.	58 months.	Three years approx.	Two years two months.

in the context of relative insight and prior experience of relapse, an individual chooses such an apparently disempowering (externalising) attribution. Weiner's attribution theory argues that perceived causes of an event differ on the dimensions of internality, stability and controllability. Birchwood suggests that to label early signs as relapse is to make an attribution that is internal, stable, global and, for most, uncontrollable. Internality and controllability dimensions are thought to be involved in the genesis of esteem-related emotion. The relapse attribution, according to Birchwood, is therefore likely to arouse guilt and lowered self-esteem: externalising attributions may be self-esteem-preserving as well as inherently more controllable (e.g. through the use of avoidance). Birchwood argues that this attributional process and the negative affect it generates are instrumental in either accelerating or arresting the process of relapse. For example, dysphoric symptoms could be regarded as arising out of fear of impending relapse, or a failure to explain disturbing and dangerous symptoms and experiences. Thus Birchwood hypothesises that symptom exacerbation occurs (or is prevented) via two routes. First, the tension, uncertainty and danger inherent in some attributions could accelerate the relapse process in line with the stress vulnerability model – which highlights the relationship between stress and its impact on the threshold for expression of vulnerability as symptoms (Clements and Turpin 1992). Second, symptoms could be exacerbated through an externalising attribution process which, while preserving self-esteem and control, drives delusion formation. This two-process theory suggests that the co-existence of internal and external attributions gradually alters and an attribution develops which is purely external. Furthermore, this model hypothesises that those individuals with extensive prior experience of relapse and its associative negative repercussions would respond with high levels of fear and perhaps helplessness leading to depression and withdrawal. On the other hand, it suggests that those with less experience may respond with puzzlement, confusion and perplexity (Gumley et al. 1999). However, Birchwood's cognitive explanation of early relapse omits to detail how an individual's attributional processes (and therefore relapse signature) may develop and change as the individual experiences more and more psychotic breakdowns.

Birchwood's model highlights the role of an individual's attributions for, and meanings ascribed to, symptoms and internal experiences. This cognitive analysis of early psychosis is structural as opposed to functional in nature. Observed behaviour is seen as a sign or symptom of the illness. Taking this view, the behaviour itself is relatively unimportant. It is only important as an index of those unobservable constructs that are believed to be the cause of the clinical problem. Thus the purpose of cognitive assessment is to uncover the cognitive schemata and perceptual biases that the client has. These non-observables are given special status as the underlying cause of the client's problem (Sturmey 1996).

In contrast, behavioural assessments are functional in nature. Functionalist approaches emphasise the purposes that behaviours serve for the person (Goldiamond 1974, 1975a; cited in Sturmey 1996). Functionalist approaches emphasise an idiographic approach to the assessment of each problem. That is, they are interested in the analysis and treatment of the behaviour of the individual, rather than assigning a person's behaviour to a number of predetermined types, such as paranoid schizophrenia.

Bandura (1977) hypothesised that behaviour results from the interaction of persons and situations, rather than from either factor alone. Personal and environmental factors do not function as independent determinants – rather, they determine each other. The experiences produced by behaviour also partly determine what a person becomes and can do, which, in turn, affects subsequent behaviour. Thus we have the social learning theory of interaction, analysed fully as a process of reciprocal determinism, behaviour and other personal and environmental factors, which all operate as interlocking determinants of each other (Bandura 1977). Furthermore, the relative influences of these independent factors differ in various settings for different behaviours. Therefore there are times when environmental factors exercise strong constraints on behaviour and other times when personal factors are the determining regulators of the course of environmental events. Individuals are neither driven by inner forces (covert behaviour) nor buffeted by environmental stimuli. Rather, psychological functioning is explained in terms of a continuous reciprocal interaction of personal and environmental determinants. Within this approach symbolic, vicarious and self-regulatory processes assume a prominent role (Bandura 1977).

Virtually all learning resulting from direct experience occurs on a vicarious basis: that is, from observing other people's behaviour and its consequences for them. Some complex behaviours can be produced only with the aid of modelling (i.e. learning from others). The ability to use symbols (cognitive processing) provides individuals with an effective means of dealing with their environment. Through symbols individuals process and preserve experiences in 'representational' forms. This information then guides future behaviour. Furthermore, through the use of symbols, individuals can solve problems, anticipate the probable consequences of different actions and alter their behaviour accordingly. Indeed, without symbolising powers individuals would not be capable of 'reflective thought'. Furthermore, individuals have self-regulatory capacities. By arranging environmental inducements, making cognitive supports and producing consequences for their own actions, individuals are able to exercise some measure of control over their own behaviour. However, although self-regulatory functions can be supported and shaped by environmental factors, self-influence partly determines which actions an individual performs (Bandura 1977).

A social learning theory approach to understanding human interaction explains how patterns of behaviour are acquired and how their expression is continuously regulated by the interplay of self-generated and external sources of influence. Thus functional relationships are not static; rather, they are developmental in nature and can therefore vary over time (Gresswell and Hollin 1992). In contrast, cognitive assessments generally place little emphasis on the situation or context of behaviour and assume a reasonable degree of trans-situational consistency (Sturmey, 1996). Indeed, Birchwood's cognitive analysis places no emphasis on the situation or context of behaviour, and his theory of the relapse signature assumes trans-situational consistency.

The usefulness of the relapse signature concept and the ESS

The relapse prodrome, when analysed in social learning theory terms, is not the static phenomenon Birchwood's relapse signature theory suggests; rather, it is developmental in nature and can change in content, experience, pattern of development and duration, from relapse to relapse. A generalised clinical assessment tool such as the ESS could not predict or capture the evolution of an individual's relapse prodrome.

As an individual does not follow the same sequential prodromal pattern each time he/she relapses, it is reasoned that a more idiographic, detailed approach is needed to understand the development of prodromal behaviour in its environmental context. It is proposed that multiple sequential functional analysis (MSFA; Gresswell and Hollin 1992) can be applied to understand further an individual's prodrome and predict relapse. A case example is presented to illustrate how this methodology can be used to predict relapse. The names and personal details of the individual in this case study and his family have been changed to preserve anonymity.

USING MSFA TO EXPLORE AND PREDICT THE PRODROME TO PSYCHOSIS: A FORENSIC CASE STUDY

Jon has experienced two psychotic episodes. The development of his illness is summarised in three stages of analysis: the initial prodrome, the onset of frank psychosis/duration of untreated psychosis and first treatment, and the relapse prodrome. Each stage of analysis consists of an A:B:C sequence, as described earlier in this chapter. Key learning is included for each stage of the analysis and the behaviour category is separated into overt (directly observable behaviours) and covert (thoughts, feelings and physiological activity) sections. Information was obtained from Jon and members of his family. Medical notes, court reports and discussions with his treating clinical psychologist were used to check the reliability and validity of the qualitative data.

Jon's initial prodrome (5–15 years)

The initial prodrome was defined as the illness onset, the first appearance of any psychiatric symptoms (Rabiner *et al.* 1986), and the period between normal functioning and frank psychosis (Yung and McGorry 1996).

Jon was five years old when his father became bankrupt. The family subsequently moved from their town home to a council house in a rural area. Jon recollects an incident when he was six, when his mother was extremely upset and his father, for some reason, was very annoyed with her. Jon claims this was when he first heard a voice (unknown female) asking him questions about the incident. The atmosphere at home subsequently became very tense and awkward and communication became very strained. From this point onwards Jon claims his parents gave him little support or guidance. Jon states that his father started to misuse alcohol. Jon began to rely on his voices (several females and occasionally some males) for explanations of events and feelings. However, the voices often added to his confusion by asking him questions, which he could not answer. Several years later Jon found out that the change in his home life had been triggered by his mother having an affair.

Jon was put into a special class at school, because he was experiencing difficulties with concentration, comprehension, reading and writing. He claims he became highly sensitive to other people's feelings and emotions. Jon alleges that from an early age he was different from the other children at school. His mother's fashion sense was ahead of the times and Jon's bleached hair and pierced ears made him look and feel different. Jon was also embarrassed about his poor, shabby home, and was conscious about not being a local boy. He also suffered from an illness which required him to wear a leg calliper as a child. Apart from being teased about the calliper, it also prevented him from participating in physical activities. The amalgamation of these factors made it difficult for Jon to strike up relationships with other schoolchildren, so he made friends outside school with older boys who were involved in crime, violence, drugs and women.

At school he became mischievous and was often in trouble. His delinquent behaviour escalated throughout his teens. Jon soon learnt that petty thieving would get him into trouble with the police, which would result in his father having to pay him some attention. In addition, Jon stole things for his family. It appears that his crimes were rewarded with affection by his mother.

In his teens Jon played truant. He was also often suspended from school for disruptive and aggressive behaviour. He describes how he was afraid of the teacher making him the centre of attention by asking him a question. Jon claims he was encouraged by the voices purposefully to get into trouble in order to be dismissed from the classroom.

As a teenager Jon was building up his reputation for crime, fighting and abusing alcohol and drugs. He was also taking a keen interest in girls. Even with other members of the gang Jon professes he had communication problems and was often awkward and argumentative. He also claims he was continuously low in mood, anxious and had too much physical and sexual energy, which made him feel uncomfortable. Consequently Jon could not sleep and spent most nights engaged in criminal activity.

Jon claims the voices became more complicated and confusing throughout adolescence, continuously pressurising him into engaging in sexual activity. Jon became increasingly promiscuous and sexually disinhibited. Indeed, his reputation for one-night stands reinforced his delinquent image, which increased his self-esteem.

When at school Jon spent a lot of time day-dreaming, looking through the classroom window, as he claims this intensified his perception of colours. Jon also began to fantasise about sex, violence and crime against an intense background colour. Background colours subsequently became symbolic. Blue represented crime, yellow goodness and red sex. Jon states he purposefully got into trouble to maintain the blue-coloured background because he claims it symbolised his image as a criminal, which not only gave him prestige but enabled him to make sense of what other people thought of him.

At the age of 15 Jon was expelled from school because his behaviour had become increasingly disruptive, aggressive and problematic. In particular, Jon was bullying several of his female classmates. He subsequently spent more time in public houses, drinking, which helped to dampen the voices. Table 5.3 summarises Jon's initial prodrome.

Offset of initial prodrome/onset of frank psychosis/ duration of untreated psychosis and first treatment (16–25 years)

The offset of the initial prodrome and the onset of frank psychosis was defined as the first point in time when the operational criteria of *The Diagnostic and Statistical Manual of Mental Disorders*, fourth edition (*DSM-IV*; American Psychiatric Association 1994) were fulfilled. As these criteria were applied retrospectively, the onset of frank psychosis was considered to be at the beginning of the one month of active phase symptoms. This definition attempts to apply a measurement of severity and provides clear boundaries between the offset of the initial prodrome and the onset of frank psychosis. The duration of untreated psychosis (DUP) was defined as the time from the onset of frank psychosis to the time when first adequate treatment was received (McGlashan and Johannessen, 1996).

Jon believes that at the age of 16 years he had his first real experience of paranoia, which he claims was triggered by taking cannabis. He became fearful that his friends would physically assault him, or would let him down in

Table 5.3 Initial prodrome – Jon (5–15 years)

A
Family stresses and parental conflict
Liberal parenting
Childhood illness and leg calliper
Rejected and teased at school; associates with older peer group

B: Covert
Voices give guidance/support; increasingly confusing over time
Difficulties with reading, writing, concentration
Highly sensitive to others' feelings
Feels different from other schoolchildren
Frightened of being centre of attention
Continuously low in mood and anxious
Increasing physical and sexual energy
Visual hallucinations; intense background colours
Fantasies re sex, violence, crime

B: Overt
Withdrawn and mischievous at school
Truanting
Increasingly disruptive and aggressive
Physically abusive towards female classmates
Escalating delinquent behaviour
Communication problems; awkward and argumentative
Disrupted sleep pattern
Sexually disinhibited behaviours: running around streets naked

C
Expelled from school at 15 years
Loss of support systems
Drug and alcohol misuse as coping strategies

Key learning
1 Voices provide him with all the support/guidance he needs.
2 Crime reduces pressure from voices, and is financially, socially and personally rewarding.
3 Sexual intercourse reduces uncomfortable physical energy and reinforces his delinquent image.
4 He has no respect for the opposite sex.

other ways. Feeling threatened, Jon left home and became nomadic. This was arguably the offset of the initial prodrome and the onset of frank psychosis. In accordance with *DSM-IV* he fulfils the criteria for a diagnosis of schizophrenia as he is experiencing two active phase symptoms – hallucinations and delusions – which are severe in nature, for at least one month, and attenuated symptoms of psychosis for at least six months.

Within a year Jon returned to live with his parents, where he spent the next 18 months as a recluse, too frightened to engage in criminal activity as he had no friends in the area to support him. Instead he became obsessed with writing about crime, sex and violence, which enabled him to manage the voices and retain the rewarding blue visual hallucination.

In his early twenties, Jon left home and found work on a building site. However, he was unable to concentrate at work, was dangerous in his operation of the machinery and was soon sacked for his incompetence and thieving of building materials. He subsequently moved into a squat, re-established contact with his former gang friends and returned to his past delinquent lifestyle.

During this period of his life Jon had his only serious sexual relationship, which lasted several months. As he became more emotionally involved he claims the voices told him his girlfriend was having an affair with his best friend. It appears that his use of amphetamines at that time intensified these beliefs and led to him physically assaulting his girlfriend on several occasions. This relationship subsequently terminated.

Weeks later Jon was invited to stay at his best friend's house for the weekend. This friend's sister, who was under 16 years of age, was also staying. Jon claims this young woman made sexual advances towards him. He responded, but did not have intercourse. A few days later, this girl informed the police that Jon had sexually assaulted her. Frightened, Jon returned to live with his parents.

Jon was subsequently convicted of indecent assault on a minor and sentenced to community service. He became extremely worried that people would find out about this offence. He became more violent and out of control, and tried to commit suicide through dangerous driving. In his endeavour to cope with increasing paranoia and the continuous torment from the voices, Jon again turned to crime in an attempt to regain control and restore some self-esteem. Jon was subsequently accused of several armed robberies and was held on remand in prison. Here Jon claims he was bullied into not giving evidence against his co-accused, who knew about his conviction for indecent assault and threatened to spread it around the prison. Jon was subsequently charged for two robberies and sentenced to nine years' imprisonment. His co-accused was acquitted of all charges. Thereafter Jon's paranoia escalated; he was in contact with the prison healthcare services on a frequent basis and was diagnosed as suffering from a psychotic illness.

Jon was treated with major tranquillisers but did not take his medication regularly for fear of not being able to fend for himself in the prison environment. Because he was not aware that his experiences were abnormal, Jon did not talk to the medical staff about them. He was unable to rest in his shared cell; he was too paranoid to go to sleep in case his cellmate attacked him. Jon again returned to stealing, which in a prison environment may have had several functions, one of them being an attempt to reduce the torment from his voices and to recreate the blue background hallucination which had a calming effect on his condition. Jon soon learnt that the punishment for these crimes was being sent to the isolation block. After several days Jon would return to the main wing, feeling more in control. He would recommence writing stories, which he claimed he sold to the other inmates for drugs. In due course his paranoia would increase and he would find himself back on the hospital wing, or in the isolation block. This continued until he eventually told the doctor about his experiences and was referred to a psychiatric hospital.

In hospital Jon's condition was stabilised. Uncomfortable at being in a psychiatric hospital, he requested to be returned to prison as soon as he could to complete his sentence. At this stage Jon did not understand that he was suffering from a severe mental illness. His key learning predicts that because he has experienced being in a psychiatric hospital, in the future he will be less fearful of seeking external help when he feels he is losing control. Also, on his return to prison Jon is likely to become increasingly concerned yet again about others finding out about his sex offence conviction. Table 5.2 summarises the onset of psychosis, DUP and treatment of Jon's first breakdown.

Second prodrome and breakdown (25–29 years)

On his discharge back to prison, Jon claims the voices commanded him to obtain legendary status in the prison system. Consequently Jon acquainted himself with the most serious of criminals and developed a harder, more violent image.

Jon took his medication irregularly and continued to misuse illicit drugs, which quickly led to a deterioration in his mental health. However on this occasion, because Jon knew the prison system, he was promptly back either on the isolation block or on the hospital wing. Thus his psychotic symptoms were not as severe or prolonged as in his first breakdown. He also relates that when he was out of isolation he was less withdrawn and more able to join in conversations about crime. This in turn helped him to keep the voices and paranoia more under control.

After several months Jon was transferred to a semi-open prison. There, a prison officer told other inmates of his sex offence. This was what Jon had feared most and immediately his paranoia escalated, which triggered his transfer to the hospital unit of his home prison. Jon had learnt not to be afraid to tell the doctors what he was experiencing and was referred more quickly to hospital. Prior to his second admission he had lost more weight, was very pale and had lost all interest in his appearance.

Jon claims this breakdown was not as serious as his first because he was less nervous about being in a psychiatric hospital; he knew what the hospital system expected of him and therefore he was more comfortable and quickly relaxed. For the first time he started to trust the medical staff and consequently he began to talk about his psychotic experiences and his sex offence. He learnt that hearing voices was not normal and he started to make sense of his condition. On this occasion Jon was well enough to benefit from

Table 5.4 Offset of initial prodrome/onset of frank psychosis, DUP and first treatment/ admission – Jon (16–25 years)

A
Sequences as in previous stage
Drug effects (cannabis and amphetamines)
Returns to live with parents
Re-establishes former contacts/returns to delinquent lifestyle
Serious relationship terminates
Charged with indecent assault on a minor
Charged for two armed robberies, sentenced to nine years' imprisonment
Bullied by co-accused in prison

B: Covert
Increasing paranoia
Highly anxious
Voices – increasing pressure and confusion
Deluded thinking
Visual hallucinations

B: Overt
Nomadic behaviour
Becomes a recluse
Obsessive writing
Dangerous, incompetent and criminal behaviour at work: sacked
Increasingly violent and aggressive
Suicide attempts
Talks nonsense, bizarre behaviour, hyperactive, disrupted sleep, taking illicit drugs
Stealing from prison guards
Neglected appearance, loses weight

C
Admitted to prison hospital; diagnosed as suffering from a psychotic illness
Punished in prison isolation block for bad behaviour
Referred to a psychiatric hospital; discharged back to prison

Key learning
1 He is increasingly concerned about people finding out about his charge for indecent assault on a minor.
2 He understands the prison system and has learnt how to obtain isolation to cope with his condition.
3 He realises that admission into a psychiatric hospital does not mean 'life imprisonment'.

various psychological therapies such as anxiety management and cognitive behavioural therapy for psychosis.

Over the last 18 months Jon's mental health has greatly improved and he is now approaching discharge. Jon has also been given the opportunity to discuss his illness at a much deeper level. He has learnt how physical exercise can reduce stress and energy levels. In addition, Jon has been attending a clinic for his past drug and alcohol problems and has learnt how illicit drugs can induce and exacerbate psychosis. Jon has also developed insight into his illness and recognises the importance of medication to keep him stable. He understands that he can become stressed over minor issues, and when stressed his voices can return for short periods of time. Jon has learnt to use a personal stereo to block out the voices and will humour or try to ignore them. At times Jon acknowledges that he does not know how to behave in certain situations and feels at a loss without the advice and guidance he claims the voices gave him. Nonetheless, he expresses great remorse for some of his past behaviour – how he threatened and humiliated people and how he had very little respect for women. However, he has also learnt that when his voices return his attitudes to women and his sexual behaviour are likely to change. Furthermore, he shows no regret for his thieving.

More recently Jon moved into a rehabilitation unit to prepare him further for discharge. Jon is currently uncertain about his future. Indeed, he is still highly sensitive to what other people think about him and his past sex offence, and has recently expressed feeling overwhelmed as he has too many things to arrange in time for discharge. He claims he may be relapsing. On discharge Jon will be moving into his own home for the first time and has stated that he wants to furnish his home only with new household goods. If he can't afford to buy such merchandise, Jon claims he will return to crime to get the money for these goods. Jon also asserts that because he is no longer guided by his voices, he will be tempted to take illicit drugs to give him the impetus to commit the first crime. It is predicted that his mental health would deteriorate thenceforth. Based on this assessment it is arguable that his current condition is prodromal in nature and moderately fragile. His condition would be exacerbated further if he rekindles his contacts with former friends and was subjected to peer pressure, or if his compliance with medication is poor. Table 5.5 illustrates the development of Jon's illness to date.

THE CLINICAL POTENTIAL OF MSFA

As illustrated in the case study of Jon, MSFA can be used to predict relapse in psychosis. This methodology may overcome many of the problems associated with the clinical implementation of the ESS. For example, Birchwood et al. (1992) acknowledge that individuals who retain very little insight, or for whom loss of insight occurs very early on in decompensation, may be unable or unwilling to complete the ESS. Birchwood also highlights the numerous disadvantages of using the ESS to self-monitor: it sensitises patients and carers to disability, promotes observations as critical responses, burdens individuals and carers with requests for repetitive information at frequent intervals and possibly increases risk of self-harm in individuals who become demoralised by an impending relapse. In addition, it is not always convenient for patients and carers to complete the ESS on a fortnightly basis, and over time individuals may become blasé in its completion. Furthermore, a patient

Table 5.5 Relapse prodrome – Jon (25–29 years)

A
Sequences as in previous stage
Voices commanding legendary status
Irregular intake of medication
Illicit drug use
Prison officer tells inmates of Jon's sex offence

B: Covert
Feels he is respected by prisoners due to bank robber status: increase in self-esteem and confidence
Less frightened to talk to doctors about his experiences
High, stable levels of anxiety
Intermittent paranoia

B: Overt
More aggressive and violent
Less withdrawn and more able to communicate with other inmates: spasmodic ability to function
Stealing to achieve isolation for rest and sleep
Losing more weight
Neglected appearance

C
Prompt admission to psychiatric hospital: more relaxed
Regular medication helps him become more amenable to other therapeutic interventions
Residual symptoms: incipient voices, low stress threshold

Key learning
1 He has developed trust in medical staff, which has enabled him to talk about his psychotic experiences and sex offence.
2 He has insight into his mental illness, recognises the importance of regular medication, has developed new coping strategies to help control symptoms and recognises prodromal signs.
3 He expresses remorse for his past sexual behaviour and has learnt that when his voices return his attitude to women and his sexual behaviour are likely to change.
4 He feels his future is uncertain and is worried about the stigma of his sex offence.
5 Crime has resolved all of his problems in the past: it is the key to his future!
6 Without the guidance of his voices he will abuse drugs to give him the impetus to return to crime.

may learn through experience the 'correct' answers to the ESS and may conceal his/her true mental state and purposely give false answers, for example to ensure re-admission to hospital or to avoid an increase in medication.

MacDonald and Mortimer (2001) found that in routine clinical practice it was not always possible for community psychiatric nurses (CPNs) to administer the ESS on a fortnightly basis, as the services in their local NHS trust were geared towards crisis resolution. CPNs therefore spent more time with individuals who were actually relapsing/psychotic than monitoring those who were relatively well.

MSFA overcomes many of these practical problems associated with the ESS. However, this in-depth, qualitative methodology is initially fairly time-consuming, as it attempts to break down a vast amount of data from multiple sources of assessment into concise manageable chunks. For example, in the case study presented, it took approximately six hours to collect the data from Jon and his family, and an additional four hours to examine Jon's case notes, court reports and other relevant documentation, before analysing the data. In the long term, however, such a methodology will arguably be more cost-effective than the ESS as it does not require fortnightly monitoring. Furthermore, the analysis can easily be updated in light of new information and additional stages added if further relapses are experienced. Such a clinical assessment tool can be used for educational purposes and can be readily accessible to the patient, carer and relevant health professionals. Unlike the ESS, MSFA can identify possible triggers of future episodes and predict the development of prodromal behaviour in its environmental context. Finally, MSFA brings a case to life. It considers the individual with psychosis in the developmental context of his/her life experiences, and attempts to understand how the function of prodromal behaviour can change in different environmental situations. A symptom-orientated approach such as the ESS lacks this sensitivity and focuses attention away from the individual and onto the illness.

CONCLUSION

MSFA can be used to explore and predict the relapse prodrome in psychosis. Using this methodology, evidence has been found to suggest that the relapse prodrome is not as static a phenomenon as Birchwood's theory of the relapse signature suggests. The same sequential prodromal pattern does not necessarily herald each psychotic breakdown. The developmental nature of the prodrome is influenced by the continuous reciprocal interaction between personal, behavioural and environmental factors over the course of the illness.

In addition, MSFA may overcome many of the practical problems associated with the ESS and can create more opportunities for clinicians to implement early intervention strategies to ameliorate a psychotic breakdown, thus reducing the risk of further relapse and/or offending behaviour.

REFERENCES

American Psychiatric Association (1994). *Diagnostic and Statistical Manual of Mental Disorders (4th edition)*. Washington, DC: American Psychiatric Association.

Bandura, A. (1977). *Social Learning Theory*. Prentice-Hall.

Birchwood, M. *et al.* (1989). Predicting relapse in schizophrenia: The development and implementation of an early signs monitoring system using patients and families as observers, a preliminary investigation. *Psychological Medicine* 19: 649–56.

Birchwood, M. (1992). Early intervention in schizophrenia: Theoretical background and clinical strategies. *British Journal of Clinical Psychology* 31: 257–78.

Birchwood, M. *et al.* (1992). Early intervention. In M. Birchwood and N. Tarrier (eds) *Innovations in the Psychological Management of Schizophrenia. Assessment, Treatment and Services*. Chichester, UK: John Wiley and Sons Ltd.

Birchwood, M. and Macmillan, F. (1993). Early intervention in schizophrenia. *Australian and New Zealand Journal of Psychiatry* 17: 374–78.

Birchwood, M. (1995). Early intervention in psychotic relapse: Cognitive approaches to detection and management. *Behaviour Change* 12: 2–19.

Birchwood, M. (1996). Early intervention in psychotic relapse: Cognitive approaches to detection and management. In G. Haddock and P. Slade (eds) *Cognitive Behavioural Interventions with Psychotic Disorders*. London: Routledge.

Birchwood, M. *et al.* (2000). Schizophrenia: Early warning signs. *Advances in Psychiatric Treatment* 6: 93–101.

Bustillo, J. *et al.* (1995). Prodromal symptoms vs. early warning signs and clinical action in schizophrenia. *Schizophrenia Bulletin* 21: 553–9.

Clements, D. and Turpin, G. (1992). Vulnerability theories. In M. Birchwood and N. Tarrier (eds) *Innovations in the Psychological Management of Schizophrenia. Assessment, Treatment and Services*. Chichester, UK: John Wiley and Sons Ltd.

Gresswell, D. M. and Hollin, C. (1992). Towards a new methodology for making sense of case material: An illustrative case involving attempted multiple murder. *Criminal Behaviour and Mental Health* 2: 239–341.

Gumley, A. *et al.* (1999). An interacting cognitive subsystems model of relapse and the course of psychosis. *Journal of Clinical Psychology and Psychotherapy* 6: 261–78.

Herz, M. and Melville, C. (1980). Relapse in schizophrenia. *American Journal of Psychiatry* 137: 801–12.

Hogarty, G. E. *et al.* (1991). Family psychoeducation, social skills training and maintenance chemotherapy in the aftercare treatment of schizophrenia, II. Two-year effects of a controlled study on relapse and adjustment. *Archives of General Psychiatry* 48: 340–1.

MacDonald, K. M. and Mortimer, A. (2001). *Implementation of Psychosocial Interventions in a Naturalistic Setting: Early Signs Monitoring – A Controlled Study*. Paper presented at the International Schizophrenia Research Conference, Whistler, Canada.

McCandless-Glimcher, L. *et al.* (1986). Use of symptoms by schizophrenics to monitor and regulate their illness. *Hospital and Community Psychiatry* 37: 927–33.

McGlashan, T. H. (1988). A selective review of recent north American long-term follow-up studies of schizophrenia. *Schizophrenia Bulletin* 14: 515–42.

McGlashan, T. H. and Johannessen, J. O. (1996). Early detection and intervention with schizophrenia: Rationale. *Schizophrenia Bulletin* 22: 201–22.

Rabiner, C. J. *et al.* (1986). Outcome study of first episode psychosis. I. Relapse rates after one year. *American Journal of Psychiatry* 143: 1155–8.

Shepherd, M. *et al.* (1989). The natural history of schizophrenia: A five-year follow-up in a representative sample of schizophrenics. *Psychological Medicine* (monograph suppl. 15).

Sturmey, P. (1996). *Functional Analysis in Clinical Psychology*. Chichester, UK: John Wiley.

Yung, A. R. and McGorry, P. D. (1996). The prodromal phase of first episode psychosis: Past and current conceptualisations. *Schizophrenia Bulletin* 22: 353–70.

Chapter 6

Can schizophrenia be predicted phenomenologically?

Frauke Schultze-Lutter, Stephan Ruhrmann and Joachim Klosterkötter

INTRODUCTION

The early detection of and thus early intervention in schizophrenia in its initial prodromal stage prior to the first psychotic episode has become a key research area during the last decade. Thereby it is intended to prevent or at least to delay the outbreak of frank psychosis and to avoid the social decline or retardation of social advancement that takes place before the first psychotic episode (Häfner *et al.* 1995; McGlashan 1998). However, sure knowledge about the nature of the initial prodrome does not exist, and different models of patterns of changes in the initial prodromal phase of schizophrenia have been suggested (see Yung and McGorry 1996).

In the epidemiological retrospective Age–Beginning–Course (ABC) study of the early course of first-episode schizophrenia (Häfner *et al.* 1998), negative and nonspecific symptoms were found in 78% of patients on average five years before the occurrence of the first psychotic symptom and 6.1 years before the first hospitalisation. Among the most frequently reported first signs of illness, nonspecific as well more specific cognitive disturbances were found (Häfner and an der Heiden 1999).

Paying tribute to the frequent observation of a prodromal phase before the onset of first psychotic symptoms, nine symptoms were emphasized as prodromal and included as diagnostic contributors in the *DSM-III-R* (APA 1987), but dismissed from *DSM-IV* (APA 1994). Their selection had been based on a retrospective conceptualization. For these symptoms, diagnostic accuracy measures were determined in a retrospective study of first-episode psychotic patients and – with specificities between 0.58 and 0.88 and positive predictive values between 0.36 and 0.48 – were found to be not pathognomonic of schizophrenic psychosis (Jackson *et al.* 1995). However, some of these nine *DSM-III-R* prodromal symptoms entered the nowadays widely-used definition of the initial prodrome of psychosis, the 'ultra-high risk' criteria as defined by attenuated and transient psychotic symptoms as well as by trait and state risk factors (Miller *et al.* 1999, 2002; Morrison *et al.* 2002; Philips *et al.* 2000; Yung *et al.* 2003). Studies of 12-month transition rates to psychosis in samples fulfilling these ultra-high risk criteria – though measured with different instruments – reported development of frank psychosis in 40.8% (Yung *et al.* 2003), 35.7% (McGorry *et al.* 2002), 54% (Miller *et al.* 2002) and 16% (Morrison *et al.* 2002) of potentially prodromal patients not receiving any special treatment. The majority of patients in these studies had shown attenuated psychotic symptoms at inclusion. It was concluded that it is possible to recruit patients with an imminent risk of developing psychosis that justifies targeted intervention (Yung *et al.* 2003). However, it is still unclear what symptoms or risk factors are the best predictors of psychosis.

In the Cologne Early Recognition project (CER; Klosterkötter *et al.* 2001), patients in a possible prodromal phase prior to first psychotic episode were studied prospectively for the schizophrenia-predictive value of another group of potentially prodromal symptoms. The study aimed to examine the prognostic accuracy of initial prodromal symptoms as assessed with the Bonn Scale for the Assessment of Basic Symptoms (BSABS; Gross *et al.* 1987) – that is, basic symptoms (Huber and Gross 1989; Klosterkötter 1992). It showed that certain basic symptoms might indeed predict a subsequent psychotic development surprisingly well, yet potential prodromal symptoms and certain symptom constellations require further examination as regards their prognostic accuracy and their utilisation as inclusion criteria for intervention studies.

METHODS

Sample

The study sample was taken from 695 patients examined for basic symptoms using the BSABS in outpatient departments of German psychiatric university departments before 1991. Prior to their referral, all patients had sought help for various problems from diverse medical and/or psychotherapeutic professionals (e.g. general practitioners, psychologists or psychiatrists). Referrals had been made due to difficulties arising in the diagnostic and therapeutic procedure. Thus patients presented at the specialized outpatient departments for a general diagnostic clarification and/or for clarification of a possibly incipient schizophrenic disorder and were examined with the BSABS and the ninth version of the Present State Examination (PSE9; Wing *et al.* 1974).

At this examination, some patients of the 695 examined already met *DSM-III-R* criteria for schizophrenia, delusional or psychotic disorder not elsewhere classified. These subjects ($n = 189$), as well as those with a confirmed diagnosis of a substance-induced disorder ($n = 47$), organic mental disorder ($n = 34$) or mental retardation ($n = 12$), were excluded from the study. An additional exclusion criterion was age of more than 50 years at first examination ($n = 28$) to avoid a high loss at follow-up due to increased rates of organic disease and death in this age group.

In all remaining 385 patients, no characteristic schizophrenia symptoms according to *DSM-III-R* and *DSM-IV-A* were found, either at first examination or at any point previously in the subjects' lifetimes. Therefore, the subjects could not yet be diagnosed as having first episodes, although a large number of them ($n = 253$) had reported basic symptoms. These patients returned to the care of their referring clinicians with only a small number ($n = 15$) keeping in sporadic contact with the relevant outpatient department. Thus, when the follow-up began in 1995, patients had to be contacted anew to be asked to participate in the study. The result of the recruitment is shown in Figure 6.1.

In all, 160 patients (41.6%) could be followed up until the conclusion of the study in 1998 (see Table 6.1). They did not differ from those lost to follow-up in mean age, distribution of gender, tentative diagnosis or presence of any basic symptom (see Figure 6.2), and thus can be regarded as representative of the whole sample.

At first examination, all 385 patients in the sample received tentative diagnoses – according to the prominent clinical picture – mainly of axis-I disorders and personality disorders (see Figure 6.2). In addition, 110 of these DSM-diagnosed patients had reported disturbances at first examination that met the definition of basic symptoms (see Figure 6.3).

Despite statistical trends ($p < 0.10$) towards more frequently diagnosed hypochondriasis in the followed-up group, and more frequently diagnosed schizotypal personality disorder in the lost to follow-up group as well as in those followed up with basic symptoms, there were no significant differences in the distribution of gender, age or tentative diagnosis either between followed-up patients and those lost to follow-up or between followed-up patients with and without basic symptoms at first examination (see Figures 6.2 and 6.3).

According to DSM-IV criteria (A–E), 79 patients (49.4%) developed

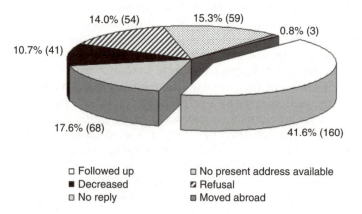

Figure 6.1 Results of follow-up recruitment.

Table 6.1 General data of sample (*n* = 160)

	Females (n = 76) Mean ± SD Median	Males (n = 84) Mean ± SD Median	Total (n = 160) Mean ± SD Median
Age at first examination (in years)	29.7 ± 11.4 25.0	28.9 ± 8.7 26.0	29.3 ± 10.0 26.0
Age at follow-up (in years)	38.4 ± 12.4 35.0	40.6 ± 11.4 37.5	39.6 ± 11.9 37.0
Follow-up period (in years)	8.6 ± 7.5 5.5	10.5 ± 7.6 10.0	9.6 ± 7.6 7.8
Duration of prodromal phase (in years)	4.3 ± 3.7 3.0 (n = 35)	6.7 ± 5.8 4.0 (n = 42)	5.6 ± 5.1 4.0 (n = 77)*

* Two individuals developed a frank psychosis without any assessable prodromal phase (time between first self-reported prodromal symptom meeting BSABS-criteria and first self-reported psychotic symptom meeting PSE9-criteria).

schizophrenia in the follow-up period, whereas 81 patients (50.6%) had not (Klosterkötter *et al.* 2001). In 77 of the 79 patients who became schizophrenic, basic symptoms had been found at first examination that persisted until outbreak of the illness. On average, a transition to schizophrenia in women occurred 4.3 years after the onset of the initial prodrome, and in men after 6.7 years (see Table 6.1). Furthermore, with one exception, no significant difference between the two outcome groups was found regarding the general data or the *DSM-IV*-adapted tentative diagnoses. Only the initial diagnosis of a schizotypal personality disorder had a significant positive correlation with the outcome of schizophrenia (phi-coefficient 0.191, $p < 0.05$).

Whereas 77 of the 79 patients who went on to develop schizophrenia had definitely reported at least one of the 66 basic symptoms at first examination and only two had not (percentage of false negative predictions, %FN = 1.3), 33 of the 81 patients without subsequent schizophrenia had also shown at least one definite basic symptom (percentage of false positive predictions, %FP = 20.6) and only 48 had not. Thus outcome was correctly predicted by the presence or absence of at least one basic symptom at first examination in 78.1% of cases (χ^2 = 59.9; *df* = 1; $p < 0.0001$). Accordingly, basic symptoms predict subsequent schizophrenia with a specificity of 0.59, a sensitivity of 0.98, a positive predictive value of 0.70, a negative predictive value of 0.96, a positive diagnostic likelihood ratio of 2.39, a negative diagnostic likelihood ratio of 0.03 and an odds ratio of 70.51 (Klosterkötter *et al.* 2001).

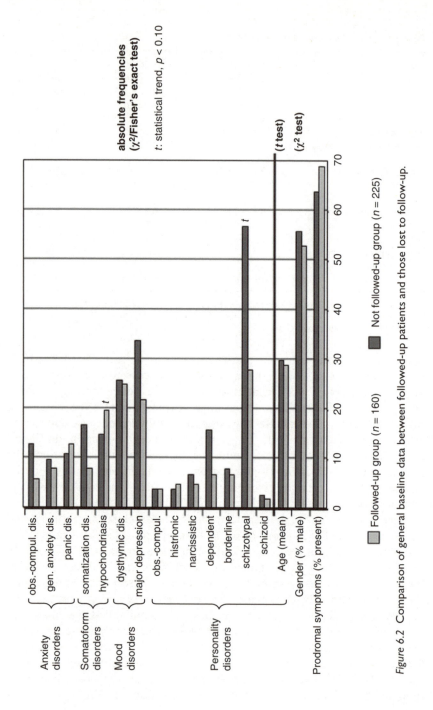

Figure 6.2 Comparison of general baseline data between followed-up patients and those lost to follow-up.

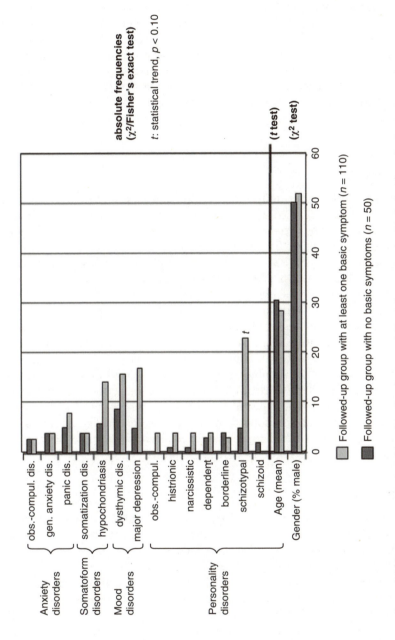

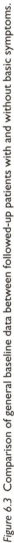

Figure 6.3 Comparison of general baseline data between followed-up patients with and without basic symptoms.

Instruments

The same two instruments, BSABS and PSE9, were applied at first examination and follow-up, and diagnoses were given according to *DSM* criteria valid at the respective assessment times: *DSM-III-R* criteria were used at first examination and *DSM-IV* criteria at follow-up. The PSE9, which includes 140 items grouped together in 20 partly overlapping sections, includes all characteristic symptoms relevant for *DSM-IV* diagnosis of a schizophrenic disorder. To evaluate basic symptoms, a shortened version of the BSABS with 66 items in five subsyndromes (Klosterkötter *et al.* 2001) was used that mainly differs from the original BSABS in being devoid of central-vegetative disturbances.

Procedure

The time interval between first examination and follow-up was 9.6 years on average (see Table 6.1). After giving their informed written consent, patients were re-examined by two members of our group, all of whom had undergone thorough training in the BSABS and the PSE9. Prior to follow-up, inter-rater reliabilities for the BSABS-subsyndromes and PSE9 sections had been tested on 10 remitted inpatients with a *DSM-III-R* diagnosis of schizophrenic disorder and received satisfying bias-corrected κ values (Schouten 1982) between 0.72 and 0.78 for pairwise agreement. At follow-up, interviewers and diagnosticians were blind to the patients' initial results and diagnoses. Diagnoses at follow-up were given by two experienced senior psychiatrists taking all available results and information about the clinical course into account. Transition to a first schizophrenic episode was assumed only if it could be assured that the *DSM-IV* criteria for schizophrenia had been met during the catamnestic period. The onset of the prodrome was assumed as being the time the patient had first noticed subtle changes that met any BSABS criterion; the onset of frank psychosis was defined as the time when PSE9 criteria for psychotic symptoms were first reported.

Data analysis

Our main purpose was to examine basic symptoms and certain basic symptom constellations with regard to their prognostic accuracy for schizophrenia. Values typically used to evaluate the diagnostic or prognostic accuracy of binary variables are sensitivity, specificity, positive and negative predictive values (PPV and NPV), percentage of false positives and of false negatives (%FP and %FN) and, recently, positive and negative diagnostic likelihood ratios (PDLR and NDLR; Leisenring and Pepe 1998) and odds ratio (OR; Kraemer 1992). These are not independent of each other; yet, there is no general rule to their usage but there are different rules of thumb (Boyko

1994). Whereas sensitivity, specificity and diagnostic likelihood ratios are thought to be independent of the prevalence of the disorder in the sample, positive and negative predictive values as well as odds ratios are not. Furthermore, the odds ratio tends to be over-optimistic, choosing the best quality of the test or symptom and ignoring its weaknesses, thus generally exceeding the positive diagnostic likelihood ratio (Kraemer 1992).

The overall prognostic accuracy of ordinal or metric variables independent of the choice of cut-points is typically assessed by a geometric approach: the area under the 'receiver operating characteristic' (ROC) curve, c. A nonparametric technique used for related samples was expressed as the sum of symptoms present; it was expected that a number of symptoms would only rarely be present but, taken together, might show good prognostic accuracy.

In the absence of general criteria for either minimally acceptable values of diagnostic accuracy measures (Kraemer 1992) or for the choice of the leading quantity in symptom selection (Boyko 1994), emphasis has previously been put on both sensitivity and PPV, and the minimally acceptable value of both quantities defined by two studies of diagnostic/prognostic accuracy of symptoms in schizophrenia (Andreasen and Flaum 1991; Jackson *et al.* 1995). Thus a sensitivity value of 0.25, a slightly more liberal value than that required for symptoms of an acute episode (Andreasen and Flaum 1991), and a PPV of at least 0.70, regarded as already high in a retrospective study of *DSM-III-R* prodromal symptoms (Jackson *et al.* 1995), were chosen as selection criteria, leading to a selection of ten cognitive and perceptive disturbances (Klosterkötter *et al.* 2001) – see Table 6.2. Furthermore, in a methodological study using the same data (Schultze-Lutter 2001), a cluster of nine mainly peculiar cognitive basic symptoms, therefore called 'cognitive disturbances' (see Table 6.2), was repeatedly selected as the most predictive of all seven clusters.

These two symptom selections will be compared and discussed for their symptom and general accuracy and their utilization as inclusion criteria for intervention studies.

RESULTS

Predictive accuracy of symptom selections

The two symptom selections have five cognitive basic symptoms in common: thought interference, thought pressure, thought blockages, disturbance of receptive language and unstable ideas of reference (see Table 6.2). Except for disturbance of abstract thinking and captivation by details of perception, all symptoms were present in at least 20% of later schizophrenic patients at first examination. Furthermore, all symptoms were highly specific, had a good to excellent positive and a moderate negative predictive value and a rate of false

Table 6.2 Predictive accuracy of basic symptoms included in selection criteria

Basic symptom	Sensitivity	Specificity	PPV	NPV	PDLR	NDLR	OR	% FP	% FN
Thought perseveration	0.32	0.88	0.71	0.57	2.67	0.77	3.45	6.3	33.8
Decreased ability to discriminate between ideas and perception, fantasy and true memories	0.27	0.95	0.84	0.57	5.40	0.77	7.03	2.5	36.3
Derealization	0.28	0.90	0.73	0.56	2.80	0.80	3.50	5.0	35.6
Visual perception disturbances*	0.46	0.85	0.75	0.62	3.07	0.64	4.83	7.5	26.9
Acoustic perception disturbances*	0.29	0.89	0.72	0.53	2.64	0.80	3.30	5.6	35.0
Thought interference	0.42	0.91	0.83	0.62	4.67	0.64	7.32	4.4	28.8
Thought pressure	0.38	0.96	0.91	0.62	9.50	0.65	14.71	1.9	30.6
Thought blockages	0.34	0.86	0.71	0.57	2.43	0.77	3.16	6.9	32.5
Disturbance of receptive language	0.39	0.91	0.82	0.61	4.33	0.67	6.46	4.4	30.0
Unstable ideas of reference	0.39	0.89	0.78	0.60	3.55	0.69	5.17	5.6	30.0
Inability to divide attention	0.20	0.91	0.67	0.54	2.22	0.88	2.53	4.4	39.4
Disturbance of expressive speech	0.23	0.94	0.78	0.56	3.83	0.82	4.68	3.1	47.5
Disturbance of abstract thinking	0.04	1	1	0.52	–	0.96	–	0	50.6
Captivation by details of the visual field	0.09	1	1	0.53	–	0.91	–	0	50.6

PPV: positive predictive value; NPV: negative predictive value; PDLR: positive diagnostic likelihood ratio; NDLR: negative diagnostic likelihood ratio; OR: odds ratio; %FP: % false positive predictions; %FN: % false negative predictions.
– is displayed where figures cannot be calculated because of division by 0 due to specificity equal 1.
* Rated as binary variable: 'at least any one present' versus 'none present'.
Lines coloured white: symptoms only included in the selection according to sensitivity and PPV ('1 of 10 most predictive'; Klosterkötter et al. 2001).
Lines coloured pale grey: symptoms included in both selections.
Lines coloured dark grey: symptoms included only in 'cognitive disturbances' cluster ('2 of 9'; Schultze-Lutter 2001).

positives well below 10%, yet the false negatives rate was between quarter and half of the sample: that is, half to nearly all of the patients who went on to develop schizophrenia were missed. The positive diagnostic likelihood ratio, PDLR, and odds ratio, OR, varied greatly and couldn't be calculated for disturbance of abstract thinking and captivation by details of perception, because a division by zero occurred due to specificity being equal to one. Replacing one by a slightly lower number x causes PDLR/OR $\to \infty$ with $x \to 1$. The negative diagnostic likelihood ratios were between 0.96 and 0.64, indicating a reduction in the post-test probability of going on to develop schizophrenia to between 96% and 64% of the pre-test probability. Thus, all selected symptoms performed quite well as regards prognostic accuracy.

General predictive accuracy of symptom selections

As regards general predictive accuracy, the two symptom selections hardly differed (see Figures 6.4 and 6.5). Whereas the ten predictive basic symptoms with a sensitivity of at least 0.25 and a PPV of at least 0.70 showed a highly significant area under the ROC curve (c) of 0.83 (95% Cl: 0.76/0.90; $p <$ 0.000) with a standard error of 0.33, the nine basic symptoms of the cluster 'cognitive disturbances' had an equally highly significant c of 0.82 (95% Cl: 0.75/0.89; $p <$ 0.000) with a standard error of 0.34. The most favourable cut-off was one symptom of the ten-symptom selection with a sensitivity of about 0.87 and a specificity of about 0.54, and two symptoms of 'cognitive disturbances' with a sensitivity of about 0.67 and a specificity of about 0.83.

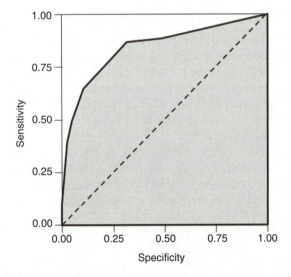

Figure 6.4 'I of 10' predictive basic symptoms: general prognostic accuracy (area under the ROC curve, c; $n = 160$).

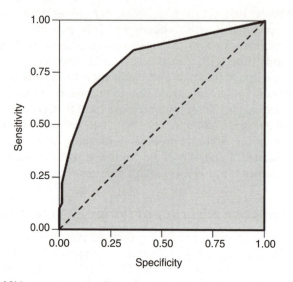

Figure 6.5 '2 of 9' basic symptoms of 'cognitive disturbances': general prognostic accuracy (area under the ROC curve, c; n = 160).

At these cut-offs, the two selection criteria showed satisfying accuracy values with the '2 of 9' selection tending to be more conservative than the '1 of 10' selection (see Figure 6.6).

Comparison of symptom selections

All 67 patients who would be identified as at risk for schizophrenia by the '2 of 9' selection reported at least one of the five symptoms shared by both criteria and thus would also be identified as at risk by the '1 of 10' selection, which would identify 106 patients as prodromal. Of this overlap, 56 of 67 patients would still fulfil both criteria in a selection restricted to the shared items, because they reported at least two of the five symptoms common to both selections (see Figure 6.7).

Of the 67 patients fulfilling both criteria at first examination, 14 did not develop schizophrenia in the follow-up period; nine of them had reported at least two of the five symptoms common to both criteria. However, 10 patients who later developed schizophrenia were missed by both criteria (see Figure 6.8). In all, the '2 of 9' selection made fewer false predictions (n = 40; 25.0%) than the '1 of 10' selection (n = 47, 29.4%), and in particular made fewer false positive predictions (see Figure 6.8).

With regard to the time from retrospectively-reported first onset of basic symptoms to that of psychotic symptoms, about 28% reporting at least one of the ten predictive basic symptoms (n = 30) and 37% of those reporting at

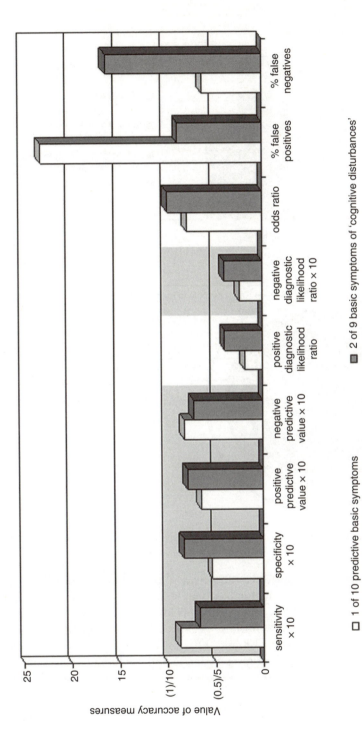

Figure 6.6 Diagnostic (i.e. prognostic) accuracy measures of criteria.
Note: Shaded portions indicate measures that are generally given in values between 0 and 1; for the purposes of this graph they have been multiplied by 10.

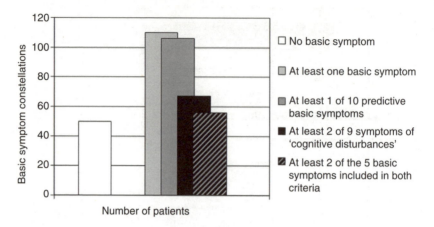

Figure 6.7 Overlap by criteria (*n* = 160).

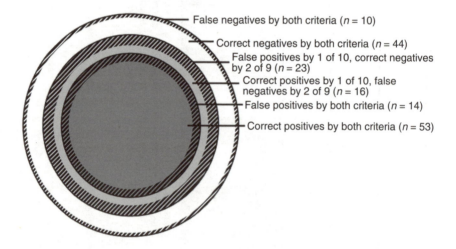

Figure 6.8 Distribution of false and correct predictions by inclusion criteria; visible area equals number of patients (*n* = 160).

least two symptoms of 'cognitive disturbances' (*n* = 25) developed positive symptoms of schizophrenia within less than 36 months, one of them within the first 12 months after the occurrence of the first basic symptom. However, in terms of correct positives and false negatives, the numbers differed less: about 30% not meeting '1 in 10' and 30% not meeting '2 in 9' developed positive symptoms during this time, and 43.8% of those fulfilling the '1 of 10' selection criterion and 47.2% of those fulfilling the '2 of 9' selection criterion did so (see Figures 6.9 and 6.10).

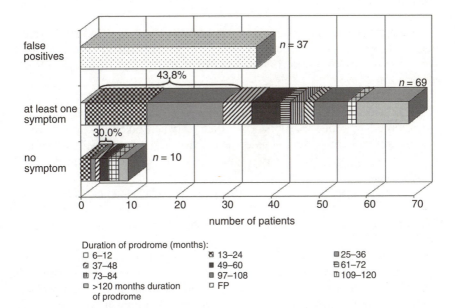

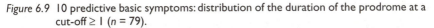

Figure 6.9 10 predictive basic symptoms: distribution of the duration of the prodrome at a cut-off ≥ 1 (*n* = 79).

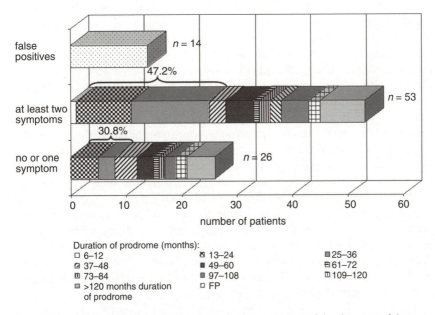

Figure 6.10 BSABS cluster 'cognitive disturbances': distribution of the duration of the prodrome at a cut-off ≥ 2 (*n* = 79).

DISCUSSION

It was earlier stated that prodromal symptoms as listed in *DSM-III-R* were found to possess a low to modest accuracy of prediction of a first episode of schizophrenia (Jackson *et al.* 1995; McGorry *et al.* 1995) and it was therefore suggested that:

> [W]e also need to assess the performance of prodromal symptoms as proposed by other researchers . . . that . . . when taken in concert with one another, may have greater sensitivity and specificity, and more importantly, greater positive and negative predictive powers for psychosis.
>
> (Jackson *et al.* 1996: 503)

Such an alternative symptomatology is offered by the basic symptom concept.

The predictive accuracy of basic symptoms for schizophrenia was first evaluated in the Cologne Early Recognition project (CER; Klosterkötter *et al.* 2001). Although the first prospective study with an observation period that easily covers the mean duration of the initial prodrome of five years (Häfner *et al.* 1995), a limitation of this study is that no repeated measures were carried out as is usually done in prospective studies. Consequently, possible changes in symptoms or symptom profiles in the longitudinal course could not be appraised reliably, and survival analyses to assess time-to-event dependencies could not be carried out (Klosterkötter *et al.* 2001).

Furthermore, only 41.6% of the initial sample could be followed up. Therefore, regarding the overall transition rate of 49.4% that reached 70% for patients with initial prodromal symptoms, the question arises of a selection bias for especially seriously disturbed patients at follow-up. But since no significant differences between followed-up patients and those lost to follow-up occurred in the presence of prodromal symptoms, tentative diagnoses, age or gender, no indication of an additional selection, work-up or verification bias at follow-up is given, and the follow-up sample seems fairly representative. On the other hand, the presence of an initial referral bias can be neither negated nor affirmed (Klosterkötter *et al.* 2001). However, current early detection and intervention services do not aim at identifying and treating persons with an increased risk for schizophrenia in the general population, but rather among those already seeking help for mental problems; thus they operate explicitly with an initial referral bias. Therefore, the presented data of the CER study might well be representative of the clientele of such specialized services; still, they will require replication.

Additional general problems in early detection research arise from the definition of predictive accuracy measures themselves and the provisional status of current diagnostic criteria in psychiatry. Despite the shortcomings associated with the four main measures used to evaluate the accuracy of a binary symptom rating – sensitivity, specificity, positive and negative predictive value – and the different rules of thumb advocated for their use (Boyko 1994; Sackett 1992), they are still typically used in medical decision-making (Leisenring and Pepe 1998) along with odd ratios (e.g. Verdoux *et al.* 1998). Applying rough guides from other fields of medicine, such as pneumology (Jaeschko *et al.* 1994) or otorhinolaryngology (Leisenring and Pepe 1998), to psychiatry in a one-to-one manner seems unadvisable, because there appears to be a much closer connection between aetiology and syndrome in somatic medicine than in psychiatry.

Consequently, as Jablensky pointed out, in psychiatry, 'the majority of the current diagnostic criteria remain provisional (and some of them are frankly arbitrary)' (Jablensky 1999: 138), with classifications not precluding multiple category membership on the basis of the same data set. Cloninger summarized this dilemma: 'No-one has ever found a set of symptoms, signs, or tests that separate mental disorders fully into non-overlapping categories' (Cloninger 1999: 176). Or to put it in statistical terms: No-one has ever found a set of symptoms, signs or tests that possess perfect sensitivity, specificity, positive (PPV) and negative predictive values (NPV), 0% false positive or false negative prediction rates, or an infinitely high positive diagnostic likelihood ratio (PDLR) or odd ratio (OR) for certain mental disorders. This is also true for schizophrenia, which can be only incompletely separated from other disorders by the distribution of symptoms (Andreasen and Flaum 1991; Cloninger 1999; Peralta and Cuesta 1999; Verdoux *et al.* 1998). Unfortunate as the situation might be, researchers and clinicians have to work with the current classifications of mental disorders as best as they can, which also means that we cannot expect to find greater diagnostic accuracy in symptoms preceding a disorder than was found in diagnostically relevant symptoms of the disorder itself (or better and more accurate criteria for the disorder would have been found). Instead the prognostic accuracy of potentially prodromal symptoms should be evaluated in relation to what has been found for diagnostically relevant symptoms of the acute disorder and – as was done for these – further measures should be added, such as duration, severity, symptom pattern or exclusion criteria, to improve their accuracy (David and Appleby 1992).

In a recent study (Peralta and Cuesta 1999), the diagnostic accuracy of Schneiderian first rank symptoms of *DSM-III-R* schizophrenia in a sample of psychotic patients reached (positive diagnostic) likelihood ratios between 0.96 (OR = 1.0) and 1.97 (OR = 2.0), and only 1.23 for at least one symptom (OR = 1.7). These numbers would have been higher, had schizophrenics been compared to patients with non-psychotic disorders, as done in the CER study. In another study (Verdoux *et al.* 1998), patients in general practices were examined via questionnaire for the lifetime presence of delusions or auditory hallucinations. Comparing psychotic patients with patients with other psychiatric diagnoses, the odds ratio was highest for 'hearing voices conversing' (OR = 7.0), and comparing psychotic patients with patients with no psychiatric history highest for 'conspiracy against you' (OR = 15.2; PDLR = 6.1) and 'hearing voices conversing' (OR = 11.4; PDLR = 7.7).

Comparing these results with those found for the 14 basic symptoms included in the two selections, basic symptoms with ORs between 2.53 and 14.71 performed as well as self-rated positive symptoms in patients seeking help for mental problems. Furthermore, nearly all these 14 symptoms satisfied the criteria of a sensitivity of about 0.30 (Andreasen and Flaum 1991) and a PPV greater than 0.70 (Jackson et al. 1995). And, according to a rough guide for using diagnostic likelihood ratios in somatic medicine (Jaeschko et al. 1994), with all PDLRs exceeding 2.0, they indicated small but possibly important changes in the pre-test probabilities of going on to develop schizophrenia. Yet their NDLRs, which did not go below 0.64, altered the pre-test probabilities only to a very small and rarely important degree.

This picture changed when the symptom selections were looked at in terms of the diagnostic likelihood ratios. Not having any of the ten predictive symptoms decreased the disease probability to 24% of its pre-test estimation, whereas having at least any one increased it by nearly two times; having fewer than two of the nine symptoms of 'cognitive disturbances' decreased it to 40%, whereas having at least two increased it by nearly four times, thus indicating – even from the somatic disorders point of view – small, but probably important, shifts from pre-test to post-test probabilities.

Thus both symptom selections, with their chosen cut-off, might well serve as inclusion criteria for intervention trials. However, weighing the costs of missing false negatives and unnecessarily treating false positives (McNeil et al. 1975), with the rather high number of false positives, as well as not quite satisfying specificity, but achieving high sensitivity, the '1 of 10' criterion should only be applied when a fairly safe treatment is available not causing undue harm if administered to false-positive patients – for example, a psychotherapeutic treatment focusing on improvement and monitoring of individual symptoms.

The opposite is true for the '2 of 9' criterion: It had shown high specificity and only moderate sensitivity along with a rather low number of false positives. Thus, according to McNeil and colleagues' (1975) rule of thumb, it would justify even a pharmacological treatment with its potential side-effects in order to avoid serious and permanent harm, such as the recently discussed neurotoxic effects of first-episode psychosis (Copolov et al. 2000; Pantelis et al. 2001). If this criterion is refined by the additional condition that basic symptoms should be present for at least a year, only the one person who transited within 12 months after the onset of basic symptoms would have to be regarded as a false negative instead of a correct positive. Applying this additional time restriction to the whole sample, thus reducing the time to transition by the 12 months by which meeting the refined criterion would have been delayed, 35.8 per cent of all fulfilling the '2 of 9' criterion (i.e. correct and false positives) and 45.3 per cent of those fulfilling it and actually developing schizophrenia (i.e. correct positives) had transited in less than 24 months, 18.9 per cent in less than 12 months. This is comparable to the 12-month transition rate from first examination to psychosis reported for attenuated symptoms by Morrison and colleagues (2002).

SUMMARY

In research on early detection and intervention in psychosis, attenuated and transient psychotic symptoms or a combination of risk factors and functional loss are widely used. An alternative approach is given by the basic symptom concept. Within the Cologne Early Recognition (CER) project, two predictive constellations of cognitive-perceptive basic symptoms were identified using different methodological procedures and were compared for their prospective accuracy measures. Although both constellations possessed excellent predictive accuracy overall, their application should be guided by considerations of the potential harm of treatment and imminence of psychosis.

REFERENCES

American Psychiatric Association (APA) (1987). *Diagnostic and Statistical Manual of Mental Disorders* (3rd rev. ed.) *(DSM-III-R)*. Washington, DC: APA.

American Psychiatric Association (APA) (1994). *Diagnostic and Statistical Manual of Mental Disorders* (4th ed.) *(DSM-IV)*. Washington DC: APA.

Andreasen, N. C. and Flaum, M. (1991). Schizophrenia. The characteristic symptoms. *Schizophrenia Bulletin* 17: 27–49.

Boyko, E. D. (1994). Ruling in or ruling out disease with the most sensitive or specific diagnostic test: Short cut or wrong turn? *Medical Decision Making* 14: 175–9.

Cloninger, C. R. (1999). A new conceptual paradigm from genetics and psychobiology for the science of mental health. *Australian and New Zealand Journal of Psychiatry* 33: 174–86.

Copolov, D. *et al.* (2000). Neurobiological findings in early phase schizophrenia. *Brain Research Reviews* 31: 157–65.

David, A. S. and Appleby, L. (1992). Diagnostic criteria in schizophrenia: Accentuate the positive. *Schizophrenia Bulletin* 18: 551–7.

Gross, G. *et al.* (1987). *Bonner Skala für die Beurteilung von Basissymptomen [BSABS; Bonn Scale for the Assessment of Basic Symptoms]*. Berlin, Heidelberg: Springer.

Häfner, H. and an der Heiden, W. (1999). 'The course of schizophrenia in the light of modern follow-up studies: The ABC and WHO studies. *European Archives of Psychiatry and Clinical Neuroscience*, 249 (suppl. 4): IV/14–26.

Häfner, H. *et al.* (1995). When and how does schizophrenia produce social deficits? *European Archives of Psychiatry and Clinical Neuroscience* 246: 17–28.

Häfner, H. *et al.* (1998). The ABC schizophrenia study: A preliminary overview of the results. *Social Psychiatry and Psychiatric Epidemiology* 33: 380–6.

Huber, G. and Gross, G. (1989). The concept of basic symptoms in schizophrenic and schizoaffective psychoses. *Recenti Progressi in Medicina* 80: 646–52.

Jablensky, A. (1999). The nature of psychiatric classification: Issues beyond ICD-10 and DSM-IV. *Australian and New Zealand Journal of Psychiatry* 33: 137–44.

Jackson, H. J. *et al.* (1995). Prodromal symptoms of schizophrenia in first episode psychosis. Prevalence and specificity. *Comprehensive Psychiatry* 36: 241–50.

Jackson, H. J. *et al.* (1996). The inter-rater and test–retest reliabilities of prodromal symptoms in first-episode psychosis. *Australian and New Zealand Journal of Psychiatry* 30: 498–504.

Jaeschko, R. *et al.* (1994). User's guides to the medical literature. III. How to use an article about a diagnostic test. B. What are the results and will they help me in caring for my patients? *Journal of the American Medical Association* 271: 703–7.

Klosterkötter, J. (1992). The meaning of basic symptoms for the development of schizophrenic psychoses. *Neurology, Psychiatry and Brain Research* 1: 30–41.

Klosterkötter, J. *et al.* (2001). Diagnosing schizophrenia in the initial prodromal phase. *Archives of General Psychiatry* 58: 158–64.

Kraemer, H. C. (1992). *Evaluating Medical Tests. Objective and Quantitative Guidelines.* Newbury Park, CA: Sage.

Leisenring, W. and Pepe, M. S. (1998). Regression modelling of diagnostic likelihood ratios for the evaluation of medical diagnostic tests. *Biometrics* 54: 444–52.

McGlashan, T. H. (1998). Early detection and intervention in schizophrenia: Rationale and research. *British Journal of Psychiatry* 172 (suppl. 33): 3–6.

McGorry, P. D. *et al.* (1995). The prevalence of prodromal features of schizophrenia in adolescence: A preliminary survey. *Acta Psychiatrica Scandinavica* 92: 241–9.

McGorry, P. D. *et al.* (2002). Randomized controlled trial of interventions designed to reduce the risk of progression to first-episode psychosis in a clinical sample with subthreshold symptoms. *Archives of General Psychiatry* 59: 921–8.

McNeil, B. J. *et al.* (1975). Primer on certain elements of medical decision making. *New England Journal of Medicine* 293: 211–5.

Miller, T. J. *et al.* (1999). Symptom assessment in schizophrenic prodromal states. *Psychiatric Quarterly* 70: 273–87.

Miller, T. J. *et al.* (2002). Prospective diagnosis of the initial prodrome for schizophrenia based on the Structured Interview for Prodromal Syndromes: Preliminary evidence of interrater reliability and predictive validity. *American Journal of Psychiatry* 159: 863–5.

Morrison, T. *et al.* (2002). Early detection and intervention for psychosis in primary care. *Acta Psychiatrica Scandinavica* 413: 44.

Pantelis, C. *et al.* (2001). The timing and functional consequences of structural brain abnormalities in schizophrenia. *NeuroScience News* 4: 36–46.

Peralta, V. and Cuesta, M. J. (1999). Diagnostic significance of Schneider's first rank symptoms in schizophrenia. Comparative study between schizophrenic and non-schizophrenic psychotic disorders. *British Journal of Psychiatry* 174: 243–8.

Phillips, L. J. *et al.* (2000). Identification of young people at risk of psychosis: Validation of the Personal Assessment and Crisis Evaluation Clinic intake criteria. *Australian and New Zealand Journal of Psychiatry* 34 (suppl.): S164–9.

Sackett, D. I. (1992). A primer on the precision and accuracy of the clinical examination. *Journal of the American Medical Association* 267: 2638–44.

Schouten, H. J. A. (1982). Measuring pairwise agreement among many observers. Some improvements and additions. *Biometrics* 24: 431–5.

Schultze-Lutter, F. (2001). *Früherkennung der Schizophrenie anhand subjektiver Beschwerdeschilderungen: Ein methodenkritischer Vergleich der Vorhersageleistung nonparametrischer statistischer und alternativer Verfahren zur Generierung von Vorhersagemodellen.* Available online at http://www.ub.uni-koeln.de/ediss/archiv/2001/11w1210.pdf

Verdoux, H. *et al.* (1998). A survey of delusional ideation in primary-care patients. *Psychological Medicine* 28: 127–34.

Wing, J. K. *et al.* (1974). *Measurement and Classification of Psychiatric Symptoms. An Introduction Manual for the PSE and Catego-Program.* London: Cambridge University Press.

Yung, A. R. and McGorry, P. D. (1996). The prodromal phase of first-episode psychosis: Past and current conceptualizations. *Schizophrenia Bulletin* 22: 353–70.

Yung, A. R. *et al.* (2003). Psychosis prediction: 12-month follow up of a high-risk ('prodromal') group. *Schizophrenia Research* 60: 21–32.

Chapter 7

Phase-specific group treatment for recovery in an early psychosis programme

Jean Addington and Donald Addington

INTRODUCTION

The Calgary Early Psychosis Program (EPP) in western Canada is a well-established comprehensive programme for individuals experiencing a first episode of psychosis, offering treatment to patients and their families for three years (Addington and Addington 2001). EPP serves a population of 930,000 through a publicly funded healthcare system and receives approximately 100 referrals per annum. The EPP is situated in the department of psychiatry in one of the acute care facilities in the city. The programme, which began in December 1996, was specifically designed to meet the needs of those young people diagnosed with a first episode of psychosis.

This chapter describes the group therapy component that is embedded in the larger EPP programme. The overarching concern of the group programme is to support the concept of recovery from psychosis. According to *Webster's Dictionary*, the formal definition of the word recovery means 'to get back: regain' or 'to restore (oneself) to a normal state'. The term 'recovery' has been used to include concepts such as awareness of the toll of the illness; recognition of the need to change; insight as to how this change can begin; and the determination it takes to recover. In a review of the recovery literature, Ralph (2000) identified four dimensions of recovery. These include internal factors, self-managed care, external factors, and empowerment. Internal factors are factors within the individual, such as awareness of the toll the illness has taken, recognition of the need to change, insight as to how this change can begin, and the determination it takes to recover. Self-managed care is an extension of the internal factors in which individuals describe how they manage their own mental health and how they cope with the difficulties and barriers they face. External factors include interconnectedness with others, the support provided by family, friends, and professionals, and having people who believe that they can cope with, and recover from, their mental illness. Finally, empowerment is a combination of internal and external factors where internal strengths are combined with interconnectedness to provide self-help, advocacy and caring about what happens to us and to others (ibid.).

The goal of recovery can be addressed by first considering the developmental issues and problems facing these young patients. Group intervention can have an impact on the developmental tasks that have been delayed by the onset of psychosis. The Early Psychosis Program offers a range of groups including a psychosis education group, a recovery group, a substance use group, and a family group. The major focus of this chapter is on groups that have been specifically designed to help the individual to manage different phases of illness and of recovery following the first episode. The interventions offer education about the illness, help to develop an understanding of the impact of the illness, and aid in adjusting to the illness and making future plans. As the individual moves further into recovery the relevant group moves from being educational to cognitive-behavioural and eventually encompasses some aspects of interpersonal therapy.

THE IMPACT OF PSYCHOSIS ON THE DEVELOPMENTAL TRAJECTORY

The onset of psychosis may complicate or interfere with many of the developmental tasks that the young adult is attempting to accomplish at this time (Erikson 1950; Muuss 1988). Typical developmental tasks of early adulthood include individuating from the family, developing interests, hobbies, and skills, discovering and experimenting with sexuality, forming and maintaining relationships, and engaging in further and/or higher education and vocational activities.

Identity formation is one of the first major tasks of young adults. According to Erikson (1950), developing a meaningful self-concept is central to identity formation. A vital component of this process is social interaction with significant other people (Muuss 1988). It is through such interactions that the young person is able to obtain some sense of how they are perceived by others. As the young person approaches adulthood he or she becomes more dependent on peers than on family members for these interactions. Clearly, for people experiencing a first episode of psychosis, these important social interactions are often missed if, because of psychosis, the individual begins to withdraw from friends and peers.

A second important component in the development of a positive identity is good self-esteem and sense of self-worth (Erikson 1968). Poor self-esteem is typically characterized by low confidence, a sense that others have poor opinions of one, and often sensitivity to criticism. There is then no consistent frame of reference within which to accommodate and assimilate experiences of self and others. Such negative affects and cognitions may result in avoidance of the very situations that could potentially enhance self-esteem.

A third step towards developing a positive identity is role formation, which often means determining one's vocational or career path. Role diffusion is not unusual for the adolescent struggling with these developmental tasks – a problem that again is compounded by the onset of psychosis.

It is not difficult to envisage the often devastating effects that psychosis and even the early pre-psychotic phase can have on the normal struggle with adult developmental tasks. When these young individuals develop a psychosis they often fall out of step with their peers, become socially isolated, have an altered self-perception, and are unable to complete their education. The potential for achievements is reduced and, as the gap between these individuals and their peers widens, catching up becomes more difficult. The potential for achievements is further reduced if these individuals delay completion of education or vocational training because of difficulties resulting from their illness. Thus, failure or difficulty in accomplishing these developmental tasks, along with any experiences of stigma, has a major impact on the young person over and above the psychosis itself. The group programme is designed to address these issues in order to support recovery from psychosis.

VALUE OF GROUPS IN EARLY INTERVENTION

Group intervention is valuable as it can help to overcome disruption to the developmental trajectories due to psychotic illness (Albiston *et al.* 1998). For young adults, the peer group is the major source of a sense of belonging and acceptance and it offers an environment in which to take risks and explore options. Many individuals experiencing a first episode of psychosis feel alienated from their previous social contacts and networks and have fewer and more limited contacts (Breier and Strauss 1984). This situation can be compounded by a longer duration of untreated psychosis (DUP; Larsen *et al.* 1998). Even after recovery, previous social withdrawal and isolation makes it very difficult to rejoin social groups, leading to longer-term social difficulties. Consequently, interventions that focus on social recovery during the early phase or critical periods of psychosis are extremely important. Group work offers an opportunity to begin or continue to work on the developmental tasks that are helped by social interaction with others and thus can potentially aid completion of these tasks.

The Early Psychosis Prevention and Intervention Centre (EPPIC) delineates many of the positive aspects of group work for those who have recently experienced a first episode of psychosis (EPPIC, 2000). Participating in groups encourages the development of a positive social role. They promote self-awareness and identify skills and abilities to enhance the development of identity, especially when self-esteem is low. Communicating with peers who are having similar experiences of psychosis, in combination with opportunities to explore alternative explanatory models of illness, can assist with the development of a personal model of psychosis that enhances, rather than hinders, a positive self-esteem. The group provides the opportunity to develop and maintain social skills, improve social relationships, and develop an understanding of the illness in order to adequately address the impact of the psychosis. Additionally, participation in groups can provide support and encouragement to take an active role in personal and group decision-making and thus help with the establishment of realistic and practical life goals. It is valuable to have contacts with others who may be at different points in the recovery process. Support and hope can be offered to those who are feeling stuck, lost, or demoralized that recovery is taking too long (Albiston *et al.* 1998; EPPIC 2000).

The early stage of recovery includes the remission of positive symptoms after a first episode, which is often marked by a move to more active involvement in treatment. The early recovery phase may include an initial exploration of explanatory models of psychosis and coping strategies. As the positive symptoms improve, secondary morbidity from the experience of psychosis, such as depression, anxiety, and substance use, may emerge. Changes may become slower, which often leads to frustration. Group interventions can help with these changes and alleviate the associated frustration. Group work needs to take into consideration that recovery, including rates, level, and style, will vary amongst individuals, particularly with issues such as 'sealing over' versus 'integration' (McGlashan and Johannessen 1996).

The later stages of recovery involve re-establishing the developmental tasks of early adulthood and accomplishing the tasks of recovery as described by Ralph (2000). This can be complicated by those who are described by Edwards *et al.* (1998) as having a prolonged recovery with respect to symptoms. Prolonged recovery involves the persistence of positive and negative symptoms and affective disturbances. Such issues need to be addressed to distinguish between prolonged recovery and sub-optimal treatment, relapse, and the persistence of pre-existing characteristics (Edwards *et al.* 1998).

Thus, groups are a potentially valuable intervention for the young person who has had a first episode of psychosis. They should be designed to offer specific interventions that can help these young adults to develop mastery over the illness through education, coping strategies, and self-management (Birchwood and McMillan 1993). More specifically, groups should be developed so that individuals can learn about the processes and the course of the psychotic illness, and subsequently learn coping strategies that will enhance their ability to manage the psychosis. The sense of acceptance and understanding from those who have had similar experiences is an extremely valuable component of the group programme.

RELEVANT MODELS OF GROUP INTERVENTION THEORY

Group therapy is a therapeutic intervention that can complement other interventions such as individual and family work. Since there is a range of theoretical models from which a group leader may choose that might best meet the identified needs and goals of the clients, group leaders need to know and understand the practical application of the range of theories underlying group programmes. Group process describes the 'life' of the group: what is happening in the group and how this changes over time. Group processes include such aspects as phases of group development, communication patterns, group composition, energy level, group roles, themes, and leadership style (Block and Crouch 1985; Yalom 1995). Group processes are a function of group dynamics (the behaviour of people within a group context). Group process can be considered from an individual perspective, focusing on the individual within the group, and from a group perspective. This is seeing the group as a whole and considering it an entity in and of itself (Yalom 1995).

The types of groups we are considering for work in early psychosis are unlikely to make use of group dynamics and processes to affect therapeutic change for clients. Nevertheless, group leaders should have an understanding of group dynamics and group processes, and the skills needed to manage these processes so that group objectives can be achieved. These are basic tools of group work in any group environment, regardless of the theoretical framework or type of group. Additionally the therapist should consider key implicit factors of group work such as universality, instillation of hope, cohesion, altruism, interpersonal learning, imitative behaviour, socialization, catharsis, and corrective recapitulation of the primary family group (Yalom 1995). There are several relevant texts that address group theory, which is beyond the scope of this chapter (Block and Crouch 1985; Corey and Corey 2002; Yalom 1995).

Selection of the appropriate theoretical framework for a specific group programme should be guided by clearly defined objectives. This framework, in conjunction with the stated goals and behavioural objectives, will determine the kinds of interventions to be used in the group. The groups we use in our Early Psychosis Program range from psychoeducational to cognitive-behavioural and finally encompass some aspects of interpersonal therapy.

Psychoeducation groups

Through psychoeducation we can give information about symptoms, etiology, and treatment of psychosis. This is a technique used in clinical practice with the goals of increasing understanding and changing behaviour. Individuals have the right to be fully informed about the nature of their illness. This way they can gain knowledge that helps them understand and integrate the experiences of themselves and their world. This understanding is empowering as it helps clients to take an active role in the management of their illness. Thus psychoeducation is an integral part of the overall therapeutic process.

Psychoeducation in early psychosis is particularly important, as at this point individuals and their families probably have little experience with or knowledge about psychosis. There are several principles of psychoeducation in early psychosis. First, it should be provided for all clients and their families. In addition to the information given by the therapist or group leader, we have to include the client's own explanation of illness and recovery style. A comprehensible, explanatory model for understanding psychosis involving both the individual's and group leader's accounts should be developed. The origins of and factors influencing the illness are presented in terms of a stress-vulnerability model. It is important that psychoeducation is sensitive to cultural diversity and the individual's life circumstances and offers a positive outlook. It should always be considered as part of a broader therapeutic approach. The focus of the psychoeducation group is on support and understanding, rather than on interpretive issues as in a therapy group (Rosenberg 1984). In the psychoeducation group the leader provides guidance, advice, and information, but requires just as much training as the leader of a therapy group.

Cognitive-behavioural groups

A cognitive-behavioural therapy (CBT) group is most valuable to the goal of helping clients to develop behavioural strategies for managing and coping with psychotic symptoms (Fowler *et al.* 1995: Haddock *et al.* 1998). The focus of CBT is on an analysis of the thinking underlying the behaviour and development of behavioural changes. There are similarities and differences between a psychoeducation group and a CBT group. Change is the focus of the CBT group. A psychoeducation group may employ some CBT techniques, while a CBT group may offer some education at its beginning. However, a CBT group will focus on skills, such as social skills, problem solving, assertiveness, and coping skills, and may have a particular focus such as adjusting to psychosis, social anxiety, or depression.

ENGAGEMENT IN GROUP

Young people experiencing their first episode of psychosis may be motivated to attend groups but difficulties with engagement may emerge. Many issues can impact engagement, such as social anxiety, social stressors, lack of day-to-day routine, poor motivation, lack of self-organization, difficulty in help-seeking, and lack of social supports – often the very issues with which groups can help. EPPIC (2000) suggests that engagement problems can also result from the therapist and the service environment. Engagement problems with patients can be exacerbated by not recognizing their fears, not understanding their perspectives and level of functioning, and by placing too much pressure on them. Poorly defined aims of specific group programmes can create barriers to engagement. Practical obstacles, such as the location of the group, and cost of and access to transportation, are additional impediments. These difficulties all further support the need for effective groups that are specifically designed for young people recovering from their first psychotic episode.

There are strategies that may be useful in maximizing the potential for engagement (EPPIC 2000). The therapist could clarify goals with the client in individual meetings. Further, he or she should allow adequate time to develop first rapport with the client and then a collaborative, but not prescriptive, relationship. Clients should be allowed to engage at their own pace and even to try out the group programme at their own level of comfort. It is important that the therapist considers the individuals' explanatory models and attends to their needs and fears. Depending on the context of the group programme and how much the group's leader may know about the client, obtaining some background information prior to meeting may help. There should be an attempt to make the physical environment user-friendly, easily accessed, and comfortable.

PSYCHOSIS EDUCATION GROUP

The psychosis education group is the first group available to patients in EPP. This clearly psychoeducational group has several objectives: first, to facilitate acceptance of both drug and psychosocial treatments and to explore ways to enable the person to accept ongoing care; and second to reduce the risk of early relapse by helping clients becoming active and informed participants in the management of their illness. The psychosis education group meets first-episode clients' need for information and knowledge and complements and reinforces similar information addressed in family and individual interventions. It is a four-session group that clients are invited to participate in as soon as they are able to attend. The group is offered approximately six times per year and involves six to ten individuals for four sessions of one hour each. It covers the nature of the illness, the range of treatments offered, patterns in the course of illness and the variable nature of recovery, prospects for the future, and agencies and personnel involved in treatment.

The psychosis education group educates about:

- symptoms
- diagnoses
- theories and models of psychosis
- individual explanatory models

- impact of substance use
- use of medications
- identification of warning signs
- avoidance of relapse
- introduction to the programme.

The sessions in this group not only focus on offering information and education to clients but also on helping them make use of this information to aid their recovery. Sessions that focus on symptoms and diagnoses allow members to share their experiences of symptoms and to learn, often for the first time, that others have had similar experiences. Rather than feel they have a diagnosis, the group learns about making a diagnosis, the reason why diagnoses may be used, and what it might mean for them. A discussion of models and theories of psychosis is a way for these young people to begin the process of developing and enhancing their own explanatory models. The overview of medications focuses more on developing an understanding of why they might be receiving their medications rather than on learning about potential side effects. In this first group they begin to learn about warning signs and how to prevent relapse – topics they can work more on in later groups. Finally, the group serves to educate about the programme and the services that may be available to them. The group provides the opportunity to ask about any concerns they may have or make requests for information, and essentially serves as an introduction to future treatments and the help that is available.

RECOVERY GROUP

A recovery group is offered to EPP clients who have been in the programme for approximately three to four months, who have completed the psychosis education group, and who are experiencing at least some remission from psychotic symptoms. The goals of this group are centred on various facets of the recovery process. The group aims to facilitate the recovery of previous strengths and abilities and the development of new skills. It endeavours to improve clients' self-worth and confidence by empowering clients to cope with their illness through knowledge, understanding, and the development of coping strategies. The recovery group also seeks to facilitate positive interactions with others and to promote the development and maintenance of social networks. Together these goals are targeted at promoting recovery and preventing relapse.

The recovery group's goals are to:

- reinforce education on psychosis
- promote sharing of ideas and experiences
- increase communication about psychosis

- promote recovery
- improve coping
- decrease isolation and facilitate social reintegration
- decrease shame
- improve coping with psychosis
- help prevent relapse.

The group lasts for 12 weeks and is offered twice a year for weekly daytime sessions of one hour each. The sessions are semi-structured and focus on specific topics. These topics include recovering from a psychotic episode, adapting to symptoms, developing a daily routine, goal setting, stress management, the importance of social support in the recovery process, self-esteem, and interpersonal relationships.

The impact of illness is covered in the first six sessions, which review education on psychosis with the clients and discuss how psychosis has affected them. These sessions focus on the impact of positive, negative, and cognitive symptoms on thoughts, feelings, behaviours, and daily life. Additionally, the effect of psychosis on emotional wellbeing, manifested as depression, anger, fear, and frustration, and the process of loss and grief, are discussed. These sessions also investigate how the psychotic illness has affected self-esteem and explore the shame that may be associated with mental illness.

The next six sessions focus on coping with the illness. These involve setting short-term and long-term goals, appreciating the importance of a structured day and meaningful activities, and restoring and improving communication skills. Another focus is on problem-solving, and the role of stress in psychosis and how to cope with it. Education is provided about health and wellness, including the physical, psychological, emotional, social, and spiritual aspects of health. A focus on relapse prevention targets insight into illness and reviews precipitating, protective, and perpetuating factors with clients. Information on available community resources is provided, which may include guest speakers or outings to tour the community resource facilities.

Recovery group sessions

Sessions one to three of the recovery group look at the impact of positive, negative, and cognitive symptoms. Clients are provided with the definitions of various symptoms, then given the opportunity to describe the symptoms they are experiencing now and have experienced in the past, and to discuss what they have done to control these symptoms. These attempts at coping with symptoms are evaluated in terms of their benefits, the problems that arise, and their effectiveness. Both positive strategies, and negative strategies such as street drug and alcohol use, are considered. These sessions reinforce the education about symptoms received in the psychosis education group. The aim is to improve clients' ability to talk about their symptoms, and help them to feel less isolated when they listen to others who have similar experiences. The education, information, and discussion provided in the group decreases the clients' sense of self-blame, and improves their insight into their illness. Importantly, the group emphasizes the seriousness of psychosis and how it affects thoughts, feelings, behaviour, relationships, and functioning in daily life. Even so, the group offers clients an increased sense of hope and control over their symptoms.

The fourth session of the recovery group deals with the emotional impact of psychosis on the individual and his or her significant others. The group discusses the stages of grief, helplessness, and dependency. The goal is to normalize the negative emotions felt by individuals and the difficulty encountered when an individual is stuck in a stage of recovery, such as denial, anger, or depression. Group members are encouraged to review their present emotional stage, where they have been, and what stages they have yet to negotiate. Acknowledging that this process is not linear and that not everyone goes through it in the same way is an important feature. In the group, clients have an opportunity to talk about their emotional state. Clients and group leaders also discuss feeling helpless and hopeless, and how to regain control. These varied emotional states are normalized.

In the recovery group's fifth session, the impact of psychosis on relationships is considered. Various developmental stages of relationships are presented and clients are encouraged to look at their present relationships and observe how they have changed since the onset of their psychosis. It is common for many clients to experience changes in their relationships. For example they may have lost friends or friends may see them as different, thus changing the nature of the relationship. For some, independence is lost with increased dependency on relatives. Caregivers are at times viewed as overprotective, intrusive, or even adversarial. The group works to combat the resulting stress by helping clients to understand their caregivers' concerns and work towards re-establishing trusting, independent relationships, and developing and using formal and informal resources.

In session six the group works on the definitions of self, self-esteem, and self-concept and how these have been affected by having a psychosis. Many clients blame themselves for the psychosis and feel shame. The issue of shame is dealt with by helping group members recognize that the individual is not the illness. Clients are encouraged to regain their confidence and self-esteem and are given ways to work on their self-concept, self-esteem, and feelings of confidence and competence. Issues of shame and stigma are addressed. The group also looks at the similarity and differences between physical illness and mental illness and how the general public views these different types of illness. The aim of this discussion is to reduce the stigma associated with the perception of mental illness by showing how it is analogous to physical illness. The group members discuss the possibility of blame now that they are aware they have an illness. Knowing what can help and what can exacerbate the illness is emphasized. The clients are asked to reflect on whether they are responsible or to blame for the consequences of neglecting their illness.

The sessions in the second half of the recovery group focus on coping with a psychotic illness. Session seven of the group deals with goal setting. Many clients experiencing a psychosis have had their personal, academic, and vocational goals affected by the onset of their illness. This part of the group is designed to help them understand their frustration and the resulting stress of having their goals delayed or postponed. In this session clients are encouraged to formulate short-term and long-term goals. The characteristics of realistic goals are discussed as well as general suggestions for implementation of these goals. Realistic goals are seen as balancing aspirations with an acknowledgement of limitations and combating depression and lack of drive.

The eighth session features discussion of a structured day and meaningful activities. Negative symptoms are sometimes the major concern for someone recovering from a psychotic illness. Many clients need to be encouraged to take steps towards regaining aspects of their previous levels of functioning at school or work. The group maintains the importance of a structured day, especially with regard to the importance of work or school. As psychosis can decrease an individual's independence and increase his or her dependence on caregivers, the group discusses important ways of taking steps to re-establish independence. Clients are made aware of the dangers of isolation.

In session nine communications skills are explored, as psychotic illness can affect one's ability to communicate through loss of confidence and self-esteem, and the impact of negative symptoms. The psychosis can also hinder one's ability to read and pick up subtle communication cues that others may take for granted. The group attempts to get group members to describe present difficulties in communication and to see the importance of regaining or improving the quality and frequency of their communication. Topics include the importance of communication, verbal and nonverbal forms of communication, how to increase clarity, and how illness can affect interaction with others.

The effect of stress on illness is the focus of the tenth session. Since the stress-vulnerability model recognizes the importance of stress on psychosis, the group looks at the various stressors in the clients' lives and the importance of coping with stress efficiently and effectively. The group is encouraged to understand how the same event may be seen as both a positive and negative stress. For example, a new baby may be a positive event but it may cause many stresses. Substance use may be seen as a way with coping with negative affects, but abuse can create new interpersonal, financial, and illness-related stresses. Additionally, clients are provided with problem-solving strategies to help them to decrease stress effectively.

The emphasis in session eleven is on the health of the individual. Negative symptoms may affect hygiene or desire to look after oneself. Health may suffer due to risky behaviours or lack of maintenance. Weight gain, a medication side effect, increases the chance of diabetes and can pose other significant problems. This group discusses the concept of health and its physical, social, psychological, emotional, and spiritual elements. Clients are encouraged to examine parts of their health in need of attention. Realistic goals are set by clients to work on the areas of their health that require consideration.

In the final session the various issues that have been addressed are reviewed. Throughout the course of the recovery group many clients may have improved their insight into their illness and their knowledge base of psychosis. The group examines their insight into illness and observes whether any changes have taken place since beginning the group intervention. It is valuable for the members to have worked on their own personal model or formulation of the illness. Here they need to have developed a good understanding of their illness's precipitating factors, perpetuating factors, and protective factors. At this time, it is important to reinforce clients' participation in the group and to acknowledge their progress.

INTERPERSONAL SKILLS GROUP

The six-session interpersonal skills group is for clients who experience symptoms of social anxiety, lack of confidence in social interactions, or relationship difficulties. Many individuals with a first episode of psychosis report experiencing changes in their relationships and decreased confidence in social situations. The aim of these sessions is to learn and practice strategies to cope with anxieties in social situations in a safe and supportive environment.

The interpersonal skills group's goals are:

- to increase understanding of social anxiety
- to learn strategies for coping with social anxiety
- to decrease level of anxiety in social situations
- to increase confidence in social interactions
- to improve level of social skills and confidence in social situations
- to reduce social alienation and isolation.

Interpersonal skills group sessions

This group attempts to explore, educate, and provide an understanding of social anxiety and relationships. The group gives members an opportunity to explore and understand their anxiety. The group offers a cognitive-behavioural approach and skill-building that group members are expected to work on in and outside of the group. In the first session, engagement is a major challenge as group members are socially anxious and fearful of social situations. Both long-term and short-term consequences of avoiding a regular commitment to the group are addressed. Education about and discussion of social anxiety is offered in this first session. Structured techniques to facilitate participation are used.

In the second session clients talk about their personal theories of why they are experiencing social difficulties, and begin to learn about a range of improved communication skills. The third session reviews the different treatments for social anxiety and their effectiveness and drawbacks. Formal treatments that are considered include medication, behavioural therapy and cognitive therapy, and changing beliefs. Furthermore, clients coping with the problem of social anxiety assess the effectiveness of their attempts to cope. In the two subsequent sessions the group is involved in developing techniques and strategies that have proved to be most effective while decreasing the use of those that are least effective and may create new problems. Practicing new techniques can begin in group. The final session of the interpersonal skills group focuses on aspects of relationships. A developmental approach is taken. Changes in previous relationships are explored and plans for developing new relationships are made.

SUBSTANCE USE

We offer a substance use group that is part of a more comprehensive approach to address substance use (Addington 2002; Addington and Addington 2001). The goals of the substance use group are:

- to educate about effects of substances and the interaction of substances and psychosis
- to develop a commitment to achieve reduction or abstinence
- to develop awareness of barriers to reduction
- to learn strategies to reduce or be abstinent.

Details of this group have been well documented elsewhere (Addington 2002; Addington and Addington 2001).

The sessions run as follows:

1   Education of effects of substances
2   Relationship between substances and psychosis
3   Goal setting
4   Barriers to quitting
5   Learning problem-solving skills
6–9 Relapse prevention.

SUMMARY

The Early Psychosis Program in Calgary, Canada, offers a group programme embedded within a comprehensive programme for early psychosis. Groups are phase-specific, time-limited, flexible, and relevant to the needs of individuals recovering from their first episode of psychosis. In this chapter we have focused on our psychosis education group, our recovery group, and our interpersonal skills group, which are the core groups focusing on different phases of recovery. In addition, there is a need for the development of groups with a special focus, such as substance use, voices, and health issues, that are designed specifically for the client recovering from a first episode of psychosis.

Given the many issues that an individual experiencing a first episode of psychosis must confront, group interventions are an important therapeutic tool to deal with all phases of the illness. Groups can promote education, aid in the transition to recovery, help with interpersonal skills, and address comorbid problems such as substance use. The next stage in group development for early psychosis would be a comprehensive evaluation of the effectiveness of such groups. This would determine whether they are effective, for whom they are effective, and at what time in the recovery process they are most useful.

REFERENCES

Addington, J. (2002). An integrated treatment approach to substance abuse in an early psychosis program. In H. Graham *et al.* (eds) *Substance Misuse in Psychosis: Approaches to Treatment and Service Delivery*. Chichester, UK: Wiley.

Addington, J. and Addington, D. (2001). Impact of an early psychosis program on substance use. *The Journal of Psychiatric Rehabilitation* 25: 60–7.

Albiston, D. J. *et al.* (1998). Group programes for recovery from early psychosis. *British Journal of Psychiatry*, 172 (suppl. 33): 117–21.

Birchwood, M. and McMillan, F. (1993). Early intervention in schizophrenia. *Australian and New Zealand Journal of Psychiatry* 27: 374–8.

Bloch, S. and Crouch, E. (1985). *Therapeutic Factors in Group Psychotherapy*. Oxford: Oxford University Press.

Breier, A. and Strauss, J. S. (1984). The role of social relationships in the recovery from psychotic disorders. *American Journal of Psychiatry* 141: 949–55.

Corey, M. S. and Corey, G. (2002). *Groups: Process and Practice* (6th ed.). New York: Brooks-Cole Publishing.

Early Psychosis Prevention and Intervention Centre (EPPIC) (2000). *Working with Groups in Early Psychosis: No. 3 in a Series of Early Psychosis Manuals*. Victoria, Australia: Psychiatric Services Branch, Human Services.

Edwards, J. *et al.* (1998). Prolonged recovery in first-episode psychosis. *British Journal of Psychiatry* 172: 107–16.

Erikson, E. H. (1950). *Childhood and Society*. New York: Norton.

Erikson, E. H. (1968). *Identity, Youth and Crisis*. New York: Norton.

Fowler, D. *et al.* (1995). *Cognitive Behaviour Therapy for Psychosis*. Chichester, UK: John Wiley and Sons Ltd.

Haddock, G. *et al.* (1998). Individual cognitive-behavioural interventions in early psychosis. *British Journal of Psychiatry* 172 (suppl. 33): 101–6.

Larsen, T. K. *et al.* (1998). First-episode schizophrenia with long duration of untreated psychosis. *British Journal of Psychiatry* 172 (suppl. 33): 45–52.

McGlashan, T. H. and Johannessen, J. O. (1996). Early detection and intervention with schizophrenia: Rationale. *Schizophrenia Bulletin* 22: 201–22.

Muuss, R. E. (1988). *Theories of Adolescence*. New York: McGraw-Hill, Inc.

Ralph, R. O. (2000). *Review of Recovery Literature: A Synthesis of a Sample of Recovery Literature 2000*. Alexandria, VA: National Technical Assistance Center for State Mental Health Planning.

Rosenberg, P. P. (1984). Support groups. *Small Group Behavior* 15: 173–86.

Yalom, I. (1995). *The Theory and Practice of Group Psychotherapy* (4th ed.). New York: Basic Books.

Chapter 8

Phase-specific psychosocial interventions for first-episode schizophrenia

Rachel Miller and Susan E. Mason

INTRODUCTION

In the United States 50,000 new cases of schizophrenia are diagnosed each year and between two and four million people have the disease (Lieberman 1993). Most of those newly diagnosed are young, usually in their late teens to mid-twenties. Some deteriorate over a long period of time, while others will suddenly, overnight, enter psychosis (Sheitman *et al.* 1997). Whichever the case, the diagnosis and hospitalization of patients experiencing a first episode of schizophrenia is a crucial period in treatment. The clinician who has a comprehensive understanding of the phases of the illness and the difficulties affecting patients and families during each phase will be better prepared to help patients with phase-specific interventions.

In this chapter we will review the phases of schizophrenia and discuss the interventions that we find work well for first-episode schizophrenia. These interventions are based on our experience with 68 first-episode patients in a psychiatric hospital-based treatment facility. We refer to the first episode of schizophrenia as the pre-acute period, also known as the prodromal or pre-psychotic stage, and the first five years after onset of the illness (Lieberman *et al.* 1996; Munich 1997). It is during this five-year period that behavioural functioning shows the most severe deterioration. Ideally, patients experience a disease course that moves from florid symptoms to a time of healing and then onto remission. However, progress is often uneven and unpredictable; patients may progress from psychosis in the acute phase onto healing and maintenance, only to suffer unexpected setbacks to previous phases. In this context we work with a model that delineates three phases: the acute phase, the healing phase, and the maintenance phase. The literature on schizophrenia acknowledges the concepts of acute and maintenance phases (Carpenter 1996; Drury 1994). We have identified the healing phase as separate and equally in need of particular interventions. Others have referred to this time of healing as the residual or reconstituting phase (Kopelowicz and Liberman 1998) or sub-acute and convalescent phase (Munich 1997).

The timeliness of psychosocial interventions, recognized by many experts as crucial for effective schizophrenia treatment (Edwards *et al.* 1994; Hogarty *et al.* 1995; Kopelowicz and Liberman 1998), is in need of detailed, clinical description, especially as it relates to first-episode patients. Currently, there are no reliable guidelines for the expected length of time most patients will remain in any one phase. For this reason these phase-specific psychosocial interventions are targeted toward patients' symptoms and levels of functioning rather than on time frames. A phase-specific personal therapy regimen was developed and tested by Hogarty *et al.* (1995), who treated a mixed group of chronic and first-episode outpatients in an attempt to reduce relapse rates for schizophrenia. Although our work differs from Hogarty's in technique and structure, we also propose that interventions should be based on patients' clinical states and that treatment protocols can be constructed to match phases of the illness. In this chapter we describe the phase-specific interventions that we have found to be successful in keeping first-episode patients and families supported and connected with treatment.

Concurrent with the concept of treatment phases is the matching of suitable services with patients' needs. Typically, patients suffering from the acute phase of schizophrenia are treated in the inpatient unit of hospitals. Healing and maintenance phase patients are treated in day-treatment programmes, outpatient clinics, or private offices. Patients' needs and sites of service are not always accurately matched. This makes it crucial that clinicians apply phase-specific psychosocial interventions regardless of setting.

PHASES AND PSYCHOSOCIAL TREATMENT FOR FIRST-EPISODE SCHIZOPHRENIA

The acute phase

The acute phase of schizophrenia occurs when psychotic symptoms become florid and levels of functioning indicate a steep decline. Prior to this there may be a long pre-acute phase during which patients struggle to cope with the beginning of symptoms. Then, as symptoms worsen, there are often as many as 12–24 months of psychotic experiences before individuals enter hospital (Fenton 1997; Sheitman *et al.* 1997), usually in a state of crisis. Newly hospitalized first-episode patients experience the symptoms associated with the acute phase: delusions, hallucinations, thought disorders, and bizarre behaviours (all of them or a combination). About 70% of first-episode patients will sustain lasting impairment and residual symptoms and 25% will be so impaired that they will require custodial care (Lieberman 1993). Although there is no general time frame for remission of psychosis for first-episode patients, Lieberman and colleagues found the mean and median times to be 35.7 weeks and 11.0 weeks respectively (Lieberman *et al.* 1993).

During this early stage standard psychosocial interventions are best accomplished by using two parallel processes: beginning work with patients, and beginning work with families. Both patients and families require emotional support, psychoeducation, and assistance in understanding the necessity of medication treatment. Treatment modalities used are individual treatment, family treatment, psychoeducation, and group work.

Treatment modalities

Individual treatment

The primary interventions of the acute phase focus on providing support and psychoeducation. Emphasis is on dealing with the immediate problem of beginning treatment for schizophrenia rather than on patients' past traumas or family dysfunction. Support for patients requires communicating the belief that there is hope. It also demands a respectful attitude, and empathy for patients' loss of recognizable self. As with all supportive therapy, the first step in treatment is building a therapeutic alliance. This may begin as simply as sitting quietly with a catatonic patient, or saying to an agitated patient: 'Good morning Tom. I heard you had a rough night.' Reflection and empathy are essential interventions at this point. For example, to the patient who wants to leave the hospital the therapist would state in an empathic manner: 'It's very difficult to be in the hospital.'

Once an initial alliance is in place, supportive therapy is then guided by a psychoeducational approach that is timed and appropriate to patients' capacity for understanding. Psychoeducation is in itself supportive when it offers patients hope and a feeling of some control over the illness. Most patients are frightened at being hospitalized for the first time and do not understand what is happening to them. Early in hospitalization, therefore, patients benefit from being told that they are having symptoms of an illness and that they will feel better with treatment.

Work with Jane illustrates the blend of supportive therapy and psychoeducation that reinforces the concept of the illness as a biological one. Jane has been hospitalized for ten days. She feels hopeless and discouraged that she does not see an improvement in her symptoms. In an empathic manner she is reminded of other illnesses, like a bad cold or flu, that she thought would never get any better but did.

This combination of supportive therapy and psychoeducation is also essential for addressing treatment compliance issues. In an overwhelming majority of patients there is resistance or ambivalence toward medication and continued therapy. During this phase, common reasons patients give for resistance are fear of being changed, fear of their brain being controlled, a life-long abhorrence of medications, fear of side-effects, and denial that there is any problem requiring treatment with medication. A working therapeutic alliance has been shown to increase compliance rates (Fenton *et al.* 1997). With psychoeducation, encouragement, and the opportunity to explore, verbalize, and reality-test their negative (and positive) feelings, patients are often able to overcome resistance to ongoing treatment.

Patients with severe paranoia and no insight into their illness require special sensitivity. The initial interventions are first to form an alliance and then to encourage compliance. Since paranoid patients are less trusting, building an alliance requires more time and patience. Without insight into the illness patients may rebuff empathic statements; however, they generally will not reject interest in themselves as people. As early as the alliance allows, psychoeducation is introduced in a simple and unchallenging manner: 'You have symptoms of an illness, just like any other illness, and it needs treatment.' This is straightforward and honest and this candor will be valued later in treatment. It is also the foundation of subsequent supportive and psychoeducational interventions. When introducing the issue of medication to paranoid patients, focusing on the paranoid symptoms is avoided; emphasis is placed on other symptoms such as poor sleep or anxiety. Challenging fixed beliefs is introduced gradually, only after an initial alliance is in place. This is illustrated in work with William.

William is a 19-year-old black male who believed the FBI and staff were plotting to kill him and his family. His delusions caused him to be extremely fearful, agitated, and anxious. During the first week the emphasis was on helping him remain in the hospital and to take medicine to reduce his anxiety and sleeplessness. The idea that he was suffering from a biological illness was introduced early in the week. As expected, he maintained his false beliefs. When he spoke about these beliefs the therapist's response was non-challenging and empathic but avoided validating the false belief:

William:　The FBI is going to kill my mother.
Therapist:　It must feel terrible to think the FBI is going to kill your mother.
William:　Well they are. I know it.
Therapist:　It has to be a horrible feeling. It's going to get better. Can you hang on? How about your sleep last night?

Due to the pervasiveness of his paranoia it was necessary the following week to reinforce his trust in the alliance:

Therapist:　Does it feel like I'm part of the plot against you?
William:　Sometimes.
Therapist:　What do you think now?
William:　Well. I don't know. No.

As the symptoms lessened it was possible gradually to increase his understanding of the illness and the need for ongoing treatment.

As a last resort, when psychosis prevents patients from accepting medication, treatment may be enforced by the judicial system. There has been some discussion as to whether it is ethical for clinicians to participate in forcing patients to take medication (Schwartz *et al.* 1988; Rosenson 1993). Among mental health professionals, consensus holds that irrational thoughts are symptoms and do not constitute patients' true wishes. The clinician's role includes discussing this decision with families if forced medication becomes a possibility. When psychosis remits the therapeutic alliance is re-established.

In addition to therapeutic interventions, help with concrete services such as insurance, housing, treatment site changes, and referrals to outpatient and rehabilitation services are required for first-episode patients. Their needs for such services cannot be emphasized enough since they often do not have insurance, benefits, or the ability to obtain essential services.

Family therapy

In recent years work with families of patients with schizophrenia has received increased attention. This is largely due to recognition of the fact that families need support if they are to help in the treatment and rehabilitation process (Goldstein 1994; Lam 1991). Concurrent patient/family treatment for persons with schizophrenia has been shown to reduce relapse rates (Carpenter 1996). We have found that family treatment during the acute phase is best when it includes: support for adjusting to the patient's illness, psychoeducation, and help with accepting the need for medications. A respectful attitude and empathy for the family's anguish are essential. The protective distancing used by staff requires monitoring to prevent misunderstanding and tension between staff and families (Hough 1995). In addition, support for families is more effective when there is recognition of cultural diversity (McGoldrick *et al.* 1982).

During the first months of illness, families are often in crisis. This may exacerbate any already-existing individual psychological or family system problems. However, during this period families are generally more receptive and open to psychoeducation and family sessions. Referrals to support groups such as those sponsored by the Alliance for the Mentally Ill are offered. Such referrals are made with care since families in this early period are frequently frightened and resist identifying with families of the chronically ill. A further difficulty with working with families occurs when there are other family members who have mental illness. Family members may feel guilt and shame – guilt that they caused the illness and shame that they are 'not normal.' Occasionally, family members who previously functioned adequately develop transient symptoms. In all instances, sensitivity and patience are required as families work through their pain and loss. In some cases referrals for individual counseling are offered.

Cultural differences often affect families' perceptions of mental illness and the usefulness of available support systems. The clinician ascertains what it means to have a family member with a mental illness in the patient's culture or country of origin. It is helpful to know whether a culture assigns blame to families for mental illness and what the treatment modalities are for that specific environment. In one case, 19-year-old Michael's elderly parents, born and raised in China, were unable to accept his symptoms as caused by an illness until they could speak about Chinese attitudes towards the mentally ill. In their experience, mentally ill people brought great shame and secrecy to their families. They were sent away, chained to beds, and usually never seen again. In the USA the cloud of previously-held theories that blamed families for schizophrenia continues to cause families to feel guilt and shame, feelings which diminish their availability to accept the illness (Schooler and Keith 1993).

Providing support and psychoeducation to families generally leads to acceptance and support of treatment requirements. Families are advised of the treatment team's recommendations and available options; the clinician works toward developing a plan with family members.

Psychoeducation with patients

Psychoeducation is an essential building block for compliance with treatment and has been shown to help prevent relapses (Kopelowicz and Liberman 1998). The clinician is presented with various dilemmas in the case of first-episode patients. First, the diagnosis is often unclear for a period of time. Patients may present with symptoms consistent with the beginning stages of schizophrenia, but DSM-IV criteria mandate a six-month period during which there are definitive indications of the illness (American Psychiatric Association 1994). Second, many patients have limited or no insight and do not believe they have a problem with their thinking, feeling, or behaviour. Unfortunately, without an understanding of the illness and its treatment requirements, patients are unlikely to follow treatment recommendations that will help them rebuild their lives.

Patients' fears, sensitivity, and cognitive difficulties at this early stage suggest that information should be presented gradually and expanded upon as their condition improves. One effective way of presenting psychoeducation is for the clinician to acknowledge patients' psychotic symptoms and difficulties in functioning and clearly state that these are caused by an illness of the brain. Presenting the psychotic disorder as a biological illness akin to heart disease or diabetes is helpful: 'After all, the brain is an organ just as is the heart or the lungs, and can also get sick.' If patients have at least some insight into the illness as a biological disorder, being told that there is treatment available is therapeutic, educational, and potentially more acceptable. For patients whose insight is limited, psychoeducation presents an alternative understanding of symptoms which patients are helped to integrate as their thought processes become clearer. This reality-testing can be viewed as a cognitive approach to treatment wherein we are asking the patient to evaluate distortions in thinking (Miller and Mason 2002).

Psychoeducation with families

Psychoeducation for families in this early phase is presented using the biological illness model. Again: 'The brain is an organ and can get sick.' We explain that the patient is suffering with a psychotic illness, possibly schizophrenia, which is difficult to diagnose definitively at this early point. For most families psychosis is a difficult concept and requires explanation. In simple terms families are told that when the chemistry of the brain is not functioning properly, thinking, feeling, and behaviour are affected. The information that comes in through the five senses is interfered with and people may then hear voices, see visions, smell or taste strange things, and believe something is on their skin. Confused perceptions may bring about behavioural changes. Families need help to understand that aggressive or unusual behaviours are symptoms of the illness; they are not volitional or changes in character. If there is a substantial mood component, this too is explained as being caused by the chemical dysfunction in the brain.

Families are frequently seeking a diagnosis, etiology, and prognosis. The difficulty making a diagnosis at this stage is explained. Families are reminded that a diagnosis does not determine how well patients recover. With schizophrenia there are no clear answers regarding etiology and prognosis. We emphasize how little we know about the causes but that we do not believe schizophrenia is caused by 'bad parenting.' The stress-diathesis model is discussed in simple terms: 'Each of us has a predisposition or vulnerability that, when combined with other factors such as trauma, drug use or even a virus, may result in illness.' The metaphor utilized to assist in understanding this is that each person's heart is different. One person may have a predisposition to heart problems but is never challenged because of the luck of life circumstances. Another person may have the same predisposition, climbs a mountain, and becomes ill. Whatever the cause, what is occurring is a chemical process within the brain. The important message is that this is a serious illness but it can be treated. Questions about prognosis are difficult to answer because of the wide diversity of symptoms and recovery rates. Balancing hope with the real problems to be faced is essential. Focus is on the fact that each person is unique, but with medication and therapy many patients do well, return to school or work, and have a social life.

The role of families in medication compliance has been shown to be critical (Solomon *et al.* 1996). It is essential that parents, involved siblings, spouses, and others closely aligned with patients understand and support the need for compliance. In the early stages of illness it is often the case that families are wary of medications. This may be due to cultural issues, family denial, religious beliefs, or fear of side-effects and dependence. Again, the clinician's alliance with families and the psychoeducational process will assist in overcoming family resistance.

Sometimes families and clients need to experience the outcome of non-compliance in order to understand the need for treatment. This is not viewed as a failure but as part of the process of accepting the disease and its treatment. This is illustrated by the case of Peter.

Peter, a 17-year-old single male, responded quickly to antipsychotic medications. While he was in both inpatient and outpatient treatment his family avoided family sessions. His mother believed Peter had suffered a drug reaction from marijuana use that would resolve itself. After four months he discontinued antipsychotic medication and went off to college. In a short time negative symptoms worsened and Peter stopped attending classes. When brought in by his mother he was thin, oddly dressed, lethargic, and depressed. This time he and his mother agreed to a treatment plan which included medication and group therapy.

Group therapy

During the acute phase patients are often isolative and reluctant to attend groups. For patients who have never been in a psychiatric hospital, the illnesses that surround them are overwhelming. Patients may not be ready to relate to others who appear impaired. Whenever possible, patients are encouraged to attend groups on the unit in order to decrease isolation. Ideally first-episode patients are invited into groups with other first-episode patients who are further along in their treatment. These peer groups are very supportive and offer hope as well as first-hand advice. In addition, open discussion of acute symptoms with peers in the context of psychoeducation frequently helps people examine and reality-test their own symptoms. For example, it is not unusual for a patient to recognize that a group member's thoughts are delusional and begin to wonder about his or her own delusions.

The healing phase

The healing phase follows the acute phase; it is when patients' psychotic symptoms begin to diminish and stabilize. Insight is improving and motivation to return to health is high. This presents a unique window of opportunity to bring patients to readiness for ongoing treatment.

At this phase patients are usually transferred to a day-treatment or outpatient clinic. This transition is especially difficult for this group of patients, who may be fearful, paranoid, and isolated, or in denial of the illness. Family support and a strong therapeutic alliance are especially useful in assisting patients to make the transition to continued treatment.

Specific issues generally arise as patients progress through the healing phase. Particular attention to the following problem areas is vital:

- compliance with treatment
- adjustment to role changes
- reasonable vocational/educational expectations
- reframing the illness from psychological to biological
- abstinence from drug and alcohol use.

Modalities of treatment again focus on phase-specific issues.

Treatment modalities

Individual treatment

Individual treatment is offered when patients refuse group treatment. It is our clinical experience that patients who receive group treatment during the healing phase have a significantly lower drop-out rate than patients who are only in individual treatment (Miller and Mason 2001). However, some patients refuse because of fearfulness or inability to attend. In such cases individual treatment is provided in the hope that patients will be integrated into group treatment at a later date. An alliance with patients is once again the first step in treatment and treatment compliance the second step. The alliance continues to require a respectful attitude, empathy for the loss of recognizable self, and conveyance of hope.

Resistance to psychotherapy and medication management is an ongoing issue for most patients in the healing phase. Although many patients appear to have an attitude of compliance with medication during the earlier acute stage, they may become increasingly resistant as symptoms decrease. Uncomfortable side-effects often lead to decreased medication compliance. In our experience patients have the most difficulties with tardive dyskinesia, sedation, restlessness, constipation, sexual dysfunctions, and weight gain. Young male patients are especially upset by impotence. During this stage patients often believe that they can control their symptoms without medication, that the medications are ineffective, or that taking medication defines them as mentally ill. Some patients are secretive while others openly refuse medication. Patients are encouraged to discuss and complain about all side-effects. Often simply verbalizing frustration with medication is sufficient to allow patients to comply. Exploration of resistance, reality-testing, psychoeducation, encouragement, adjustment in medication by the psychiatrist, and support from clinicians and family members are often successful means of overcoming resistance to medication treatment.

As psychotic symptoms remit, patients become aware that their functioning is adversely affected by the disease. They experience changes in their roles as students, employees, friends, spouses, daughters, or sons. For the adolescent or young adult diagnosed with schizophrenia, social development often stalls at the point of illness. Patients describe themselves as becoming increasingly dependent upon family members. Families, in their wish to help, become understandably over-protective. The diminished role of 'patient' is viewed as temporary; they are encouraged to return to more normalized roles within the family.

Realistic planning for vocational/educational functioning prevents patients from experiencing failure and unnecessary stress that may lead to decompensation. Depending on the duration and severity of symptoms, some patients will want to return to school or work quickly. This should be promoted within limits that allow for successful role performance experiences. Other patients require more intensive outpatient programmes to manage their symptoms and to help with a slower re-entry into work, school, or training. Once more, if patients are helped to understand recovery as a process similar to that from any other serious physical illness, they are better able to accept the need to take one step at a time.

Family treatment

The healing phase is an understandably difficult one for families. Patients are not fully recovered but need to be independent and must begin to take responsibility for their health. It is at this point that patient, family, and clinical team are encouraged to begin the process of becoming a collaborative unit. Family sessions, which now include patients, can be supportive in nature but focus on issues that impede recovery. Most often these issues concern non-compliance, denial, and family over-involvement. Additional problems emerge such as conflicting patient and family expectations, the need for drug and alcohol abstinence, persisting symptoms, and medication side-effects. Families require support and guidance from the clinician as they address the possible need to lower their hopes and expectations for the patient (Zerbe and Larson 1988). Calling upon the concept of the biological model of illness helps the clinician keep patients and families directed toward treatment goals.

Psychoeducation with patients

Patients in the healing phase of illness are ready for additional information. Emphasis is on reframing the illness as a medical rather than an emotional disorder. Psychoeducation is provided using analogies that are easy to conceptualize. Patients can often begin to understand, for example, that there are chemical messengers that carry impulses from one brain cell to the next, and that if, as in the example of a child's electric train set, too much energy is delivered the brain will go off-track. When this occurs, messages between neurons in the brain become faulty. Thinking, feeling, and behaviour are then distorted, resulting in symptoms such as auditory hallucinations, delusions, bizarre behaviours, and confused thinking. Any of the five senses – sight, touch, hearing, smell, and taste – may be affected. It is emphasized that these are symptoms in the same way fever and coughing are symptoms of pneumonia. In this way patients can continue to question and test cognitive distortions of reality. To assist with the psychoeducation process we designed and use *Diagnosis: Schizophrenia* (Miller and Mason 2002), a book written specifically for patients.

The need for abstinence from drugs and alcohol is also approached from the biological and psychoeducational perspective. Patients can usually understand that these substances change the chemistry of the brain, thereby putting them at risk of relapse. The concept that many people use substances because they are attempting to treat overwhelming feelings of anxiety or depression by self-medication is introduced. When this has indeed been the case, patients are helped to see that this did not work for them. Patients with symptoms of depression may require additional information about alcohol's effect in increasing depression. Those who have a serious history of drug or alcohol dependence are encouraged to seek specialized treatment modalities. However, first-episode patients often refuse to go into special programmes, many of which have a confrontational approach to treatment. With the exception of patients who are putting their lives at risk by abusing substances, patients in this phase can be helped by maintaining the therapeutic relationship and compliance with medication while working gradually to increase motivation for abstinence from substances. The complexity of treatment for schizophrenia with substance abuse requires significant levels of support from consistent family involvement in treatment.

Psychoeducation with families

Family psychoeducation during the healing phase also places emphasis on the biological nature of the illness. More detailed information is provided, with diagrams of neurons and dopamine receptors. Once families have an adequate understanding of schizophrenia, preventing relapse becomes a primary goal of psychoeducation. Without a doubt relapse affects self-esteem and is a significant setback for patients and families. Statistics regarding noncompliance and relapse rates are shared. Families are advised that occasionally patients will relapse even when they have been compliant. This may be due to the course of the illness, which cannot always be controlled (Steingard *et al.* 1994), or when medications are ineffective or require adjustments to lessen side-effects. Families are informed that recent research indicates that with each relapse patients may run the risk of additional impairment to the brain (Lieberman 1993). This indicates that compliance with the treatment protocol is essential. The metaphor of multiple episodes of pneumonia causing increased damage to the lungs is often helpful in understanding the importance of preventing relapse.

Families are frequently ready for additional educational materials. The need of families for understandable, sophisticated technical information cannot be underestimated (Budd and Hughes 1997). Interventions that can provide families with some peace of mind, including the knowledge that they are not to blame, can be enhanced with the use of helpful books designed for the lay-person such as *Surviving Schizophrenia* (Torrey 1995) and *Coping with Schizophrenia* (Mueser and Gingerich 1994). Families often report that reading materials are frightening and must, therefore, be reminded that authors frequently address the most problematic patients and do not always take into account recent treatment advances.

Group treatment

Making connections with others and achieving mastery of social skills are essential for all adolescents (Malekoff 1997), and become especially important to patients who are often feeling isolated due to the illness. Using a modified model of support groups for medical illnesses, the clinician integrates pyschoeducation, coping skills training, and social/emotional support (Miller and Mason 1998; Spira 1997). Groups of between three and eight patients are open-ended, and, when possible, are organized with patients at similar levels of functioning. A cohesive group structure is fostered to focus on relapse prevention and symptom management. All issues addressed in the individual treatment of the healing phase are amenable to group treatment. The following illustrates integration of treatment in the group setting.

Terry is an inpatient entering the day programme group for the first time. The other group members introduce themselves, giving their names and stating they were previously on inpatient. Several say they are diagnosed with schizophrenia and three state they used to hear voices, and thought people were following them or going to hurt them. One young man says he still hears voices but is getting better. Terry listens and then says she is an inpatient now. She does not talk about symptoms but asks what her diagnosis is. This is followed by some psychoeducation about schizophrenia provided mostly by group members who then discuss many more of their symptoms. The group then does a 'doubling' of the new patient in which they take turns pretending they are Terry in the hospital for the first time and coming to this group for the first time. They demonstrate an understanding of Terry's thoughts and feelings, which then allows Terry to say she feels better knowing she is not the only one who has these symptoms, especially the one about the television being about her. The group welcomes Terry and goes on to do their 'symptom check,' 'medication check,' and 'substance abuse check,' three closing group rituals.

The maintenance phase

The maintenance phase begins when the patient's psychosis is largely, if not completely, resolved and functioning skills are clearly on the mend. Ego functioning increases and treatment frequently moves to the outpatient setting. Judgment, insight, reality-testing, use of defense mechanisms, and maintenance of self-esteem improve but continue to require support. The previous treatment experiences of patients and their families determine the amount of psychoeducation and family therapy required in this phase. The therapeutic alliance with both patients and families remains essential.

The goals of individual, family, and group therapy, and psychoeducation, during the maintenance phase are to support treatment compliance and to promote patients' return to optimal functioning. As the work of the previous phases continues, two new issues are introduced: reintegration of identity and safe sex practices. As in the earlier stages, all issues are addressed through reframing the illness in the medical model. Special attention is paid to increasing socialization, use of rehabilitation services as needed, and return to school or work.

Treatment modalities

Individual treatment

As in the prior phase, individual therapy may be required due to logistical difficulties or patient refusal of group treatment. Individual treatment during the maintenance phase is aimed at the differing needs and capabilities of each patient. Therefore, the clinical interventions required during the maintenance phase are best described as 'eclectic as well as pragmatic,' a phrase borrowed from Coursey (1989: 352). Increased coping skills, such as partializing, prioritizing, breathing exercises, and visualization, are very helpful to many patients. Cognitive-behavioural interventions are used as required. For example, thinking that they are 'schizophrenics' frequently causes depressed feelings and lowered self-esteem in first-episode patients. For this reason when they refer to themselves as 'schizophrenics' they are reminded that they have a disease named schizophrenia, that schizophrenia is not an identity. Cognitive therapy, which has been shown to be effective in treating positive and negative symptoms (Beck and Rector 2000; Bustillo *et al.* 2001; Garety *et al.* 2000), is used in conjunction with psychoeducation to improve reality-testing when necessary. Dynamically-oriented psychotherapy is rarely used because it may be destabilizing. Patients' feelings regarding past traumas such as incest or rape can be validated, but the emphasis is on dealing with the here-and-now problem of coping with schizophrenia. However, there are times when immediate painful personal issues are unavoidable and require special attention. For example, both Sara's parents died within six months of each other; her father committed suicide. Len's brother was killed in a suspicious shooting. Both Sara and Len required psychotherapy for their grief, to help put words to feelings, to decrease conflicting feelings, and to increase use of coping skills.

Cognitive impairment is taken into account in all interventions. Skills to increase organization, assist memory, and help concentration are introduced. For example, Carl is a pleasant 23-year-old who missed his medication for three days. It was determined that this was due to problems with memory function. Reminder cards were designed for his refrigerator and bedroom doors, family assistance was requested, and a daily medication dispenser was provided. Another patient, Susan, is performing well in college but requires help organizing her work assignments.

As patients recover, reintegration of identity emerges as an important issue. This is a gradual process of accepting and redefining the self. As with any other serious, chronic illness, patients now feel 'different' and vulnerable. However, rather than being unable to trust the body, individuals with schizophrenia are in the terrifying position of being unable to trust the mind. This is compounded when families and friends relate to individuals as 'mental patients.' Frequently, patients have their own preconceptions about people who have mental illnesses. Most of our patients report that before becoming ill they believed that people with schizophrenia had split personalities or were dangerous. These preconceptions often determine how they then perceive themselves. Some patients will deny their illness. Others become angry, depressed, homicidal, or suicidal, which needs to be addressed in treatment. To assist in the process of reintegration of identity patients require extensive amounts of psychoeducation, support, and cognitive restructuring. This is provided in a manner that is accepting of the person as a unique individual who suffers from a biological illness of the brain.

During the maintenance phase most patients are able to discuss issues of safe sex. Patients with schizophrenia are particularly vulnerable and this issue is therefore addressed as soon as possible in treatment. Safe sex practices are addressed in a straightforward manner and as a necessary medical issue (Mason and Miller, 2001). There is documented evidence showing that patients with schizophrenia are likely to practice safe sex only when they are convinced that there is a connection between behaviour and risk of HIV infection (McDermott et al. 1994). The danger of unwanted pregnancy is also an important concern. Information about AIDS testing and birth control measures is provided.

Many first-episode patients use alcohol and drugs prior to hospitalization. This is frequently a result of inadequate judgment or attempts to self-medicate. Once symptoms subside patients may be tempted to resume prior behaviours. Therefore, pre-emptive work with patients is key to preventing a return to drug or alcohol use. A good starting point for treatment is Prochaska et al.'s (1992) motivational model. Ziedonis and D'Avanzo

(1998) provide a thorough explication of the treatment of schizophrenia and substance abuse – especially helpful for patients with an extensive history of drug/alcohol use.

Family treatment

Although family therapy during the maintenance phase is generally offered on an as-needed basis, an on-going relationship with the family is funda-mental. As symptoms remit families are frequently reminded that they are essential to sustaining compliance. This is especially true for families of resistant and memory-impaired patients. Family members can be extremely helpful in advising the treatment team of patients' progress or problems. Often changes must be made in medications, and this requires full family cooperation.

With the absence or stabilization of acute positive symptoms, the family's focus moves to problems with side-effects, negative symptoms, and cognitive deficits. Among the more pronounced side-effects concerning parents are the large weight gains experienced with use of the newer medications, and tardive dyskinesia caused by older medications. Families are helped to express their uneasiness regarding the significant changes in patients' appearance. Possible future adjustments in medications are discussed.

Negative symptoms and cognitive deficits are equally difficult for families to accept. Understanding negative symptoms and cognitive deficits as being part of the illness helps families to provide appropriate support to patients. It decreases feelings of frustration and anger and increases realistic expec-tations. In our experience, a sound understanding of all symptoms helps fam-ilies to moderate their levels of expressed emotions. This is important because high levels of expressed emotions have been shown to affect patients nega-tively (Hogarty et al. 1997). Some families are extremely sensitive to blame; therefore, when explaining the need for decreased expressions of criticisms, hostility, and emotional over-involvement, we are careful to underscore that family stressors are not responsible for the illness. However, once patients have schizophrenia they are more sensitive to stress.

Psychoeducation with patients

In the maintenance phase patients assume increased responsibility for their own care. Psychoeducation centers on expanding patients' understanding of schizophrenia. Information regarding diagnosis and etiology is now grad-ually introduced. Additional psychoeducation regarding positive and nega-tive symptoms is provided. Understanding negative symptoms helps patients to feel they can get some control over symptoms of low energy, little interest or enjoyment, low motivation, isolation, and depressed mood. Diagrams of neurons and dopamine receptors are used to help patients symbolize and explain the disease in accord with the medical model of schizophrenia. Often we share research findings in order to provide patients with information on which they can make their own decisions. For example, we advise them that 80% of the patients in our institution's study of first-episode schizophrenia relapsed within five years but the risk of relapse was five times greater when they stopped medication (Robinson *et al.* 1999). Psychoeducation regarding the connection between drugs/alcohol and psychosis or depression is reviewed. This is especially important at times of vulnerability such as holidays. Because patients continue to struggle with the necessity for treatment, medication and side-effects remain important subjects for psychoeducation.

When patients begin to accept their diagnoses they appear better able to learn the coping skills needed. They learn to identify warning symptoms such as sleeplessness, anxiety, refusal to eat, isolation, referential ideation, rumination, irritability, or confusion. They learn how and where to get help if necessary. They learn that although stress did not cause their illness, they are now more stress-sensitive. This knowledge contributes to reducing feelings of powerlessness. Many patients suffer from cognitive deficits and request reassurance that these symptoms will remit. Unfortunately, we can only tell them that for many patients who are compliant with treatment, symptoms such as confusion, disorganization, and poor concentration do improve over time.

Psychoeducation with families

During the maintenance phase psychoeducation for families is generally the same as for patients. Families benefit from a good understanding of negative symptoms, medications, side-effects, and the effects of stress on patients. We remind families that stress affects brain chemistry, which may, in turn, affect patients' health. Families are also informed that the illness or medications may cause problems with memory, concentration, and organization skills. Like other illnesses, each person heals differently. Families are counseled that patients will need time and regular treatment.

Group treatment

Generally groups meet once weekly; however, a flexible approach is used for first-episode patients to allow for school and work schedules. During the maintenance phase patients are encouraged to learn to empathize with, respect, and help others with the same illness. This process appears to decrease self-stigmatization and improve self-esteem. Peer group power is tapped into to support abstinence from drugs and alcohol, to increase treatment compliance, and to encourage behaviours to overcome negative symptoms. The level of group discussion respects patients' improvement, their desire to obtain additional information, and their ability to address painful issues. Patients begin to address stigmatization, feelings of loss, hopelessness, disappointment, anger, and fear about the future, who to tell about the illness, frustrations with medication, persistent symptoms, and problems with dating or family. Medication compliance continues to be tenuous for many patients and is a frequent group issue. The case of Lisa illustrates how maintenance phase group therapy helped get a patient back on track so she could continue to work toward stabilization.

Lisa, a 19-year-old college student, was described as becoming increasingly 'spacey' during the three years prior to her hospitalization for acute psychotic symptoms. She had a history of drug and alcohol abuse. Lisa's family was well educated and had a good understanding of mental illness. Both sides of the family have a history of schizophrenia. Lisa's family attended family sessions and supported group and individual treatment as recommended. Gradually Lisa returned to college part-time and took a part-time job. The group successfully supported her abstinence from alcohol and drugs. After one year of steady progress she began to doubt her diagnosis and skipped doses of medication in order to be more like her college friends. When she subsequently had strange thoughts and disorganized behaviour, Lisa's group helped her to recognize her symptoms as such, and accept her illness and its treatment.

Group techniques are varied and are integrated according to patient needs. Role-play, mirroring exercises, psychodrama, cognitive-behavioural interventions, and psychoeducation are each adapted for individuals' strengths and deficits in cognition and interpersonal skills.

Chester had a history of multiple hospitalizations for psychotic and depressive symptoms. His functioning was extremely poor and he suffered marked cognitive impairments. Psychoeducation regarding alcohol use was regularly provided to Chester's day-hospital group. Chester continued to drink until his group instituted a ritual to help him to stay alcohol-free. Each session before the group ended members tried to convince Chester to have a drink. 'Just one,' they would good-naturedly cajole. After several months Chester was proud to say: 'No thanks. Alcohol makes my symptoms worse.' The group provided much-deserved congratulations and support for his real and role-played abstinence.

The group modality is also very effective for social skills training (Bellack et al. 1997). Poor eye contact, difficulty communicating, and poverty of speech are common problems that patients work on in our first-episode groups. This is done only with the patient's permission and group members' approval. The following vignette describes the integration of social skills training.

Jill's eye contact was extremely poor. The group talked about the skills needed for communication. The therapist asked the group: 'What is it like to talk to someone who is not looking at you?' 'Like they're not paying attention to you,' they responded. 'I wonder what's going on, how come it's so hard to make eye contact?' the therapist asked. Group members replied: 'It's uncomfortable, scary to look at people after the illness.' 'I wonder,' the therapist inquired, 'if making good eye contact is something the group would like to work on?' They responded affirmatively and awareness of eye contact became integrated into the group process.

SUMMARY AND CONCLUSION

First-episode patients with schizophrenia differ from the chronic population. They and their families are coming to terms with a serious and stigmatizing diagnosis for which they have had little preparation. Clinical interventions take into consideration the newness of the change in life expectations. Table 8.1 summarizes phase-specific interventions which help patients and caregivers ameliorate the potentially devastating effects of the disease.

Clinicians may need to modify aspects of this outline based on the uniqueness of their own settings. Even where there are no additional resources for treatment of this specialized group, all or segments of this treatment plan can be used effectively by focusing on its salient theme: first-episode patients and their families require timely interventions which address their special needs.

Table 8.1 Phases and phase-specific interventions for first-episode schizophrenia

Phase of illness	Phase-specific psychosocial interventions
Acute	Providing a supportive therapeutic relationship. Conveying hope to patients and families. Introducing the concept of biological illness. Helping patients accept medication. Engaging the support of the family.
Healing	Reinforcing the concept of biological illness. Emphasizing the need for abstinence from drug and alcohol use. Building compliance with medication and treatment. Helping clients adjust to role changes. Encouraging realistic vocational and educational plans. Engaging patients and families in a collaborative process.
Maintenance	Continued support for treatment compliance. Furnishing in-depth psychoeducation emphasizing positive and negative symptoms. Teaching coping skills. Providing opportunities for reduced social isolation with group treatment. Helping clients regain self-esteem. Providing social skills training. Supporting educational and vocational options. Teaching safe sexual practices. Encouraging abstinence from drugs and alcohol.

ACKNOWLEDGMENTS

We are grateful to all of the patients and families who have contributed to our understanding of the treatment needs of first-episode patients. Portions of this chapter appeared in Miller, R. and Mason, S. E. (1999), Phase-specific psychosocial interventions for first episode schizophrenia, *Bulletin of the Mennninger Clinic* 63: 499–519. Copyright © Guilford Publications. We would like to thank the *Bulletin of the Menninger Clinic* for permission to use these sections.

REFERENCES

American Psychiatric Association (1994). *Diagnostic and Statistical Manual of Mental Disorders* (4th ed.). Washington, DC: APA.

Beck, A. T. and Rector, N. A. (2000). Cognitive therapy of schizophrenia: A new therapy for the new millennium. *American Journal of Psychotherapy* 54: 291–300.

Bellack, A. S. *et al.* (1997). *Social Skills Training for Schizophrenia*. New York: Guilford Press.

Budd, R. J. and Hughes, I. C. T. (1997). What do relatives of people with schizophrenia find helpful about family intervention? *Schizophrenia Bulletin* 23: 341–7.

Bustillo, J. R. *et al.* (2001). The psychosocial treatment of schizophrenia: An update. *The American Journal of Psychiatry* 158: 163–75.

Carpenter Jr., W. T. (1996). Maintenance therapy of persons with schizophrenia. *Journal of Clinical Psychiatry* 57 (suppl. 9): 10–8.

Coursey, R. D. (1989). Psychotherapy with persons suffering from schizophrenia: The need for a new agenda. *Schizophrenia Bulletin* 15: 349–53.

Drury, V. (1994). Recovery from acute psychosis. In M. Birchwood and N. Tarrier (eds) *Psychological Management of Schizophrenia*. Chichester, UK: John Wiley & Sons.

Edwards, J. *et al.* (1994). Early psychosis prevention and intervention: Evolution of a comprehensive community-based specialized service. *Behaviour Change* 11: 223–33.

Fenton, W. S. (1997). Course and outcome in schizophrenia. *Current Opinion in Psychiatry* 9: 40–4.

Fenton, W. S. *et al.* (1997). Determinants of medication compliance in schizophrenia: Empirical and clinical findings. *Schizophrenia Bulletin* 23: 637–51.

Garety, P. A. *et al.* (2000). Cognitive-behavioural therapy for medication-resistant symptoms. *Schizophrenia Bulletin* 26: 73–86.

Goldstein, M. J. (1994). Psychoeducation and family therapy in relapse prevention. *Acta Psychiatrica Scandinavica*, 382 (suppl.): 54–7.

Hogarty, G. E. *et al.* (1995). Personal therapy: A disorder-relevant psychotherapy for schizophrenia. *Schizophrenia Bulletin* 21: 379–93.

Hogarty, G. E. *et al.* (1997). Three-year trials of personal therapy among schizophrenic patients living with or independent of family, II: Effects on adjustment of patients. *American Journal of Psychiatry* 154: 1514–24.

Hough, G. (1995). A clinician with a family member with schizophrenia: A case report. *Bulletin of the Menninger Clinic* 59: 345–56.

Kopelowicz, A. and Liberman, R. P. (1998). Psychosocial treatments for schizophrenia. In P. E. Nathan and J. M. Gorman (eds) *A Guide to Treatments That Work*. New York: Oxford University Press.

Lam, D. H. (1991). Psychosocial family intervention in schizophrenia: A review of empirical studies. *Psychological Medicine* 21: 423–41.

Lieberman, J. A. (1993). Prediction of outcome in first-episode schizophrenia. *Journal of Clinical Psychiatry* 54 (suppl. 3): 13–17.

Lieberman, J. *et al.* (1993). Time course and biological correlates of treatment responses to first-episode schizophrenia. *Archives of General Psychiatry* 50: 369–76.

Lieberman, J. A. *et al.* (1996). Factors influencing treatment response and outcome of first-episode schizophrenia: Implications for understanding the pathophysiology of schizophrenia. *Journal of Clinical Psychiatry* 57 (suppl. 9).

Malekoff, A. (1997). *Group Work with Adolescents*. New York: Guilford Press.

Mason, S. E. and Miller, R. (2001). Safe sex for first episode schizophrenia. *Bulletin of the Menninger Clinic* 65: 179–93.

McDermott, B. E. *et al.* (1994). Diagnosis, health beliefs, and risk of HIV infection in psychiatric patients. *Hospital and Community Psychiatry* 45: 580–5.

McGoldrick, M. *et al.* (1982). *Ethnicity and Family Therapy*. New York: Guilford Press.

Miller, R. and Mason, S. E. (1998). Group work with first episode schizophrenia clients. *Social Work With Groups* 21: 19–33.

Miller, R. and Mason, S. E. (2001). Using group therapy to enhance treatment compliance in first episode schizophrenia. *Social Work With Groups* 24: 37–51.

Miller, R. and Mason, S. E. (2002). *Diagnosis: Schizophrenia*. New York: Columbia University Press.

Mueser, K. T. and Gingerich, S. (1994). *Coping with Schizophrenia: A Guide for Families*. Oakland, CA: New Harbinger.

Munich, R. L. (1997). Contemporary treatment for schizophrenia. *Bulletin of the Menninger Clinic* 61: 189–221.

Prochaska, J. O. *et al.* (1992). In search of how people change: Applications to addictive behaviourals. *American Psychologist* 47: 1102–14.

Robinson, D. *et al.* (1999). Predictors of relapse following response from a first episode of schizophrenia or schizoaffective disorder. *Archives of General Psychiatry* 56: 241–7.

Rosenson, M. (1993). Social work and the right of psychiatric patients to refuse medication: A family advocate's response. *Social Work* 38: 108–12.

Schooler, N. R. and Keith, S. J. (1993). The clinical research base for the treatment of schizophrenia. *Psychopharmacology Bulletin* 29: 431 46.

Schwartz, H. I. *et al.* (1988). Autonomy and the right to refuse treatment: Patients' attitudes after involuntary medication. *Hospital and Community Psychiatry* 39: 1049–54.

Sheitman, B. B. *et al.* (1997). The evaluation and treatment of first-episode psychosis. *Schizophrenia Bulletin* 23: 653–61.

Solomon, P. *et al.* (1996). The impact of individualized consultation and group workshop family education interventions on ill relative outcomes. *Journal of Nervous and Mental Disease* 184: 252–4.

Spira, J. L. (1997). *Group Therapy for Medically Ill Patients*. New York: Guilford Press.

Steingard, S. *et al.* (1994). A study of the pharmocologic treatment of medication-compliant schizophrenics who relapse. *Journal of Clinical Psychiatry* 55: 470–2.

Torrey, E. F. (1995). *Surviving Schizophrenia* (3rd ed.). New York: Harper.

Zerbe, K. J. and Larson, J. (1988). Clinical case conference: A modified psychoeducational approach with a schizophrenia inpatient. *Bulletin of the Menninger Clinic* 52: 332–8.

Ziedonis, D. M. and D'Avanzo, K. (1998). Schizophrenia and substance abuse. In H. R. Kranzler and B. R. Rounsaville (eds) *Dual Diagnosis and Treatment, Substance Abuse and Comorbid Medical and Psychiatric Disorders*. New York: Marcel Dekker.

Part III

Phase-specific treatment of psychosis

Chapter 9

The use of psychodynamic understanding of psychotic states

Delineating need-specific approaches

Johan Cullberg

INTRODUCTION

This chapter is about the need to identify the different soils within which psychosis takes place in order to offer optimum treatment. I shall demonstrate how psychodynamic thinking may be an important tool for this in different ways, depending on the kind of psychosis being dealt with and which phase of the disorder the patient is in.

During the last decade, evidence-based knowledge regarding psychodynamic treatments for psychosis has been increasingly regarded as nonexistent (Lehmann *et al.* 1998; Mueser and Berenbaum 1989). Negative findings in chronic schizophrenic states (McGlashan 1984) and the lack of studies of carefully-adapted treatments of acute psychoses have contributed to such attitudes. In contrast, we have increasing knowledge about the effectiveness of cognitive-behavioural therapies in both acute and chronic psychotic states. Since negative attitudes about dynamically-based therapies do not agree with the experiences of many pragmatically working clinicians, these attitudes need to be confronted and fresh research conducted.

Over the last few decades, the focus of my psychiatric work has mainly concerned psychotic states. During this time, my understanding of what psychodynamic understanding of the psychotic person means has changed, and I have experienced a diminishing interest in the classical formulations of psychoanalytical understanding and treatment of psychosis. Like many colleagues, I am pessimistic about the possibilities of the psychoanalytical psychotherapy of chronic schizophrenia. At the same time, my optimism has increased about the importance of a dynamic understanding of the psychotic states – not as a means of explaining the ultimate causes, but in the search for a meaning of the psychotic experiences in the person's inner world. Here we find new treatment facilities in combined dynamic-cognitive approaches. It is important to remember that the word 'psychosis' does not have a biological qualification. Psychosis is a phenomenological concept about a loss of reality sense. The background of specific biological vulnerabilities, however, also necessitates a concurrent and approximative medical view of the phenomena.

There is one primary fact that I consider important when discussing the appropriateness of dynamic approaches: namely, the acute psychotic state has a self-healing capacity provided the individual is given an optimal psychological and social milieu. Psychiatry may facilitate the healing processes; however, in my experience, this capacity is often obstructed by traditional psychiatric care conditions that are counterproductive to these processes. I will highlight this theme later in the chapter.

THREE CLINICAL TYPES OF PSYCHOSIS

For practical reasons we may differentiate between three types of non-organic ('functional') psychoses:

- the acute mainly one-episode psychosis in a seemingly normal person
- the recurring psychoses in a person who sometimes may suffer from an early personality disorder
- long-term psychotic or near-psychotic states with an increasing personality change/disability.

These three types need very different understanding and handling, regardless of the amount of positive, negative, disorganised, etc. symptoms. Thus, we avoid the often non-productive diagnostic differentiation between schizophrenic and other psychoses. I shall discuss the possibilities of dynamic understanding of each of these three types.

The acute first-episode psychosis

Of course, we cannot know for sure whether a first-episode psychotic person will have just one psychotic episode. Often we hear about a seemingly normal young or middle-aged person who has reacted with a brief depression, or anxiety attacks, after having experienced a significant loss or another stressful situation, be it an unsuccessful love experience or the death of an important network person. However, the symptoms deepen and suddenly paranoid ideas organise and rapidly get systematised. Sometimes auditory hallucinations are added. This state may be named brief psychosis, affective psychosis, or acute delusional psychosis, according to the symptoms. Depending on the degree and quality of symptoms, it may also be named a schizophreniform psychosis. However, the clinical validity of the diagnostic terms is low.

Traditionally an acute psychotic state is immediately treated with neuroleptic medication. Since the patients often do not accept hospitalisation and medication, the treatment will be compulsory. In the acute psychiatric ward, the patient is exposed to a milieu characterised by high expressed emotion (HEE). The patient's anxiety and psychotic symptoms are increased, resulting in higher neuroleptic doses, and the side effects make the patient feel even worse. As we may understand, to start a treatment in such a milieu – where medication is experienced as a violation, and no meeting is offered to try to connect the psychosis with the preceding life problems – is a primitive and counterproductive way of working. The most obvious result is a patient who promises him or herself never again to turn to psychiatry if he or she gets out of hospital.

A dynamic understanding stresses the necessity of quite a different approach to an acute problem. Besides questioning the wholesomeness of the typical in-patient-ward milieu, there are problems to be highlighted with the patient and the patient's family – if there is one. What has happened during the previous months, and what do the family members perceive to be the main problems? The psychosis may be explained as a deep-seated crisis reaction which, in many ways, has a logical and understandable course and treatment. This means trying to give a new kind of understanding, meaning and hope to the events. You can work surprisingly effectively even in the presence of an acutely psychotic family member. I will give a rather typical example of the problems.

A 30-year-old woman fell ill after a period of acute marital problems that were accompanied by almost total sleeplessness for several weeks. She developed a delusional psychosis with a brief period of hallucinating voices. The paranoid psychosis lasted for more than nine months. At hospitalisation she was treated with increasing doses of neuroleptics including depot injections, but without effect. ECT was ordered but the patient refused. After four months her case was taken over by our project for first-episode psychotic patients – due to a mistake the patient had not been reported to us from the beginning. After I had met the patient, her medication was discontinued, as was her compulsory care, with an agreement that I would see the patient at regular and frequent intervals. She was greatly relieved not to suffer the side effects of the drugs any longer. That was also helpful to our therapeutic alliance. The patient came to our meetings in spite of being very paranoid about my identity, believing the ward was a disguised police station and that there were hidden microphones, and so on.

From the beginning I was working with her anxiety about being the object of systematic persecution. I told her that there were two possibilities as I understood it: first, that her anxious ideas about being locked up as a victim of unjust prosecution were correct, in which case she urgently needed protection. The second working hypothesis was that, in a state of sleeplessness and despair, she had gradually started to misinterpret her surroundings. My task, as I suggested to her, was to be her consultant in investigating these hypotheses. I also told her that I realised that she at least had to pretend to rely on my honesty in order to co-operate. This intelligent patient, who was a dedicated diary-writer, gradually produced much material describing her earlier and ongoing experiences in the hospital. This was a description of terror, humiliation and loneliness. It was also an intricate mixture of her being exposed to stereotypical and incoherent treatment ambitions, and her psychotic interpretations of why this humiliation would continue. I discussed possible alternative interpretations of the events but without pleading for the truth.

Parallel with this, we talked about her marital life. She had married her husband at a very young age, partly as an effort to separate from her parental home. There were no children, and there had been no sex life for several years; in fact, psychologically, the relationship had been finished for a long time. Her husband had behaved in an increasingly threatening way during the previous year. The patient, however, had not believed that she could manage to live alone after a separation. Six months before her hospitalisation, she had met a woman friend who told her about feminism and about her own separation and new freedom. This was when the patient's nightly quarrels with her husband started, followed by the sleeplessness – she wanted her husband to 'allow' and support a separation she otherwise did not dare to undertake. This resulted in an increasing feeling of unreality and of being exposed to a gigantic experiment. Paranoid ideas, together with her suicidal behaviour, resulted in her compulsory admission to the locked psychiatric ward.

Our meetings, which started four months after admission, continued over the following four months until the paranoid system started to loosen and she could accept joint meetings with her husband, her parents and her work colleagues where she could discuss their former 'strange' behaviour. The patient did not return to the marital home and instead rented a flat of her own. She gradually regained full insight and psychic strength and went back to her job. She was recommended a private psychotherapeutic contact to investigate further and work on her low self-esteem.

This intelligent but neurotic patient could have been spared a prolonged and deep suffering if her psychological predicament had been observed from the beginning. It was evident that her problems emanated from her inability to solve the conflict between her need to leave her husband and her not daring to stand on her own feet. Her psychosis was triggered by the sleeplessness and enforced by the strange and anxiety-provoking milieu. Our psychotherapeutic work was guided by a clinical feeling that behind the paranoia the patient had a possibility for full recovery.

I have discussed this patient in some detail because she is typical of a good prognosis case where a dynamic understanding is important in order to provide a need-specific treatment. It also shows the combination of dynamic and cognitive methods which is often quite necessary when working with psychosis.

A seemingly normal person may sometimes react to significant traumas with a psychosis, which may be difficult to recognise if one does not know the person well. One may observe the symbolic provocation of memories of a very specific early trauma which here serve as an Achilles heel. That may be an early sexual offence, the early death of a brother or a sister, or a similar trauma which is suppressed and 'forgotten'. Here specialised psychotherapy may be needed after the psychosis is over.

Strauss (1989) has talked about the 'low turning point' when, as a consequence of rather ordinary relational provocations, rigid and defensive personality traits burst into psychotic disintegration. In order to make a real turning point, the person must have the time and the support to reintegrate and to grow after the psychotic crisis. Such psychotherapy does generally not imply 'symbolic' psychoanalytic interpretations, but rather a dynamic understanding of the patient's actual and phase-specific life problems. This must include support for his/her return to society and to self-esteem. In such cases we may sometimes have reason to say that the psychosis carried a new opportunity for the person. Otherwise psychosis is not an experience one would recommend for therapeutic reasons.

In more complicated cases the psychosis may present itself when a partially immature and dependent person tries to separate from the parental home. Such vulnerability expresses the patient's thin emotional 'skin' which may also be regarded as their genetic endowment. The prognosis may be better, provided the family can get help, both to co-operate in the separation process and to regard the psychosis as a meaningful crisis reaction. Often, but not always, a neuroleptic medication in low doses is helpful. Such is the case when there are painful psychotic symptoms or when the psychosis in spite of good caring conditions continues for weeks without lowering in intensity. Because of this vulnerability, such a psychosis also may recur at a new provocation.

Recurrent psychosis with no personality deterioration

We may encounter the second type of psychosis, with recurring psychotic crises, in a person with a more prominent personality disorder living a self-destructive or 'borderland' existence. In these cases, we not only meet the sequels of early childhood trauma but often there are one or two family members who have also suffered a psychotic disorder, indicating a genetic or other vulnerability. Working psychotherapeutically with severe personality disorders is both time- and energy-consuming and many therapists only have one or two such patients in their caseload that have been treated successfully, and several others with less successful results. According to the major Wallerstein study (1989), these double diagnosis patients may best be treated with supportive dynamic and respectfully confrontational methods. In practice, the main therapeutic goal must often be similar to those for other personality disorders. This means helping the patients to get optimal psychiatric support during psychotic relapses, supporting them in not committing suicide, becoming addicts being overmedicated, and waiting for the late maturation to come, hopefully by their fourth decade.

There are many cases with recurring psychosis where a biological vulnerability must be hypothesised. Today these patients are mainly treated with antidepressants or mood-stabilising medication, which often may be good alternatives. Sometimes the best psychotherapeutic results are achieved with an unorthodox combination of cognitive and dynamic approaches, which does not mean that the therapeutic frames are abolished.

In one psychotherapy research project Sonja Levander and I interviewed a 40-year-old woman who started severe acting out, including suicide attempts, at the age of 16 (Cullberg and Levander 1991). At 25 she was attributed a schizophrenia diagnosis for the first time. Between her psychoses, she was likeable and did not show any cognitive or affective defect. She had been offered psychotherapy several times but did not accept it because, as she put it, 'I had to be in the very bottom to allow myself psychotherapy.' When she eventually accepted treatment, this was the beginning of a six-year-long intensive out- and in-patient treatment with many dramatic incidents and an initial aggravation of her disorder. She refused neuroleptic medication. Her very complicated parental relations and incestuous experiences were dealt with in the treatment. When we met the patient she had not been psychotic for five years; she had a meaningful job, and she could talk about her experiences in a very subtle and realistic way. She described her psychotherapy as life-saving.

Sometimes we can find the mood swings of a typical bipolar disorder accompanying or releasing the psychotic relapses. Even here I have found psychotherapy important in working with specific personal vulnerabilities, in connection with a mood-stabilising long-term medical treatment.

Psychosis with long-term personality change

Now we reach a difficult point in the dynamic understanding of psychoses: the third type of psychosis with long-term personality change, according to my simplified nosology. Here we may find years of prodromal symptoms with a gradual and frightening experience of undergoing a deep and enduring change of the self. This is accompanied by a steady decline in social capacity, as has been demonstrated by Möller and Husby's naturalistic study of first-episode schizophrenia patients (2000). When the psychosis appears it is just a way of expressing the subjective experiences of ongoing inner changes of the self – and the person starts to project the experiences as originating outside him/herself. This way of trying to get an explanation for what is happening inside is transformed into a delusion and confirmed by hallucinatory voices, which are perceived as emanating from the outside world. I have met many of these young men and (less often) women over the years and I have tried psychotherapy of different kinds with many of them. I have supervised colleagues' treatments, or I have just been an on-looker. When ambitions are too high and supervision too low, the psychotherapists often finally do not want

to work at all with psychotic patients. But when goals are set more realistic-
ally, to help the patient adapt to his/her disability, then the psychotherapeutic
success is more evident.

These cases – perhaps 10% of all first-episode psychosis patients – may
represent a special subgroup of the schizophrenic psychoses to which the term
'illness of the self' may be appropriate. The most malignant early features are
the slow illness progression, low energy, and lack of will and interest. In these
cases, conventional dopamine receptor-suppressing medication is often rather
useless or negative, suggesting a different biological aetiology. Every year new
research data indicate specific genes, specific morphological changes in the
brain and so on, but later on the findings are rejected. Nevertheless, I would
not be surprised if we witnessed some kind of breakthrough in the biological
research into this subgroup of schizophrenic patients during this decade.

Negative therapeutic experiences with these cases have falsely been
extrapolated to all schizophrenic patients. This may explain the simplified
'evidence-based statements' which today block the psychodynamically
informed psychotherapy of psychoses. However, we know – thanks to the
research of Ciompi, Bleuler, Harding and others – that with the right care
and thoughtful rehabilitation there is good hope for the majority, even for
chronic schizophrenic patients. In the long run the damage to the self, namely
the chronic personality change, will heal to a large extent.

In such cases, psychodynamic understanding is important, in order better
to understand the patients' reactions to their vulnerability. Working with
vulnerable near-psychotic people we often observe protective mechanisms
which are inhibited when the person is exposed to a situation that may
provoke aggression or fear: these mechanisms are autistic withdrawal and
delusional thinking.

In my experience, some of these patients also have a predisposition, which
is analogous to the alexithymic reaction first described by Peter Sifneos in
psychosomatic patients (Sifneos 1973). This means that they have a low capacity for the verbal expression of their aggressive feelings. Instead, they react
according to their high vulnerability with withdrawal and delusions. This is, I
believe, one of the reasons why it is so easy to make a chronic patient out of a
person with schizophrenia. It may also explain the psychosis-inducing effects
of the phenomenon of HEE.

A young schizophrenic, well-functioning medical student was provoked by
his fiancée in a discussion and developed paranoid thoughts in the same
moment. He was able to control his psychosis and when he visited me the
following day I asked him what he felt during the discussion with his fiancée.
He denied any feelings. When I rephrased my question, he suddenly became
pale and asked in a whispering tone if there were any microphones in my
office. The patient's ego fragility was high and I decided that I would not try
to work with his threatening aggression problems. Instead his needs were met
with the increase of his medication over a few weeks.

THE 'HEROIC' PSYCHOTHERAPIES

How do we understand the dramatic and often heroic cases of psychotherapy, which many have heard or read about, where a long-term schizophrenic person is rescued and returned to normal life after years of deep involvement and struggle? We must not forget, however, that the majority of such patients show very little benefit, or even get worse, with intensive psychoanalytic therapy. Again the crude schizophrenia diagnosis is quite invalid for predicting outcome and therapeutic method. Several of the successful cases I have met or read about have been patients who would originally have had a good prognosis, but due to early institutionalisation, too much medication and lack of human relations, they had given up their hope and withdrawn into their inner world. This withdrawal also gave a protection against the deep hatred and aggression collected during several years of sufferance. When the therapist at a later moment enters into this person's life he or she is taking a large risk in possibly releasing these forces when helping the patient to get closer to his/her feelings. Having the ability to create an understanding and confidence, enduring all the relapses, standing the aggression and believing in the humanity behind the chronic patient's sometimes inhumane manifestations is a job for a few dedicated and naturally talented people. In my experience, this is nothing you can teach as 'normal' psychotherapy. It is the highest level art of psychotherapy and it is often performed on a tightrope.

I believe there is a difference between a secondary giving-up/withdrawal into chronicity, and the malignant primary withdrawal which we encounter in those core schizophrenic persons I described earlier. But there must be quite an overlap. Will it be possible to learn to differentiate better at an earlier stage?

Finally, skilled and sensible psychotherapists can have little effect if their work is not supported by the psychiatric organisation aiming to be need-adapted for these patients, and not primarily adapted for the needs of an outdated one-sided hospital-centred psychiatry (Alanen 1997). A really effective organisation would put an emphasis on family and network relations, crisis support, self-confidence, continuity, and skilful psychotherapeutic and pharmacological treatment. If we wish to accomplish this, a dynamic understanding is pertinent. Then, the most important aspect of the dynamic understanding will be made possible: that every member of staff working with psychotic patients will have the knowledge, training and supervision for creating and maintaining a therapeutic relationship with their patients.

REFERENCES

Alanen, Y. O. (1997). *Schizophrenia. Its Origins and Need-Adapted Treatments.* London: Karnac Books.

Cullberg, J. and Levander, S. (1991). Fully recovered schizophrenic patients who received intensive psychotherapy. A Swedish case-finding study. *Nordic Journal of Psychiatry* 45: 253–62.

Lehmann, A. *et al.* (1998). The schizophrenia Patient Outcome Research Team (PORT) treatment recommendations. *Schizophrenia Bulletin* 24: 1–10.

McGlashan, T. H. (1984). The Chestnut Lodge follow-up study: II. Long-term outcome of schizophrenia and the affective disorders. *Archives of General Psychiatry* 41: 141–4.

Möller, P. and Husby, R. (2000). The initial prodrome in schizophrenia: Searching for naturalistic core dimensions of experience and behavior. *Schizophrenia Bulletin* 26: 217–32.

Mueser, K. T. and Berenbaum, H. (1989). Psychodynamic treatment of schizophrenia: Is there a future? *Psychological Medicine* [Editorial] 20: 253–62.

Sifneos P. E. (1973). The prevalence of 'alexithymic' characteristics in psychosomatic patients. *Psychotherapy and Psychosomatics* 22: 255–62.

Strauss, J. S. (1989). Mediating processes in schizophrenia: Towards a new dynamic psychiatry. *British Journal of Psychiatry* 55 (suppl. 5): 22–8.

Wallerstein, R. S. (1989). The psychotherapy research project of the Menninger Foundation: An overview. *Journal of Consulting Clinical Psychology* 57: 195–205.

Chapter 10

A cognitive analytic therapy-based approach to psychotic disorder

Ian B. Kerr, Valerie Crowley and Hilary Beard

INTRODUCTION

The past decade has seen renewed interest in the role of psychosocial factors in the development and outcome of psychotic disorders, even from previously hard-line biological researchers and despite the dominance over recent years of a predominantly biomedical and pharmacological paradigm in addressing these disorders (see reviews by Csernansky and Grace 1998; Hemsley and Murray 2000; Martindale *et al.* 2000; Wykes *et al.* 1998). Overall, the 'stress-vulnerability' paradigm (Nuechterlein and Subotnik 1998; Zubin and Spring 1977) positing genetic and/or biological vulnerability to such disorders in the context of psychosocial stressors (both developmentally and contemporaneously) has generated a greater consensus among all workers whether they are predominantly of a biomedical or psychosocial orientation. Thus clinical research questions have come to be centred around which aspects of which treatment models will be most effective in addressing the variety of psychological difficulties and symptoms which may lead to, perpetuate or exacerbate these disorders.

Although family therapy and cognitive behavioural therapy (CBT) have been demonstrably efficacious in controlled trials for many patients with many kinds of difficulties, it is clear that they are not a panacea, neither in terms of effectiveness nor in terms of engaging some of the more 'hard to help' or 'resistant' patients. Given this situation, a small group of workers using the cognitive analytic therapy (CAT) model have been exploring, on a preliminary basis, the development of a model of psychosis as well as its applicability and usefulness, with encouraging results (Kerr 2000; Kerr *et al.* 2001; Pollock 2001; Ryle and Kerr 2002). Although collective experience is limited so far to a few dozen cases and this approach requires more extended, systematic evaluation, it would appear that this recently developed, integrative model could have a useful role to play in extending our conceptual and therapeutic repertoire. It would apply both as a model of developmental psychopathology and as a treatment aimed at individual patients as well as staff teams and others involved such as friends and families. Prior to summarising the development and articulation of such a CAT-based model of psychosis and illustrating and discussing its possible applications, a brief overview of the CAT model and its background will be offered.

CAT – BACKGROUND

CAT is an integrative model of psychotherapy developed in the UK by Anthony Ryle (Ryle 1990, 1995; Ryle and Kerr 2002). It was initially developed as a brief, time-limited model of therapy for a range of 'neurotic' disorders but it has been extended well beyond this with its application to more 'difficult' groups of patients such as those with severe personality disorders and its application as a model informing, for example, group therapy and day hospital or community mental health team work as well as consultative work not involving patient contact. It has roots in Kellyian personal construct theory, cognitive and developmental psychology, psychoanalytic object-relations theory and, more recently, has been further transformed by Vygotskian activity theory (Ryle 1991) and concepts of a 'dialogic' self inspired by the work of Bakhtin (Leiman 1997).

In this model, early, socially meaningful experience is seen to result in the internalisation of a repertoire of 'reciprocal roles' (RRs) which come to form part of the structure of the self. This process is understood to occur on the basis of our innate predisposition to intersubjectivity and joint sign-mediated activity as described and stressed by contemporary developmental psychologists (see Trevarthen and Aitken 2001). The development of a repertoire of RRs is also seen as being partly influenced and determined by individual temperament. These RRs and their procedural enactments (reciprocal role procedures or RRPs) are understood to determine subsequent interpersonal behaviours and self-management and are, importantly, understood always to anticipate or elicit the role of literal or historic other(s). They therefore effectively represent a template through which interpersonal experience is interpreted. An RRP is understood to comprise a complex of intention, affect, procedural memory, action and subsequent evaluation. A role is also understood to be associated with an internalised (partly cultural) dialogic 'voice'. An important feature of the model is that both ends of a reciprocal role are internalised and may be subsequently enacted, frequently in internal self–self procedures.

Abnormal development is understood in CAT in terms of the internalisation of dysfunctional role procedures (which can be seen as avoidant, defensive or symptomatic) and failures or disruptions of their integration as self processes. These may be the result of difficult or traumatising developmental experience determined in part by biological vulnerability. CAT thus differs increasingly from its sources in its greater emphasis on the social formation of mind.

CAT – PRACTICE

The practice of CAT, influenced increasingly by post-Vygotskian activity theory, is based on an explicitly collaborative therapeutic position involving the active participation of the patient. Its central aims are to create with patients both narrative and diagrammatic reformulations of their difficulties. The written reformulation identifies and describes maladaptive role procedures and their enactments in the context of an explicit retelling of, or 'bearing witness' to, the patient's life story (in itself seen as important: see discussion by Holmes 1998), while the diagrammatic reformulation aims to depict them and their consequences in the here and now.

The work of therapy is aimed at the recognition and revision of dysfunctional RRPs both in the outside world and as experienced within the therapy relationship. Therapeutic change is seen to depend on the creation of a non-collusive relationship with the patient informed by the joint creation of the mediating tools of letters and diagrams within a phased, time-limited relationship. This includes articulation of target problem procedures and related therapeutic aims which are worked on and monitored. The general validity of this reformulation process has been evaluated positively by process research (Bennett and Parry 1998). In the case of more disturbed and damaged patients, such as those with severe personality and many psychotic disorders, diagrammatic mapping will also involve the recognition and description of dissociated 'self-states', each of which embodies one RRP. Therapy also aims to help the patient to be able to reflect on these at a meta-procedural level. This is normally a particular difficulty for patients with severe personality disorders or in psychotic states.

A CAT MODEL OF VULNERABILITY TO AND DEVELOPMENT OF PSYCHOTIC DISORDER

From the perspective of the stress-vulnerability paradigm (Zubin and Spring 1977), it is generally accepted that psychotic disorders represent the outcome of a process of development whereby psychosocial stressors impact on vulnerability factors (usually conceived of as genetic and/or biological) to result in psychotic states and also to determine their subsequent course. Vulnerability factors differ for the range, currently poorly validated, of diagnostic categories of psychotic disorder. They range from neurocognitive, information-processing and motivational impairments in many schizophrenic-type disorders through to liability to lability of mood and disinhibition in those described as bipolar affective. However, it is generally accepted that the impairment of consensual reality-testing and of executive function associated with and characteristic of all psychotic disorders will be generated by both vulnerability factors and psychosocial stressors. From a CAT perspective, the extent to which current models conceptualise the internalisation of such stress would, however, be seen to be in general seriously deficient, characterised on the whole by a simple, additive approach, and predicated on a less radically social understanding of human psychology.

We suggest that the CAT model of development and psychopathology may have much to offer in extending such conceptualisations as well as subsequent approaches to treatment. From the fundamentally social view of mind implicit in the current CAT model of development and psychopathology, all mental activity is heavily determined by and rooted in a repertoire of RRs. It can therefore be seen that disordered mental function, as occurs in psychotic states, can be similarly understood in part as disordered enactment and dissociation of RRs. In normal development, by contrast, the outcome would be the internalisation of an adaptive and integrated repertoire of RRs and consequent metaprocedural integration of the executive functions of the self. This little-emphasised aspect of psychotic disorders has been stressed by some authors (Davidson and Strauss 1992) and has been postulated to be a consequence of impaired information processing (Hemsley 1998) and also to be related to a core inability to generate a theory of mind (Frith and Corcoran 1996). A CAT model suggests that many apparently incomprehensible psychotic phenomena, whether relating to longstanding symptoms such as delusions or acute behavioural disturbances, may be interpreted in terms of disordered or distorted enactments of underlying RRs and disruption of the normally integrated self into dissociated self states. Each of these self states will be characterised by one RR with dissociation resulting in impairment of the ability to self-reflect, as occurs for different reasons in borderline personality disorders (Ryle and Golynkina 2000). Clinical experience using CAT has so far borne out the validity of such a conceptualisation (see also the example below).

Thus the origins of psychotic disorders can be understood from this CAT perspective as lying in the acquisition and enactment of neurotic and maladaptive RRs through the process of internalisation of early experience and in the context of probable neurocognitive abnormalities related to information processing, including social cognition. It can be seen that such individuals may well be experienced as difficult due to their neurocognitive disabilities and, as children, elicit difficult or harsh reactions; or, they may simply experience and misperceive the behaviour of others as critical, hostile or hard to interpret. Such an adverse 'non-shared family environment' could ironically contribute in those already vulnerable by virtue of neurocognitive deficiencies to further stress, and in a 'knock-on' fashion to further possible internal stress and possible neurodevelopmental damage long-term (see Fox *et al.* 1994). In vulnerable individuals it can be seen that maladaptive RRs could be enacted in muddled, amplified or distorted forms in states of stress and contribute to the development of psychotic states. What is more, acquisition of maladaptive and 'self-stressful' RRs in a vulnerable individual could thus in dialectical fashion exacerbate an underlying neurobiological vulnerability due to the well-documented neurotoxic effects of early (including ante-natal: Glover 1997; Schneider *et al.* 1998) stress whether externally imposed or internally generated. It has been suggested that these could be mediated by the toxic effects of stress hormones and effects on the regulation of the neuroendocrine system overall (Walker *et al.* 1996).

From a CAT perspective we have conceived of the internal self-to-self enactment of maladaptive (e.g. harshly self-critical) roles and their associated dialogic voices as 'internal expressed emotion', by analogy with that experienced overtly in a family situation as described previously and which represents a target for therapy. Similarly, a harsh or traumatising early developmental history in reality could lead to neurotoxic effects by similar mechanisms, even in those with minimal genetic or biological loading, so contributing to a developmental vulnerability to subsequent development of psychotic states.

A CAT MODEL OF PSYCHOTIC SYMPTOMS AND EXPERIENCES

From a CAT perspective, and given the above discussion of how early interpersonal experience may be internalised to result in a repertoire of RRs which determine and influence all subsequent mental activity, it is evident that abnormalities of this process would be manifest in psychiatric disorders. It would be predicted that many apparently incomprehensible psychotic phenomena (including both positive and negative symptoms) represent muddled, distorted or amplified enactments of underlying RRs, if these can be mapped out and traced back historically as is usual practice for CAT reformulations. As we have noted previously, clinical experience (and see also the example below) bears out this hypothesis both in terms of understanding and making sense of such phenomena and working therapeutically and collaboratively with patients on them. Examples of commonly encountered internalised reciprocal roles of particular relevance in psychotic disorders include (as noted above) a 'highly (self) criticising' in relation to 'criticised' RR (associated with its dialogic voice) which might be internally enacted resulting in internal expressed emotion, an RRP of 'vengeful anger' in relation to 'abused', and a role of 'idealising help seeking' in relation to 'neglected'. The habitual enactment of these reciprocal role procedures would lead to self-stressful states and emotional isolation (perhaps in conjunction with the enactment internally of a 'coping alone/soldiering on' role), all of which may contribute and exacerbate vulnerability to and development of psychotic states. These states may frequently then be simply misattributed to biological disorder associated with neurocognitive impairments.

Likewise, historic enactments such as 'wariness and suspicion' derived from, for example, being 'treated harshly' might culminate in frank paranoia. Defensive enactments of certain RRs and the effort to make sense of such real experiences could lead to frank delusions which would represent therapeutic targets. Some such experiences might well occur through misattributions (due to neurocognitive deficits) of internalised dialogic voices to external agencies, which will be also culturally determined. Work on the nature and origins of such hallucinations and mapping them out would again represent therapeutic targets in CAT. All of these RRs represent targets therapeutically, both in terms of making sense of experience and in modifying extremely maladaptive RRs and their procedural enactments. This CAT approach may enable modification of such structures through therapy. It may also, we argue, provide a robust and coherent model of these experiences and symptoms for treating staff and therapists within the framework of an overall stress-vulnerability paradigm accounting both for biological/genetic and psychosocial factors in a dialectical mix.

We noted above that an important aspect of psychotic disorder is its systemic dimension and the reactions (as contrasted with considered responses) of staff teams and/or family and friends. They may be unwittingly drawn into unhelpful collusion with the enactments of such RRs and react, for example, by becoming over-involved or, more often, perplexed, hostile and rejecting. Clearly these reactions may in turn perpetuate and confirm the original RR being enacted by a patient. They may also result in a patient being considered 'difficult' (see Ryle and Kerr 2002 for further discussion of this concept from a CAT perspective). Such enactments would also be implicit targets of systemic therapy, although usually considered from a rather different conceptual framework. A final important implication of such a CAT-based model, in common with the hearing voices groups pioneered by Marius Romme (Romme *et al.* 1992), is that it implicitly normalises and destigmatises psychotic experience and disorder.

This model of both psychotic symptomatology and developmental psychopathology will be illustrated briefly by a description of an initial presentation of a psychotic state which demonstrates some of these various points. Use of CAT for longstanding psychotic disorder and also for post-acute psychosis on a locked ward has been described elsewhere (Kerr 2001; Ryle and Kerr 2002).

Case example

(Details have been modified considerably to preserve anonymity.) Wendy was a bright, 20-year-old student who had had a one-month hospital admission one year prior to referral for therapy for an acute psychotic episode during which she had been diagnosed as possibly having a schizo-affective disorder. On the ward she had had paranoid delusions that people were against her and had been 'difficult' and 'delinquent' (for example absconding from the ward), irritable, wary, non-compliant and non-communicative with staff, friends and family. She had gradually recovered but remained anxious and wary; she worried constantly about recurrence and pestered staff about this.

She described a rather difficult relationship with her family. Her parents were self-made business people from poor backgrounds who stressed getting on and coping. Her father frequently quoted business management phrases such as 'keep your cards close to your chest' and being able to 'think out of the box'. Mother was described as practical and only 'spontaneous by arrangement'. At family meetings, however, it transpired that Wendy had been a very intense, active and sensitive young child, in contrast to her siblings, and had always demanded attention and intimacy at the cost of irritating and alienating her family. She had been bullied at school, developed an eating disorder and taken several overdoses but had kept these to herself. She had struggled due to unhappiness with her course at university and was repeating a year when she had her breakdown. In this year she had worked very hard in isolation and had continually struggled to know, she said, what exactly was expected of her. It was at the end of this year that she had had her psychotic breakdown.

At referral she was maintained on low dose neuroleptics but was struggling to cope with the minimal support of a weekly CPN meeting and occasional review by her psychiatrist. She agreed to meet for assessment for therapy with wariness and anxiety, centred initially mostly around the nature of her 'illness' and how to understand it and cope with it, and worries about possible relapse. This was a constant 'terror' to her, as had been the episode (see Figure 10.1).

However, she engaged gradually with only an occasional missed session ('on principle'!) and worked jointly on constructing a diagrammatic reformulation of her usual ways of functioning and also depicting the experience of the psychotic episode. Interestingly, much of this was described in similar terms to the repertoire of RRs which were described and enacted ordinarily. These were clearly maladaptive, leading to internal stress and isolation and provoked incomprehension and fights and arguments with her family. On the other hand she kept her worries from her friends, and it was only when one of her formulated aims suggested that she try to communicate with trusted others (and in therapy) how she really felt, to see what happened, that things changed for the better, to her considerable surprise. She was also set the aim of challenging her 'self-critical and coping alone' voices, again with considerable effect and relief. Figure 10.1 shows her SDR (sequential diagrammatic reformulation) depicting her key RR – 'conditionally loved, criticised, unheard' in relation to 'conditionally loving, criticising' (often of self) and 'not hearing' – their enactments in a classic dilemma (broadly, either rebel or submit and strive to perform) and its consequences. These can be

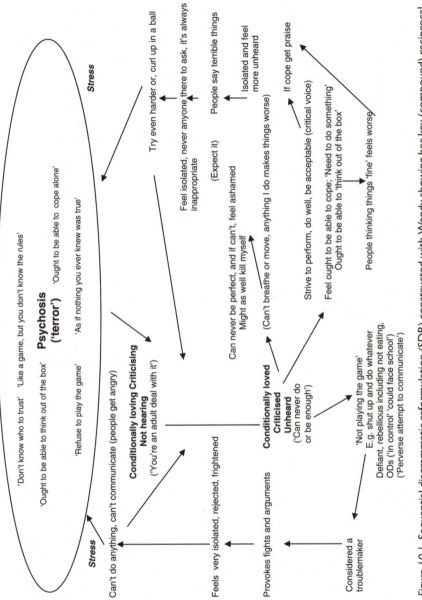

'Don't know who to trust' 'Like a game, but you don't know the rules'

Psychosis ('terror')

'Ought to be able to think out of the box' 'Ought to be able to cope alone'

'Refuse to play the game' 'As if nothing you ever knew was true'

Stress

Stress

Try even harder, or curl up in a ball

Feel isolated, never anyone there to ask, it's always inappropriate | People say terrible things

Isolated and feel more unheard

(Expect it)

Can never be perfect, and if can't, feel ashamed
Might as well kill myself

If cope get praise

Strive to perform, do well, be acceptable (critical voice)

(Can't breathe or move, anything I do makes things worse)

Feel ought to be able to cope; 'Need to do something'
Ought to be able to 'think out of the box'

People thinking things 'fine' feels worse

Can't do anything, can't communicate

Conditionally loving Criticising Not hearing
('You're an adult deal with it')

Conditionally loved Criticised Unheard
('Can never do or be enough')

Feels very isolated, rejected, frightened

Provokes fights and arguments

'Not playing the game'
E.g. shut up and do whatever
Defiant, rebellious including not eating,
ODs ('in control' 'could face school')
('Perverse attempt to communicate')

Considered a troublemaker

Figure 10.1 Sequential diagrammatic reformulation (SDR) constructed with Wendy showing her key (compound) reciprocal role with its procedural enactments and consequences. Those leading to unmanageable stress are noted as is a description of her psychotic breakdown. Many of the experiences and enactments within this are already described in the general map of her usual RRPs, dialogic voices and enactments.

seen to constitute internal stress and also to lead to isolation and friction around her, leading ultimately to her breakdown.

Work in therapy focused on revising these RRs and their procedural enactments; this also involved picking up their enactments in therapy. These included not coming to one session 'on principle', refusing initially to complete questionnaires, keeping things to herself warily and feeling she ought to cope or by turns demanding attention out of hours. This map was also used in a subsequent meeting with the family to considerable effect. Perhaps surprisingly, her parents did not feel 'got at', possibly because the origins of their 'well-meaning' actions were acknowledged, as was the role played by Wendy herself. In this way it functioned as a 'contextual reformulation' (see Ryle and Kerr 2002). This enabled better communication and acknowledgement of limits, which had previously been difficult given that she tended to persist in attempts to obtain emotional recognition from her family with whom she remained enmeshed to a considerable extent.

Other staff also noticed her improved communication and co-operation with them and apparently much diminished levels of stress. Following this intervention she remained stable, was more engaged with outside activities and was planning to resume her studies.

THERAPEUTIC IMPLICATIONS OF A CAT MODEL OF PSYCHOSIS

Given the origins of CAT and its explicitly collaborative therapeutic position, it would be anticipated that CAT will play a helpful role comparable to any generic therapy for patients suffering from a range of psychotic disorders. Garety et al. (2000) have summarised the threefold generic aims of therapy for these disorders: reducing the distress and disability caused by psychotic symptoms, reducing emotional disturbance, and helping the person to arrive at an understanding of psychosis in order to promote the active participation of the individual in the regulation of risk of relapse and social disability.

Most authors in the field stress the importance of a detailed and individual formulation of the patient's problems, ideally in conjunction with the patient. We subscribe to these aims but suggest that it is also important for therapy to offer a meaningful and idiographic account of a patient's experience and distress based on a valid account of deep psychological structures (conceived of as RRs in CAT) originating from the internalisation of early, socially-meaningful, interpersonal experience. Therapy should clearly also offer a means of changing these for the better and enabling the patient to move on and cope with them and the disorder overall. We suggest that the conceptualisation and focus in CAT on the enactment of often dissociated and distorted RRs in psychotic disorders can provide a meaningful and therapeutically helpful picture of disordered mental activity both for patients and those working with them. Its emphasis in particular on the dialogic and social nature of mind, and its explicitly reciprocal and relational approach, assist engagement of and work with more 'difficult' patients. CAT's collaborative and participative approach, in particular the use of diagrammatic reformulations, has been notably successful in achieving this in patients with borderline personality disorder (Ryle and Golynkina 2000), who constitute a similar and difficult patient group. The difficult or 'resistant' patient is recognised to constitute a challenge for all therapies, whether of a cognitive (Leahy 2001) or psychodynamic orientation (see Bateman and Fonagy 1999). Successful work with this group has appeared otherwise to depend to a considerable extent on a co-operative and motivated patient which becomes problematic when s/he enacts, as often occurs, 'therapy-interfering behaviours' (RRs).

Important therapeutic targets in psychotic disorders, from a CAT perspective, are those role enactments or RRPs (reciprocal role procedures) which are 'self-stressful' and constitute 'internal expressed emotion', and RRPs leading to emotional isolation and denial of difficulties which are in themselves stressful. This focus has similarities with the helpful descriptions of tendencies to maladaptive coping styles (such as 'sealing over') by some workers (see Birchwood and Iqbal 1998), but we suggest that CAT can usefully extend this focus to underlying internalised predispositions (RRs) to behave in these ways in a way which is meaningful and helpful to patient and therapist.

CAT also aims, like any effective therapeutic approach, to play an explicitly psychoeducational role around the nature of psychotic disorders and the stress-vulnerability paradigm which patients find on the whole reassuring and normalising.

Thus a CAT-informed approach may offer a coherent and robust account of how a patient's individual narrative and experience can be understood, both in terms of the disorder and distress being experienced and in terms of how it has an impact on vulnerability. Focus on this latter issue raises the interesting question of early intervention in such disorders, particularly given the recent interest and success in targeting not only first-episode but also 'ultra-high-risk' individuals (McGorry *et al.* 2002). The public health implications of this stress-vulnerability informed model are of course considerable for both these and other mental disorders (Albee 1998) and are explored further from a CAT perspective elsewhere (Kerr *et al.* 2003).

Last but not least, experience suggests that such a structured and explicitly mapped-out account of psychotic states can be helpful to staff teams both in working with so-called 'difficult' patients and, importantly, in not colluding with unhelpful maladaptive enactments. We suggest on the basis of recent experience that CAT may play a useful role in extending our therapeutic repertoire at the level of individual therapy, and also as part of a need-adapted, phase-oriented treatment package such as already described by various workers (see Alanen 1997; Cullberg 2001; Hogarty *et al.* 1997). CAT could also provide a conceptual framework around which to base the development and implementation of overall treatment packages (see McGorry 2000) which may also employ other treatment modalities such as pharmacotherapy or social therapy, which are of importance and which would be quite consistent with the CAT model.

Clearly such developments will require further study on a controlled basis. The model needs to be evaluated to determine which of its aspects may be more or less valid and effective in comparison to existing models and treatment modalities. However, we suggest that the preliminary articulation of such a model and its initial clinical evaluation may be a significant step towards this end and we look forward to further dialogue and collaboration with others working in this important and challenging field.

ACKNOWLEDGEMENT

We thank Anthony Ryle for his encouraging and helpful comments on this work.

REFERENCES

Alanen, Y. (1997). *Schizophrenia. Its Origins and Need Adapted Treatment*. London: Karnac.

Albee, G. W. (1998). Primary prevention of mental disorder and promotion of mental health. *Journal of Mental Health* 7: 437–9.

Bateman, A. W. and Fonagy, P. (1999). Psychotherapy for severe personality disorder. *British Medical Journal* 319: 709.

Bennett, D. and Parry, G. (1998). The accuracy of reformulation in cognitive analytic therapy: A validation study. *Psychotherapy Research* 8: 84–103.

Birchwood, M. and Iqbal, Z. (1998). Depression and suicidal thinking in psychosis: A cognitive approach. In T. Wykes *et al.* (eds) (1998) *Outcome and Innovation in Psychological Treatment of Schizophrenia*. Chichester, UK: John Wiley.

Csernansky, J. G. and Grace, A. A. (1998). New models of the pathophysiology of schizophrenia: Editors' introduction. *Schizophrenia Bulletin* 24: 185–7.

Cullberg, J. (2001). The Parachute Project: First episode psychosis – background and treatment. In P. Williams (ed.) *A Language for Psychosis*. London: Whurr.

Davidson, L. and Strauss, J. S. (1992). Sense of self in recovery from severe mental illness. *British Journal of Medical Psychology* 65: 131–45.

Fox, N. A. *et al.* (1994). Neural plasticity and development in the first two years of life: Evidence from cognitive and socioemotional domains of research. *Development and Psychopathology* 6: 677–96.

Frith, C. and Corcoran, R. (1996). Exploring theory of mind in people with schizophrenia. *Psychological Medicine* 26: 521–30.

Garety, P. A. *et al.* (2000). Cognitive behaviour therapy for people with psychosis. In B. V. Martindale *et al.* (eds) *Psychosis: Psychological Approaches and their Effectiveness*. London: Gaskell.

Glover, V. (1997). Maternal stress or anxiety in pregnancy and emotional development of the child. *British Journal of Psychiatry* 171: 105–6.

Hemsley, D. (1998). The disruption of the 'sense of self' in schizophrenia: Potential links with disturbances of information processing. *British Journal of Medical Psychology* 71: 115–24.

Hemsley, D. and Murray, R. M. (2000). Commentary. Psychological and social treatments for schizophrenia: Not just old remedies in new bottles. *Schizophrenia Research* 26: 145–51.

Hogarty, G. E. *et al.* (1997). Three year trials of personal therapy among schizophrenic patients living with or independent of family. I: Description of study and effects on relapse rates. *Journal of the American Psychiatric Association* 154: 1504–13.

Holmes, J. (1998). Narrative in psychotherapy. In C. Mace (ed.) *Heart and Soul.* London: Routledge.

Kerr, I. B. (2001). Brief cognitive analytic therapy for post-acute manic psychosis on a psychiatric intensive care unit. *Clinical Psychology and Psychotherapy* 8: 117–29.

Kerr, I. B. *et al.* (2000). Cognitive analytic therapy (CAT)-based approaches to psychotic disorders: A preliminary model. *Acta Psychiatrica Scandinavica* 102 (suppl. 404): 6–7.

Kerr, I. B. *et al.* (2003). Clinical and service implications of a cognitive analytic therapy (CAT) model of psychosis. *Australian and New Zealand Journal of Psychiatry* 37: 515–23.

Leahy, R. L. (2001). *Overcoming Resistance in Cognitive Therapy.* New York: Guilford Press.

Leiman, M. (1997). Procedures as dialogical sequences: A revised version of the fundamental concept in cognitive analytic therapy. *British Journal of Medical Psychology* 70: 193–207.

Martindale, B. V. *et al.* (2000). *Psychosis: Psychological Approaches and their Effectiveness.* London: Gaskell.

McGorry, P. (2000). Psychotherapy and recovery in early psychosis: A core clinical and research challenge. In B. V. Martindale *et al.* (eds) *Psychosis: Psychological Approaches and their Effectiveness.* London: Gaskell.

McGorry, P. D. *et al.* (2002). Randomised controlled trial of interventions designed to reduce the risk of progression to first episode psychosis in a clinical sample with subthreshold symptoms. *Archives of General Psychiatry* 59: 921–8.

Nuechterlein, K. H. and Subotnik, K. L. (1998). The cognitive origins of schizophrenia and prospects for intervention. In T. Wykes *et al.* (eds) *Outcome and Innovation in Psychological Treatment of Schizophrenia.* Chichester, UK: John Wiley.

Pollock, P. H. (2001). Cognitive analytic therapy for borderline erotomania: Forensic romances and violence in the therapy room. *Clinical Psychology and Psychotherapy* 8: 214–29.

Romme, M. *et al.* (1992). Coping with voices: An emancipatory approach. *British Journal of Psychiatry* 161: 99–103.

Ryle, A. (1990). *Cognitive Analytic Therapy: Active Participation in Change.* Chichester, UK: Wiley and Sons.

Ryle, A. (1991). Object relations theory and activity theory: A proposed link by way of the procedural sequence model. *British Journal of Medical Psychology* 64: 307–16.

Ryle, A. (ed.) (1995). *Cognitive Analytic Therapy: Developments in Theory and Practice*. Chichester, UK: John Wiley and Sons.

Ryle, A. and Golynkina, K. (2000). Effectiveness of time-limited cognitive analytic therapy for borderline personality disorder: Factors associated with outcome. *British Journal of Medical Psychology* 73: 197–210.

Ryle, A. and Kerr, I. B. (2002). *Introducing Cognitive Analytic Therapy: Principles and Practice*. Chichester, UK: John Wiley and Sons.

Schneider, M. L. *et al.* (1998). Prenatal stress alters brain biogenic amine levels in primates. *Development and Psychopathology* 10: 427–40.

Trevarthen, C. and Aitken, K. J. (2001). Infant intersubjectivity: Research, theory and clinical applications. *Journal of Child Psychology and Psychiatry* 42: 3–48.

Walker, E. F. *et al.* (1996). The developmental pathways to schizophrenia: Potential moderating effects of stress. *Development and Psychopathology* 8: 647–65.

Wykes, T., Tarrier, N. and Lewis, S. (eds) (1998). *Outcome and Innovation in Psychological Treatment of Schizophrenia*. Chichester, UK: John Wiley.

Zubin, J. and Spring, B. (1977). Vulnerability: A new view of schizophrenia. *Journal of Abnormal Psychology* 86: 103–26.

Chapter 11

Cognitive remediation of patients with schizophrenia

Does it work?

Bjørn Rishovd Rund

In recent years it has been reliably demonstrated that 60–70% of patients with schizophrenia have persistent abnormalities of various types of cognitive dysfunction. It has also been shown that, to a certain degree, these abnormalities antecede the psychosis – that is, they are present during the prodromal period and are relatively specific for schizophrenia. It is therefore important to recognise routinely those with cognitive deficits and find methods of improving cognitive functioning, because these deficits influence patients' abilities to function well in the community and are related to their capabilities for social perception and learning social skills. It could be argued that attention should be given to these difficulties from the earliest phase of the illness to maximise rehabilitation potentials. This chapter will review evidence of the effectiveness of therapies that focus on these cognitive dysfunctions, describe current research and suggest where future research should be focused.

INTRODUCTION

Even though modern antipsychotics and psychosocial treatment programmes are effective in moderating symptoms and reducing the rate of relapse, most patients with schizophrenia do not function well outside structured, routine settings such as hospital wards. Outcomes other than symptom improvement and relapse prevention have not been well documented (Hogarty and Flesher 1999; Lehman *et al.* 1995). The majority of patients with schizophrenia handle ordinary social settings in a conspicuous way, and they do not manage an ordinary work or school situation very well. On average only 10–30% of patients with schizophrenia are employed at any time, and few of these are able to maintain their vocational gains (Attkisson *et al.* 1992; Hogarty and Flesher 1999). What is the reason for this?

Many clinicians now claim it is because of their serious cognitive disturbances. Several prominent researchers and clinicians have pointed out that cognitive dysfunction is the enduring core feature of schizophrenia. Some have called schizophrenia a thought disorder. Evidence from neuropsychological, neuropathological and neuroimaging studies has documented schizophrenia as a neuropsychiatric disease. Most cognitive dysfunctions seem to remain impaired to some degree when symptoms improve. Nancy Andreasen (1999) argues that the definition of schizophrenia should be rooted in basic cognitive disturbances rather than phenomenology.

The fundamental importance of cognitive deficits in schizophrenia is also substantiated by the fact that cognitive functions have proven to be of much greater significance in the prediction of prognosis and outcome than the symptoms of the illness. Patients with the most serious cognitive dysfunctions appear to have the poorest outcome. Different dysfunctions seem to relate to different functional outcomes: verbal memory, for instance, is related to all types of functional outcomes (Silverstein *et al.* 2001). Vigilance, which means the ability to focus attention over time, and poor attention span predict social problem-solving, acquisition of social skills, community outcomes and work performance (ibid.). Executive functioning – which includes functions and capabilities such as planning, abstract thinking, flexibility and the ability to make use of feedback – predicts the ability to function in the community (Sharma 1999). Impairment in cognitive processing seems to mediate the acquisition of behavioural competencies in schizophrenia. We still have limited knowledge, however, about the underlying mechanisms through which cognitive dysfunctions operate on behaviour and social functions.

What Hogarty and Flesher (1999) call social cognition – that is, the ability to act wisely in social interactions – is an important constraint on social and vocational recovery. Klosterkötter and Schultze-Lutter (2000) have shown that cognitive prodromal symptoms are the only ones with a high diagnostic efficiency: cognitive prodromal symptoms have high specificity and positive predictive powers as well as low rates of false-positive prediction. Klosterkötter claims that because of the high predictive value of these cognitive symptoms, it seems possible that a diagnosis of schizophrenia might be made during the prodromal period. He concludes that in the future an early intervention focusing on the cognitive abnormality might enable prevention of first psychotic episodes.

The fact that deviance in cognitive functions is a core deficit in schizophrenia makes them an appropriate target for treatment and rehabilitation. The obvious area to try to ameliorate is the one that is most impaired and most damaging for the person's psychosocial functioning. However, cognitive and neuropsychological deficits in schizophrenia as the basis for therapeutic interventions have so far been greatly neglected, and in spite of some promising results, attempts at cognitive remediation have been sparse. In my opinion, effective techniques for normalising or neutralising cognitive impairments would be a decisive addition to the treatment armamentarium for patients with a psychotic illness in general and patients with schizophrenia in particular.

In this chapter, a review of what has been done so far in this area will be given. Methodological problems related to therapeutic approaches and research in the field will be raised. Then a description will be given of the cognitive training programme developed at the University of Oslo and now in use at the Sogn Center for Child and Adolescent Psychiatry (SSBU). Finally, some preliminary results from a controlled study in which the effects of cognitive training are compared to a psychosocial treatment programme will be presented.

PREVIOUS STUDIES ON COGNITIVE REMEDIATION IN SCHIZOPHRENIC PATIENTS

There are two distinctly different approaches to cognitive therapy with schizophrenic patients: one focuses on cognitive content while the other is process-oriented, emphasising the correction of basic cognitive deficits.

The content-oriented cognitive approach is carried out according to the principles of cognitive therapy as described by, for instance, Beck and associates (Beck 1976, 1990; Beck et al. 1979) for the treatment of depression and other emotional disorders. However, some modifications are necessary for severely disturbed patients. Outstanding advocates of this approach in schizophrenia treatment are Perris (1989), Fowler and Morley (1989), Bentall and collaborators (1994) and Kingdon and Turkington (1994). Perris's meta-cognitive approach has been developed in small, community-based and family-style treatment centres in Sweden. Most of the treatment takes place in small groups. Bentall and associates (1994) have developed a more behaviourally-oriented treatment package that directly targets persistent auditory hallucinations. Their therapeutic programme consists of procedures for fostering attribution of hallucinations to the self rather than to external sources, and for diminishing the distress provoked by hearing voices. Kingdon and Turkington (1994) contend that people with schizophrenia are not inherently irrational, but instead suffer from a circumscribed set of irrational beliefs. Their therapeutic approach attempts to help patients in alleviating the impact of these beliefs. The treatment programme of Fowler and colleagues (Garety et al. 1994) focuses on techniques aimed at modifying psychotic thoughts.

The aim of the process-oriented approach is remediation of deficits in cognitive processes rather than changing distorted thoughts, attitudes, beliefs or hallucinations (Adams et al. 1981). This treatment strategy originated in the areas of experimental psychopathology and the neuropsychology of schizophrenia. Specific cognitive impairments detected in the laboratory are the target of change, first in the lab and later in increasingly realistic situations (Spaulding et al. 1999; Wykes et al. 1999). As such, this treatment approach has much in common with models for rehabilitation of head traumas. The present review will be limited to this approach and the empirical studies which have examined the effects of such therapeutic programmes.

There were a few clinical studies in the late 1960s and 1970s that all reported encouraging results. After this promising beginning, the research lay dormant for more than a decade.

Interest in cognitive training programmes based on empirical research was to some extent rekindled in the 1990s. A few more comprehensive training programmes have been developed, and the effects of some of them have been examined (Brenner 1989; Fowler 1992; Spaulding *et al.* 1999). In addition to these well-founded treatment programmes, there have also been several attempts to remediate more specific, elementary attentional and conceptual functions.

Brenner and colleagues (1995) have developed the most complete therapeutic programme – so-called integrated psychological therapy (IPT). IPT is a multi-element hierarchical programme in which enhancement of basic cognitive capacities is attempted before problem-solving and motor skills training is implemented. IPT is a step-by-step procedure devised for groups of five to seven patients. It comprises five subprogrammes: cognitive differentiation, social perception, communication skills, interpersonal problem-solving and social skills training. The rationale for IPT is that remediation of cognitive deficits will facilitate acquisition and maintenance of more complex skills.

A series of studies of IPT have demonstrated significant treatment effects on cognitive functions and reduction in symptomatology (Hodel and Brenner 1994). However, it has not been documented whether remediation of cognitive functions has a pervasive effect on social behaviour.

In the USA Will Spaulding has adapted and elaborated Brenner's IPT programme. Spaulding's group has published the results from a study in which 90 subjects with severe and disabling psychiatric conditions, predominantly schizophrenia, participated in a controlled-outcome trial (Spaulding *et al.* 1999). Patients receiving the cognitive training programme, consisting of the three cognitive modules in Brenner's IPT, were compared to control subjects who received supportive group therapy. Treatment was given during intensive six-month periods. All subjects also received an enriched regimen of comprehensive psychiatric rehabilitation, including social and living skills training. Patients receiving cognitive training showed incrementally greater gains than controls on the primary outcome measures. There was equivocal evidence for greater improvement in the cognitive training group on a disorganisation factor for psychiatric symptoms (the Brief Psychiatric Rating Scale), and strong evidence for greater improvement on a laboratory measure of attention processing (span of apprehension/continuous performance test). Significant improvement was also found on two measures of attention (apprehension/backward masking), memory (Rey Auditory and Visual Learning Test) and executive functioning (card sorting).

Wykes and collaborators (1999) have reported some results of a controlled trial of individual neurocognitive therapy. The effects of cognitive remediation were compared to those of a control therapy, which consisted of intensive occupational therapy to control for non-specific effects of treatment. The cognitive remediation programme is based on procedural and errorless learning, and uses targeted reinforcement and extensive practice. In a randomised control trial of 33 patients with schizophrenia, results suggest a differential effect in favour of cognitive rehabilitation for tests in the cognitive flexibility and memory subgroups, as well as for self-esteem, but not for symptoms or social functioning. However, generalised improvements in cognitive flexibility were related to improvements in social functioning.

Attempts to remediate more specific cognitive dysfunction have mainly concentrated on two areas: conceptual skills and attentional skills. Conceptual skills have been trained mostly by means of the Wisconsin Card Sorting Test. These studies all show some positive effects of training. The greatest gains have been attained by providing positive reinforcement for correct solutions. It has not been possible to demonstrate any evidence of generalisation to improved executive functions. Bellack and co-workers (1999) showed that schizophrenic patients trained on one of two problem-solving tasks similar to the WCST exhibited a marked improvement on the trained task. However, subjects trained on one test performed no better on the other instrument than subjects who received practice only.

Moving on to attentional skills, two of the most common measures are the CPT and the span task. Benedict and associates (1994) used six training tasks which all required sustained vigilance and a high degree of mental effort. An experimental group, which received sessions of guided practice on the training tasks, were compared to a no-treatment control group. Results showed improved performance on the training tasks for the experimental group. However, no significant changes on the outcome measures were observed. Benedict et al. (1994) therefore conclude that the rather substantial practice effect demonstrated did not denote an improvement in fundamental cognitive skill.

The conclusion of Benedict and associates (1994) is in accordance with the view of Bellack and collaborators (1999b). They are sceptical as to whether cognitive rehabilitation of schizophrenic patients is an achievable goal. They admit that practice can improve performance on specific tasks, but state that there is little evidence for the generalisability of such training. Thus, they claim that the task for schizophrenia researchers is to develop real-world training programmes.

However, some more positive attempts to reduce attention deficits in patients with schizophrenia have also been carried out. Kern and associates (1995) compared four groups of schizophrenic patients with regard to improved performance on a span task. Findings revealed that a combination of monetary reinforcement and instructional cues was superior to the other interventions. In the Oslo Cognitive Training Programme, which will be outlined later, we have included intensive span training with reinforcement, similar to that used by Kern and associates.

Hermanutz and Gestrich (1991) showed that it was possible to reduce the distraction of schizophrenic patients on reaction-time tasks. With training, the patients attained the same results as healthy individuals.

Olbrich *et al.* (1993) found clearly positive effects of a training module that addresses a combination of attentional, mnemonic and conceptual skills.

Van der Gaag (1992) employed a clinical rehabilitation programme and showed that although the training programme was effective in some processing domains, it did not affect tasks that rely on fast processing of information.

Medalia *et al.* (1998) assessed the impact of attention training on chronic schizophrenia patients. They found that it is feasible to use practice and behavioural learning to remediate core attention deficits in this patient group.

It should be mentioned that a few attempts have also been made to improve memory in schizophrenic patients. For instance, Koh and colleagues (1976) showed that patients were able to increase recall on a memory task to levels close to those of normal control subjects when their encoding was aided by rating the stimuli (words) in terms of pleasantness.

A recent issue of *Schizophrenia Bulletin* (1999 issue 1) was based on interventions for neurocognitive deficits in schizophrenia. Here several outstanding therapists and researchers ask pertinent questions about the results and designs of cognitive remediation research. As mentioned before, Bellack *et al.* (1999b) point out that the critical question in selecting neurocognitive targets is that of generalisability. Silverstein *et al.* also conclude that 'treating neurocognitive deficits in schizophrenia do[es] not provide strong evidence of their effectiveness or generalisability' (Silverstein *et al.* 2001: 249). They question how far-reaching the effects of training in any basic information-processing domain are. Bellack and his collaborators propose an alternative to the cognitive rehabilitation programmes mentioned above. They claim that a compensatory model is much more appropriate. Their emphasis is not on eliminating impairment as much as on minimising the resulting disability. Bellack and associates are critical of the belief that the neurodevelopmental nature of impairments defies simple solution. Further, they don't believe that rehabilitation strategies that depend primarily on repeated practice of neuropsychological tasks yield much improvement in the underlying cognitive operations or have much benefit for community functioning.

Green and Nuechterlein (1999) point out another important issue: some neurocognitive deficits in schizophrenia are rather stable over time, and it would be unreasonable to expect long-standing deficits to improve permanently with a short-lived treatment. They also point out that the key question is whether changes in neurocognition translate into changes in functional outcome.

As can be seen from this review, results from empirical research have been inconsistent. I will now elaborate on whether remediation of cognitive disorders is possible by turning my attention to a controlled treatment study in which the effects of a broad cognitive training programme are examined.

PHARMACOLOGICAL TREATMENT OF COGNITIVE DEFICITS

First, quite briefly: do we have means other than psychological techniques to reduce or remove cognitive deficits? How do neuroleptics affect cognitive dysfunctions in schizophrenia?

Current studies have provided mixed results in all the cognitive and psychophysiological areas as to the impact of conventional neuroleptics. What can be said is that there is not yet sufficient empirical evidence for dramatic effects of conventional neuroleptics, either towards improvement or impairment. Anticholinergic medication adversely affects memory and learning in schizophrenic patients (for a more thorough review, see Rund 1999).

The new antipsychotic drugs seem to have a more positive effect on cognitive functions than conventional neuroleptics. However, only a few publications have appeared so far discussing the effects of risperidone (Risperdal); the same is the case with regard to olanzapine (Zyprexa). Whether the improvement shown with the novel neuroleptics is of statistical significance only, or will prove to be of clinical significance as well, remains to be assessed (Rund 1999).

THE OSLO COGNITIVE TRAINING PROGRAMME: A CONTROLLED TREATMENT STUDY

The cognitive training programme developed at SSBU in Oslo aims to improve cognitive functioning, and develop and strengthen cognitive skills, and takes into account the specific psychopathological characteristics of schizophrenia. The Oslo Cognitive Training Programme is based on research demonstrating that the most significant dysfunctions in schizophrenia can be related to the areas of attention, memory and executive functions. In the 'Oslo Approach', we have attempted to develop a programme that covers all the mentioned areas of dysfunction.

The treatment programme is, however, also based on the assumption that cognitive impairment is a key characteristic in other psychotic disorders (see Rund *et al.* 2004). A broad spectrum of psychotic patients is, thus, included in the study (see Rund 2003; Rund and Borg 1999).

Based on the literature review presented, there are several uncertainties regarding the effectiveness of cognitive training in psychotic patients. As mentioned, no definite answer can yet be given to the main question: Can basic cognitive functions be remediated?

Another important unanswered question is: Is it possible to generalise training effects to other functions, and register this by the use of appropriate (cognitive and clinical) follow-up instruments? These are all questions addressed in the present study. However, in this chapter the focus will be on the cognitive outcome measures. Results on clinical measures are presented in Ueland and Rund (2004, 2005).

The controlled treatment study at SSBU aims to investigate to what extent this cognitive training programme can be a positive clinical supplement to a previously documented psychoeducational training programme that has proven quite effective (Rund *et al.* 1994). The psychoeducational programme was carried out at SSBU in the late 1980s and early 1990s. The outcome of this programme was compared with a standard reference treatment. Clinical outcome was assessed by relapses during the two-year treatment period, and changes in psychosocial functioning as measured by the Global Assessment Scale. Results indicated that the most effective programme measured by relapse was also the cheapest – the psychoeducational programme. Psychosocial functioning improved more in the psychoeducational group than in the group that received standard reference treatment. Patients with poor premorbid psychosocial functioning benefit most from this treatment.

In the controlled treatment study at SSBU, the question is whether a cognitive training programme can add anything to the effects of a psychoeducational programme alone: this was assessed by comparing two groups at baseline, post-treatment and at a one-year follow-up. One (Group A) received the psychoeducational programme only and the other (Group B) received the same psychoeducational treatment package and the cognitive training programme. We chose a battery of outcome measures to evaluate the effects of treatment on cognition as well as psychiatric symptoms (BPRS) and psychosocial functioning (Global Assessment Scale, GAS). Our aim was to have 15 patients in each of the two groups, all with optimal pharmacotherapy. Patients were between 12 and 18 years old; all were psychotic or had had psychotic episodes with a DSM-IV diagnosis within a broad schizophrenia spectrum area.

The training programme

The programme is arranged in four modules: cognitive differentiation, attention, memory and social perception. The first module, cognitive differentiation, is based on the supposition of a generalised impairment in verbal intelligence, abstraction-flexibility and auditory processing which is congruent with a left-hemispheric dysfunction hypothesis. Much of Brenner *et al.*'s (1995) original methodology is adapted for these tasks.

The second module addresses the area of attention and considers impairment of attention to be a central feature of schizophrenia. With the assumption that deficits in attention are part of an underlying mechanism of cognitive dysfunction, tasks aim to strengthen sustained attention over time, and to train selective attention and scanning abilities.

Memory is the focus of the third module, which is based on studies involving both verbal and visual memory. Tasks, which primarily involve short-term recall, aim to improve patients' ability to recall an increasing number of items.

The final module involves social perception, which involves the cognitive processes that allow the patient to respond and adapt appropriately to his or her environment.

Training in verbal communication, attention, memory and social perception is conducted via systematic training procedures. During the first module, cognitive differentiation, patients learn to discriminate between stimulus categories by participating in a card-sorting task. After demonstrating competence on this task, patients are introduced to a concept formation task where they are instructed to match antonyms and synonyms, distinguish concepts with different definitions and establish a hierarchy of related concepts (Brenner *et al.* 1995). Attention and memory modules are presented simultaneously with the concept formation task. Following these modules, patients participate in the social perception module where they are trained to encode social stimuli by viewing a series of slides showing actors in different social activities and demonstrating emotions of varied intensity.

In the fourth module the focus is on improving the patient's ability to attend to the statements of others; to improve the patient's ability to understand accurately what was said; and to encourage association between the patient's thoughts and the statements of those with whom they interact. This training attempts to address the lack of integration between strategies that target information processing and social learning dysfunction.

Programme structure

The four modules are systematically introduced to the patient over a period of 8–10 weeks. The training consists of 30–35 hours of individual training organised into 15-minute work sessions. The programme is developed such that the patient begins with elementary tasks and progresses to more difficult ones. The rate of progression is determined by the individual's functioning; however, a standard protocol provides the structure for progression.

In addition to the cognitive training programme outlined above, all patients in Group B participated in an intensive span of apprehension training.

In apprehension training, patients are administered the same computerised version of the span of apprehension task in six different sessions: at baseline, on three consecutive days of intervention, immediately post-test (after Session 1, 2, 3, 4 or 5), and at a 10-day follow-up (see Kern *et al.* 1995). The span task is run on an IBM computer. There are 128 test trials, consisting of 3- and 12-letter arrays. Patients are instructed to identify which of two target letters (T or F) appear on the screen by pressing one of two buttons (marked T and F, respectively) on a control pad as quickly as possible. During interventions 2, 3 and 4, patients receive both monetary reinforcement and enhanced instructions. The reward (50 øre = 5p) is given immediately following a correct response by dropping the coin into a metal container placed to the patient's right. Improved performance is reinforced; several reports have indicated that shaping is an effective method of increasing attention span (Silverstein *et al.* 2001).

Initiation of the programme

Following completion of baseline measures of the patient's current level of functioning, he/she is given a standard introduction to the training programme and develops a training schedule together with the therapist. We have chosen to implement our programme individually instead of in a group. Early on in the development of the training, it became clear that the patients themselves preferred individual sessions as opposed to group sessions. In addition, individual sessions allow the therapist to take into consideration the tremendous variation in cognitive functioning, and thus progress at an appropriate rate while adhering to the standard protocol. The cognitive training for the most part takes place in the school at the clinic. A teacher is responsible for this part of the programme. A few tasks, such as the visual scanning task 'Where is Willy', take place in the ward.

Results

Data are as yet not completely analysed. I want to stress that the number of patients is small.

The primary question asked in the present study is whether the cognitive training programme adds anything to the psychosocial (psychoeducative) programme. Results show an improvement in both groups' performance both at post-test (after five months of treatment) and at follow-up one year later, but no significant performance difference between those who have received cognitive training and those who have not. An exception seems to be early visual information processing where the remediation had a favourable long-term effect. The conclusion that can be drawn from these results is that the treatment (or the natural course of the illness) contributes to an improvement in patients' cognitive functioning. However, it is uncertain whether the cognitive training programme contributes specifically to the improvement (see Ueland and Rund 2004, 2005 for more complete results on post-test and one-year follow-up).

The second question that can be asked at the present stage of the study is this: Is it possible to improve patients' attentional performance (concentration) by intensive training over a week, and with monetary reinforcement and enhanced instructions added to the intervention? Figure 11.1 indicates that span of apprehension performance can be improved by cognitive training (see Ueland *et al.* 2004 for results from more complete data).

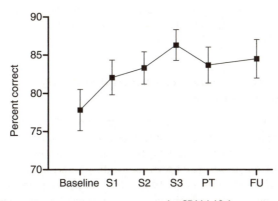

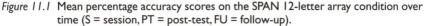

Figure 11.1 Mean percentage accuracy scores on the SPAN 12-letter array condition over time (S = session, PT = post-test, FU = follow-up).

Source: Ueland, T. *et al.* (2004). Reprinted with permission from Blackwell Publishing.

CONCLUSIONS

Taken together, the results from the studies of Brenner (Hodel and Brenner 1994), Spaulding *et al.* (1999), Wykes *et al.* (1999), and the preliminary findings in our project, point to the following answers to the questions asked in this study.

Can basic cognitive functions be remediated?

Yes, cognitive remediation works in the sense that it is possible to remediate cognitive dysfunctions in psychotic patients. What works is uncertain, however. Our preliminary results provide no basis for assuming that the cognitive training programme is more effective than the psychoeducational programme alone. This stands in a certain contrast to the findings of Spaulding and Wykes. It might be, however, that our psychoeducational therapy includes elements that are more effective at improving cognitive skills than the treatment given to the comparison groups in the two other studies. It is also possible that the number of training hours in the Oslo Cognitive Training Programme is not sufficient and need to be expanded in order to obtain significant results.

Is it possible to generalise training effects to other functions, and register this by use of appropriate (cognitive and clinical) follow-up instruments?

Our analyses as yet do not answer the question of whether cognitive training has an effect on social functions, symptoms and daily functioning. However, it is important to have realistic expectations. As already mentioned there is little evidence in the studies mentioned above for the generalisability of cognitive training.

Is it possible to improve attentional skills by intensive span training?

Yes: more intensive training sessions, combined with reinforcement, are effective in improving concentration (continuous focusing of attention). This has been shown in the present study (see Ueland *et al.* 2004 for final results), as well as in several previous studies (Hermanutz and Gestrich 1991; Kern *et al.* 1995; Koh *et al.* 1976). The challenge is to determine how to obtain lasting results which have an impact on the patient's daily functioning.

We have learned that it is difficult to carry out a systematic and consistent cognitive training programme in a clinical setting. First of all, it is difficult to be totally sure that the treatment provided to the two patient groups is in accordance with the therapy manuals. It is also very difficult to control for the effects of neuroleptics. It would be impossible, for ethical reasons, either to withdraw all patients from antipsychotic medication or to give all patients a standard dosage of medicines. Further, the researcher cannot require that all patients be on the same drug and the same dosage over a treatment period that lasts for at least 18 months.

Should the 'experiment' of cognitive remediation of psychotic patients continue? In my opinion, the answer is yes. We have sufficient positive results to do that. We have not received any reports of negative results or negative consequences of cognitive training. More data and new analyses of which variables are related to each other might throw light on which factors are influencing cognitive functions. Most likely, the improvement found in our study cannot be attributed to the inherent process of the illness alone (spon-taneous remission), independent of the treatment received. We have sufficient empirical evidence that the typical course of schizophrenia is one with many relapses, where the level of social and cognitive functioning goes up and down. With a longitudinal design such as ours, where the patient is assessed at an interval of five then 18 months, there is reason to assume that no average improvement would have been found for the group if no treatment factors had been influencing cognitive functioning.

It is important to remediate cognitive dysfunctions in patients with schizo-phrenia. Treatment programmes that do not take cognitive functions into consideration are of limited interest and value. Thus, in my opinion, there are no alternatives to cognitive training programmes today. Therefore, I think it is necessary to work hard to develop further our therapeutic inter-ventions. The only way to do this is to provide empirical evidence for what works and what does not work. From a clinical perspective, it is warranted to individualise a cognitive training programme for each individual patient, according to the deficits disclosed by baseline assessments. A related challenge is to find out which patients benefit from cognitive training and which do not (cf. Silverstein *et al.* 2001). For example, 30–40% of patients with schizophrenia do not demonstrate any significant cognitive deficits: should these patients be excluded from cognitive training programmes? Or is it more reasonable to think that these patients' cognitive performance will benefit from training programmes as well, even though they are within the normal range?

In order to answer these and related questions it may be necessary to undertake case studies. However, research based on individualised therapeutic interventions continues to be problematic. Thus, a first step towards creating an evidence-based therapy for patients with schizophrenia – to assess what works and what does not work – seems to be controlled-effect studies where the effects of therapeutic programmes/manuals are studied at a group level.

REFERENCES

Adams, H. E. *et al.* (1981). Modification of cognitive procesesses: A case study of schizophrenia. *Journal of Consulting and Clinical Psychology* 49: 460–4.

Andreasen, N. C. (1999). A unitary model of schizophrenia. Bleuler's 'Fragmente Phrene' as schizencephaly. *Archives of General Psychiatry* 56: 781–6.

Attkisson, C. *et al.* (1992). Clinical services, research. *Schizophrenenia Bulletin* 18: 561–626.

Beck, A. T. (1976). *Cognitive Therapy and the Emotional Disorders*. New York: International Universities Press.

Beck, A. T. (1990). *Cognitive Therapy of Personality Disorders*. New York: Guilford Press.

Beck, A. T. *et al.* (1979). *Cognitive Therapy of Depression*. Chichester, UK: Wiley.

Bellack, A. S. *et al.* (1999a). Generalization effects of training on the Wisconsin Card Sorting Test for schizophrenia patients. *Schizophrenia Research* 19: 189–94.

Bellack, A. S. *et al.* (1999b). Cognitive rehabilitation for schizophrenia: Problems, prospects, and strategies. *Schizophrenia Bulletin* 25: 257–74.

Benedict, R. H. B. *et al.* (1994). The effects of attention training on information processing in schizophrenia. *Schizophrenia Bulletin* 20: 537–46.

Bentall, R. P. *et al.* (1994). Cognitive behaviour therapy for persistent auditory hallucinations: From theory to therapy. *Behaviour Therapy* 25: 51–66.

Brenner, H. D. (1989). The treatment of basic psychological dysfunctions from a systemic point of view. *British Journal of Psychiatry* 155 (suppl. 5): 74–83.

Brenner, H. *et al.* (1995). *Integrated Psychological Therapy for Schizophrenic Patients*. Bern: Hogrefe and Huber.

Fowler, D. (1992). Cognitive behaviour therapy in management of patients with schizophrenia. Preliminary studies. In A. Werbart and J. Cullberg (eds) *Psychotherapy of Schizophrenia: Facilitating an Abstractive Factor*. Oslo: Scandinavian Univiversity Press.

Fowler, D. and Morley, D. (1989). The cognitive behavioural treatment of hallucin-ations and delusions: A preliminary study. *Behaviour Psychotherapy* 17: 267–82.

Garety, P. A. *et al.* (1994). Cognitive behavioural therapy for drug resistant psychosis. *British Journal of Medical Psychology* 67: 259–71.

Green, M. F. and Nuechterlein, K. (1999). Should schizophrenia be treated as a neurocogitive disorder? *Schizophrenia Bulletin* 25: 309–19.

Hermanutz, M. and Gestrich, J. (1991). Computer-assisted attention training in schizophrenics. A comparative study. *European Archives of Psychiatry and Clinical Neuroscience* 240: 282–7.

Hodel, B. and Brenner, H. D. (1994). Cognitive therapy with schizophrenic patients: Conceptual basis, present state, future directions. *Acta Psychiatrica Scandinavia*, 90 (suppl. 384): 108–15.

Hogarty, G. E. and Flesher, S. (1999). Developmental theory for a cognitive enhance-ment therapy of schizophrenia. *Schizophrenia Bulletin* 25: 677–92.

Kern, R. S. *et al.* (1995). Modification of performance on the Span of Apprehension, a putative marker of vulnerability to schizophrenia. *Journal of Abnormal Psychology* 104: 385–89.

Kingdon, D. G. and Turkington, D. (1994). *Cognitive-Behavioural Therapy of Schizo-phrenia.* Hillside, NJ: Guildford Press.

Klosterkøtter, J. and Schultze-Lutter, F. (2000). Diagnosing schizophrenia in the initial prodomal phase [Abstract]. *Schizophrenia Research* 41: 10.

Koh, S. D. *et al.* (1976). Affective encoding and consequent remembering in schizo-phrenic young adults. *Journal of Abnormal Psychology* 85: 56–166.

Lehman, A. F. *et al.* (1995). Treatment outcomes in schizophrenia: Implication for practice, policy and research. *Schizophrenia Bulletin* 21: 669–74.

Medalia, A. *et al.* (1998). Effectiveness of attention training in schizophrenia. *Schizophrenia Bulletin* 24: 147–52.

Olbrich, R. *et al.* (1993). A weighted time budget approach for the assessment of cogni-tive and social activities. *Social Psychiatry and Psychiatric Epidemiology* 28: 184–8.

Perris, C. (1989). *Cognitive Therapy for Patients with Schizophrenia.* New York: Cassell.

Rund, B. R. (1999). How do neuroleptics affect cognitive functions in schizophrenia? *Nordic Journal of Psychiatry* 53: 121–5.

Rund, B. R. (2003). Neuropsychiatric rehabilitation of schizophrenia. In P. Halligan *et al.* (eds) *Handbook of Clinical Neuropsychology.* Oxford, UK: Oxford University Press.

Rund, B. R. and Borg, N. C. (1999). Cognitive deficits and cognitive training in schizophrenic patients: A review. *Acta Psychiatrica Scandinavica* 99: 1–12.

Rund, B. R. *et al.* (1994). The Psychosis Project: Outcome and cost-effectiveness of a psychoeducational treatment programme for schizophrenic adolescents. *Acta Psychiatrica Scandinavia* 89: 211–8.

Rund, B. R. *et al.* (2004). Neurocognitive dysfunction in first-episode psychosis: Cor-relates with symptoms, premorbid adjustment, and duration of untreated psychosis. *American Journal of Psychiatry* 161: 466–72.

Sharma, T. (1999). Cognitive effects of conventional and atypical antipychotics in schizophrenia. *British Journal of Psychiatry* 174 (suppl. 38): 44–51.

Silverstein, S. M. *et al.* (2001). Shaping attention span: An operant conditioning procedure to improve neurocognition and functioning in schizophrenia. *Schizo-phrenia Bulletin* 27: 247–57.

Spaulding, W. D. *et al.* (1999). Effects of cognitive treatment in psychiatric rehabilitation. *Schizophrenia Bulletin* 25: 657–76.

Ueland, T. and Rund, B. R. (2004). A controlled randomized treatment study: The effects of a cognitive remediation program on adolescents with early onset psychosis. *Acta Psychiatrica Scandinavica* 109: 70–4.

Ueland, T. and Rund, B. R. (2005). Cognitive remediation for adolescents with early onset psychosis: A 1-year follow-up study. *Acta Psychiatrica Scandinavica* 111: 193–201.

Ueland, T. *et al.* (2004). Modification of performance on the Span of Apprehension Task in a group of young people with early onset psychosis. *Scandinavian Journal of Psychology* 45: 53–58.

Van der Gaag, M. (1992). *The Results of Cognitive Training in Schizophrenic Patients.* Delft, the Netherlands: Eburon Publishers.

Wykes, T. *et al.* (1999). The effects of neurocognitive remediation on executive processing in patients with schizophrenia. *Schizophrenia Bulletin* 25: 291–307.

Chapter 12

Finding meaning within psychosis

The contribution of psychodynamic theory and practice

Susan M. Hingley

INTRODUCTION

Hearing the person within can be one of the most important achievements for any therapist hoping to ease some of the suffering and isolation behind psychosis. Theories play their part in helping us to bridge the distance between 'psychotic' perceptions and those which are experienced by others as reflecting a more objective reality. If we can understand something of the underlying meaning and importance of a delusional or hallucinatory experience, we can begin to build a therapeutic relationship based on common humanity. Maybe the most fundamental contribution made by psycho-dynamic theory lies in its capacity to reframe the sometimes obscure disturb-ance of psychosis in terms of psychological needs and processes common to us all.

The vulnerability-stress model has proved effective in helping to integrate multiple causes of psychosis and their interaction. It is used in this chapter to express an understanding of two of the major contributions that psycho-dynamic theory can make in relation to psychosis, looking at ideas about the vulnerability of defence and the vulnerability of the self and the part they both play in the development of psychotic experience (for further details see Hingley 1992, 1997a, 1997b). The chapter then provides an example of psy-chotherapy, as it unfolded with a man experiencing delusional thinking and with a diagnosis of paranoid schizophrenia. Throughout the therapy care and attention was paid to his vulnerability and to the nature of therapeutic interventions that he was likely to be able to tolerate at each stage of the process. It was deemed crucial from the start to work at a pace that was psychologically manageable for him, and did not unhelpfully challenge his vulnerable sense of self. In this approach the stages of therapy are not pre-determined. Early stages involve building and maintaining a therapeutic rela-tionship with the client. Stages that subsequently unfold are influenced by the developing understanding of the client's preoccupations and defences, and by therapist judgements of the client's current capacities to manage more. Stages and the nature of work that takes place within them are also influenced by the capacity of the therapist and the surrounding care network to manage different aspects of the change process. It will only be possible to be clear about the stages of therapy in retrospect, after processes have unfolded.

The chapter will end with a look at the ways in which different theoretical perspectives may relate to each other, and will give a brief overview of the evidence available in support of the contributions that psychodynamic theory may make to therapeutic practice.

VULNERABILITY OF DEFENCE

Problems associated with the functioning of ego defences are of crucial importance in understanding psychosis. The capacity of the mind to enable such defences to work effectively is crucial to the security of individual development and day-to-day functioning. Defences are part of the ego, and function to protect it from painful, sometimes unbearable, affect, and from the anxiety associated with intrapsychic conflict – the conflict between impulses or wishes and their feared consequences. Defences distort experience and cause feelings to remain hidden and unconscious. The ways in which defences function throughout development influence the security of ego development and the ways in which we are enabled to experience a secure sense of self, within ourselves and in relation to others. Defences are argued to follow a maturational path during childhood and into adulthood from immature to mature types of defence. Descriptive research such as that reported by Vaillant (1971) and Cramer (1991) has attributed defences such as delusional projection, the denial of external reality and the reshaping of reality to fit inner needs as characteristic of up to the first five years of life. The functioning of mature defences is particularly characterized by the use of repression, and includes displacement, suppression and sublimation.

From Freud onwards, psychotic symptoms have been seen as reflecting the defensive functioning associated with early childhood (Freud 1894/1962, 1896/1962, 1911/1958). Klein (1946/1986) particularly elaborated on the description of early infant defences, and saw them as relating to the infant's need to cope with the overwhelming and innate terror of its own annihilation or death. She described the existence of the extreme reality-distorting defences of 'splitting' (the inability to experience both good and bad within the same object or person); the denial of outer reality; projection and projective identification; and the stifling of emotions. Other theorists see the terror of annihilation as influenced by the experience of trauma and/or inadequate care rather then being primarily innate. It is also argued that terror and fear, whatever their origin, lead to rage and anger which are unbearable and become projected onto the mother, resulting then in a fear of mother being persecutory. The only way in which terror and anger of this magnitude can be dealt with by the infant is by extreme distortions of reality. If it is these reality-distorting defences which are triggered to produce psychotic reactions in adolescents and adults, they reflect a failure of repression to fulfill its usual role in the emotional life of the individual. Various authors have seen this failure as central to the psychodynamic understanding of psychosis including Jung (1939) who saw psychosis as involving either an unusually strong unconscious forcing its way through to consciousness, or a weak conscious which could not keep back unconscious material.

But why does repression fail? It may be that the current trauma is so intense that repression is inadequate to deal with the associated emotions and inner conflicts. It may also be that the maturational environment failed the infant, so the mature development of defences was compromised. In particular it is the mother's ability to contain her infant's emotional experiences that has been argued to contribute to the healthy evolution of defences. Finally it may be that repression fails because there is a weakened boundary between conscious and unconscious mind. A strong boundary is essential for repression to function. If this were the case it would represent an underlying source of vulnerability within the structure and function of the mind, which could directly influence both the development and evolution of defences, and the way in which they are able to respond to day-to-day experiences. The origins of a weakened boundary could potentially lie in developmental experiences, be the outcome of genetic influences, or lie in an interaction between the two.

It is significant that a defect such as this in the boundary between conscious and unconscious mind has been proposed independently from within both psychodynamic theory and information processing research. Frith (1979, 1992) argued that various defects in information processing could be explained by a defect in the mechanism that controls and limits the contents of consciousness. This view was also supported by Bullen and Hemsley (1987). If present this defect would lead to problems in the cognitive capacity for defence, and could arguably have its origins in both genetic and developmental experiences. Vulnerability would then lie in the ability of defences to function effectively. Problematic experiences during development would lay the ground for personally meaningful trigger experiences to activate intense affect in adulthood, which from the start would be experienced as more intense because repression was compromised. The accelerating intensity of affect would then activate the extreme reality-distorting defences of psychosis, such as the denial of reality and the experience of persecutory delusions. Repression fails because of a cognitive defect, and the protection of the ego then requires the activation of primitive/psychotic defences. This pathway fits with Bleuler's belief that delusions were only formed under affective influence (Bleuler 1950). It is also compatible with Ciompi's affect-logic model of psychosis developed from a cognitive/constructivist perspective (Ciompi 1994).

Vulnerability   **Stress**

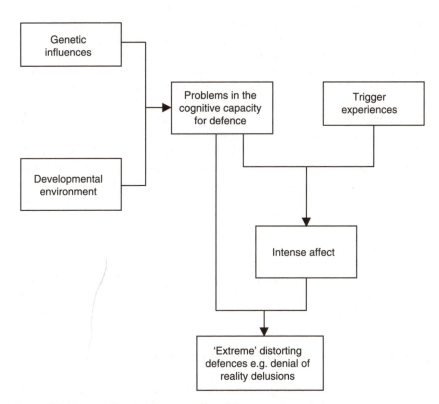

Figure 12.1 Vulnerability of defence: a vulnerability-stress formulation.

VULNERABILITY OF THE SELF

The range of ways in which the self can be seen as vulnerable in psychosis led Alanen (1994: 59) to state that schizophrenia was 'first and foremost a disorder of the ego'. The vulnerability of defence results in an ego which is unable to protect itself adaptively from the adverse impact of intense affect and internal conflict. Further difficulties include an insecure boundary between self and others, an insecure sense of identity, poor self-esteem, and difficulties in relating to others in ways which can fulfill social and attachment needs (Eissler 1954; Federn 1952; Hartmann 1953; Kernberg 1972; Robbins 1993a; Stone 1983). The weakened boundary between self and others probably plays a central role, and relates to problems in experiencing a separate identity, and the likelihood of projective identification, passivity feelings, and delusions of reference (Tausk 1933/1988). An insecure boundary plus problems in dealing with intense affect will contribute to the threats to the self inherent in intimate relationships. These aspects of psychosis clearly all bear relation to severe personality disorder, in particular narcissistic, schizoid, and borderline disorders. In all of them the development of the self has been impaired.

The evolving capacity of the child to experience a separate, cohesive, and valued sense of self is particularly relevant here. Infant–mother relationship difficulties may be experienced in terms of the symbiotic stage of development as proposed by Mahler (1968), and in terms of the need for the experience of 'positive mirroring' and 'optimal frustration' described by Kohut (1977, 1984). Some theorists have seen schizophrenia as reflecting an inability to enter into, and emerge from, the essential experience of a healthy symbiotic or merged relationship early in development (Robbins 1993b). Kohut saw psychosis as potentially being caused by a total failure of 'positive mirroring', resulting in the 'permanent or protracted breakup, enfeeblement or serious distortion of the self' (1977: 192). Early problems with intimacy could reduce the infant's opportunities to benefit from a healthy symbiotic relationship and from the 'positive mirroring' and 'optimal frustration' of effective parenting compounding its constitutional difficulties. Any deficits in the parental capacity for empathic relating would add to an already vulnerable situation. The vulnerability of defence and the vulnerability of the self both play their part in the development of psychotic processes, in the context of the challenges and stresses of life experience.

AN EXAMPLE OF PSYCHODYNAMIC THERAPY

The following case material illustrates the defence-related functions of delusional thinking, the relevance of negative emotion, the importance of identity and self-esteem, and the evolution of the relationship between therapist and client. The work was carried out in a psychiatric rehabilitation setting which was not itself guided by psychodynamic understanding. The client's name and personal details have been changed to protect confidentiality.

Tom was 35 years old and suffered intermittent delusions of grandeur, believing that he was an important political figure. He feared others having adverse opinions of him, was often afraid that his thoughts would stop, and was preoccupied with physical sensations. He had lived in residential care for ten years, had a diagnosis of schizophrenia with paranoid delusions, and was receiving regular Depixol injections.

He was an only child who experienced his parents as critical of his fears and anxieties, and as having very high expectations of him which he felt inadequate to meet. His father was headmaster of a local grammar school and his mother a successful professional musician. In early childhood Tom experienced several episodes of institutional care due to his mother's hospitalization with severe depression, and his father's inability to care for him on his own. When he was six years old, during one of these periods in care, he was physically abused by care staff. Tom was sent to boarding school when he was 14. Emotional support seemed to have failed him at many crucially stressful times, including the further experience of physical abuse in the form of severe bullying at school, and the first onset of psychosis. Tom's symptoms of severe anxiety and delusional thinking first developed while he was at university. He gained a degree in biology, worked for a year as a laboratory technician, but suffered increasingly severe symptoms resulting in long-term hospitalization.

Sessions were held every two weeks for a total of 38 sessions over 22 months. Therapy was guided by psychodynamic and self-psychology principles. Care was taken to maintain a delicate balance between accepting and exploring aspects of Tom's experience. His need for delusions was accepted; they were not directly challenged. It was left to him to make his own decisions about how to use the understanding we achieved during therapy. Empathic listening helped to validate his life experiences and their effects on him. The protective functions that his delusions may have been fulfilling for him were interpreted, and some links were made with his early experiences in order to help him understand and be accepting of his need for the delusions. At various times I chose not to confront aspects of the transference relationship between us which might involve particularly intense emotion towards me, so that the risk of exacerbating psychotic defences was reduced.

The nature of our interaction and the issues we discussed evolved over the months. There were times when Tom filled the sessions with very little space left for me. At other times our communication became much more two-way, with silences and space for my contributions. Fluctuations between these two patterns seemed to parallel the threat that therapy presented to him, a threat that could be understood as challenging his sense of security at a fundamental level. It seemed crucial that I allowed Tom to fill the therapeutic space when he needed to, and that I was not intrusive, particularly in ways that may have reflected my needs rather than his. Equally, however, it was important that I did not allow myself to be obliterated and unable to enter the relational space between us. Obliteration may have put me in the same place that he had been in during his childhood, and having no place in the relational space would have disenfranchised my capacity to help his self to develop through relation with another person. My intrusion into his space needed to be sensitive to his needs and vulnerability, and changes in my style of relating to him and the understanding I explored with him needed to be paced to match the gradual development of Tom's experience of greater security within himself.

Identity

Early on we became aware of the threat that a sense of identity posed to Tom, as if he sat on a knife-edge, terrified both of having a sense of identity and of not having one. I linked some aspects of his delusional thinking to this terror: maybe his ruminations about his body, and his fear that someone else put their thoughts into him, were both good ways of taking away both his own sense of identity and the resulting anxiety that he feared would be unbearable. In ways that were as non-threatening as possible, we discussed aspects of being himself which were problematic for him, particularly those which had been in conflict with his parents' wishes. Five months into therapy Tom felt that although he did not have a sense of his own identity, he had found 'a place in between' where he was not anxious either.

Current realities

The relevance of current realities gradually came more to the fore, and we looked at the ways in which both delusions and daydreams may have protected him from seeing the painful realities of the present. This period of therapy was accompanied by increased ambivalence about attending and some increase in reported depression. However, these experiences reflected the ways in which Tom had reached a secure enough position for us to be able to look at these realities together and be in touch with their emotional impact.

Relating to others, self-perception, emotions, and the function of delusions

After about seven months the focus of discussion shifted to issues about relating to other people, initially looking at aspects of self-esteem. Tom was now able to think about himself with me in relation to others. He talked of his fear that if he became more involved with other people he 'might not win' – he might find that others were better than he was. We looked at the role delusions might play in helping him to avoid feeling anxious and knowing that he was a fearful person. At this time the quality of our relating improved and became more relaxed. Exchanges between us were more balanced, and equal. They flowed more smoothly, and there were silences that felt comfortable. Tom described experiencing fewer delusions but feeling more anxious. We continued to look at relationships with others and the emotions which they involved. Tom revealed his negative feelings towards other people, including me. Early in therapy I had reduced the frequency of sessions from weekly to fortnightly. Tom said that this had angered him, had been behind his threats to leave therapy, and seemed similar to him to his experience of being sent to boarding school by his mother, and to her failure to support him when first experiencing psychotic problems. He revealed his fear of disastrous consequences if he had stood up to his parents and his fear of his own potential rage.

A sense of identity

Tom now started to report a greater sense of identity. He described putting himself forward more with others since they weren't 'so big now' and he 'wasn't so small'. He began to talk of identity as part of our role in life rather than something which 'came out of the blue' and we talked about the commonalities and the differences within human experience. Tom acknowledged that he had had problems before his breakdown, and that there were difficulties for him, which were not necessarily a consequence of schizophrenia.

Splitting and idealization

At around 13 months Tom said that he now realized that relationships could involve both love and hate. My experience of him changed; he seemed to become more rounded as a person to be with and more expressive of himself. Persons that he had described previously as having omnipotent characteristics were now spoken of in rather more human and fallible terms, and he was more able to accept fallibility and vulnerability in himself.

Fantasy and reality

From about 16 months into therapy, we became more involved in discussions about the distinction between fantasy and reality. Tom described his use of daydreams to avoid facing potential confrontations with other residents, in which he imagined that he had already gained his desired outcome, rather than dealing with the situation in reality. We explored the emotions that he might be protecting himself from experiencing and we identified jealousy as well as anger and rage. He came to refer to this as his 'standard reaction' at such times, and became better able to cope with such risks as perceived rejection. He described his efforts and, at times, successes in taking control of potentially powerful delusions, and fighting the temptation to dissolve into them.

Further identity and identification

During this time Tom described his sense of identity as being experienced within the interactions between us. This perhaps reflected an experience of having come to know something of who he was through an awareness of the reactions that he received from me, and who we both were in relation to each other. If this was the case it could be understood to have involved aspects of the 'mirroring' that is central to both Kohut and Winnicott's theories, as well as potential aspects of internalization, introjection, and identification (Kohut 1997, 1984; Winnicott 1960, 1974).

At this time we moved on to talk explicitly about aspects of identification, and the ways it might affect Tom's experience of himself. Initially I shared with Tom the possibility that his self-criticism might be understood as him criticizing himself as his father might have done. At around twenty months he began to feel more in touch with those aspects of himself which he saw as similar to his father, and seemed more able to identify with him in positive ways. Tom also became more accepting of the gentler aspects of himself, while clearly recognizing and expressing his angry feelings towards others. He said that in the past he had believed that only nasty people got angry and he must never do that; now he knew differently.

Our ability to talk about the experience of self in these ways reflected the progress that Tom had made towards a more secure sense of self, from which position he then had the capacity to think about his own self and inner experience in ways that had not been available to us earlier, and also to think about himself in relation to other selves.

Relating to parents

Throughout the second half of therapy Tom coped better with visits from his parents and felt less bitterness towards them, while at the same time clearly acknowledging how undermining he found their comments to be.

The end of therapy

Our therapy relationship ended when Tom moved to a rehabilitation hostel. It was arranged that another therapist would continue to work with him. Although there was a sense of loss in our therapy ending, which we acknowledged, I chose not to explore its meaning for Tom in greater depth. He appeared to transfer at least some of my importance to him onto his new therapist, who was also a woman, and it seemed appropriate not to take the risk of generating more intense emotions which may have unhelpfully triggered psychotic defences, especially at a time of major transition and other losses as Tom relocated his life. He made a successful move to the hostel.

Outcome

Tom's progress included an increased ability to assert himself and to express negative feelings; some decrease in the need to boost himself with delusions of grandeur; less bitterness towards his parents; and a greater sense of his own separate identity with an acceptance of the gentler aspects of his personality. His keyworker considered Tom to have become less sensitive to the reactions of others, less likely to respond adversely and feel hurt; he also thought Tom had become more 'integrated', more able to talk about his relationships with others, and more able to cope with visits from his parents. He considered the changes in Tom to have been of value to the ward as a whole.

Tom's grandiose delusions had supported his vulnerable self-esteem, replaced his own uncertain and feared sense of identity, and helped him to avoid the difficult realities of his life circumstances. Both grandiose and paranoid delusions helped him to avoid experiencing negative affects such as anger and jealousy and to avoid interactions with others which could trigger problematic affect. Overall, therapy reduced his fear of negative affect and enhanced his self-esteem and self-acceptance. These changes were associated with reductions in his need for immature or psychotic defences and an increased sense of and value for who he was as a person. Within the process of our time together, we had come to relate to each other as human beings who experienced something of the reality of our selves as reflected in each other.

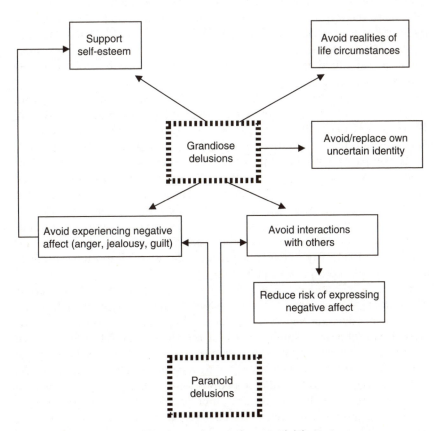

Figure 12.2 The functions of Tom's grandiose and paranoid delusions.

INTEGRATING THEORIES OF PSYCHOSIS

Since our different models of understanding can support and help each other it will be useful to look at some of the links between psychodynamic theory and other models of psychosis. Psychodynamic theory helps us to think about the vulnerability that underlies psychotic symptoms. It is in agreement with cognitive behavioural and family approaches that therapy must not be overtly challenging and confrontational, and that the level and extent of client vulnerability always needs to be taken into account. A number of similar themes can be identified across psychodynamic theory and therapy and cognitive behavioural work, including: the importance of the self, problems with ego boundaries, issues of self esteem, the defensive/protective function of delusions and hallucinations, the meaning of symptoms, and the importance of therapist empathy and rapport. All of these have been recognized as important within different examples of cognitive behavioural therapy (Bentall *et al.* 1994; Fowler *et al.* 1995; Garety *et al.* 1994; Hartman and Cashman 1983; Kingdon and Turkington 1994). Psychodynamic and self-psychology theory then have the potential to enhance and add richness to cognitive behavioural formulations, particularly in terms of the development of psychotic problems, the nature of unconscious processes, and the central importance of a therapeutic relationship that is grounded in the humanity of both therapist and client.

Cognitive approaches and associated research have also provided us with empirical evidence in support of psychodynamic processes. Kaney and Bentall (1989) showed that sufferers of persecutory delusions made excessively external attributions for negative events and internal attributions for positive events compared with normal controls and depressed participants. This evidence was taken as supportive of a self-serving attributional bias which protected individuals from self-blame, in effect supporting the increased tendency for people with persecutory delusions to rely on projection as a defence. Further research has also pointed towards the unconscious importance of the self and self-esteem in people with persecutory delusions (Kinderman 1994). Psychodynamic theory backs up the importance of all of these processes and aspects of personality.

From a family and expressed emotion (EE) perspective, the power of critical family behaviour in triggering psychotic relapses may be understood from a psychodynamic viewpoint, in terms of the sufferer's low tolerance of internal painful affect. Family behaviour may cause painful feelings, which may trigger the need for psychotic defences and exacerbate psychotic symptoms. In a similar way over-involved family members could be presenting too much of a challenge to the sufferer's vulnerability in terms of poorly defined boundaries between themselves and other people. This could then trigger psychotic symptoms which reflect the effects of that threat, and may function to restore sufficient interpersonal space.

EVIDENCE AND PRACTICE

These examples point towards various ways in which our different models may relate to each other. Taking more models into account, and working in more integrative ways which include recognition of psychodynamic ideas, has the potential to strengthen the work which we are able to offer to our clients. This view is supported by the available research evidence. Looking at the value of specifically psychodynamic therapy in practice, research reports, case studies, and reviews published over the past ten years have pointed towards a small sub-group of sufferers fulfilling *DSM-III-R* criteria for schizophrenia who can respond to intensive, often long-term, psychodynamically-oriented psychotherapy (Cullberg 1991; Cullberg and Levander 1991; Jackson 1993; Kline *et al.* 1992; Levander and Cullberg 1994; Rund 1990; Varvin 1991). This approach would seem to benefit clients who can tolerate confrontation. Good responders have been characterized by psychological mindedness, good premorbid social functioning, an absence of violence during psychotic episodes, and the experience of affect-related difficulties (McGlashan 1984). These may well be individuals who have a high loading on environmental and/or traumatogenic origins to their vulnerability, and rather less genetic predisposition.

The classic outcome study by Gunderson *et al.* (1984) supported the broader complementary value of insight-oriented (EIO) therapy to influence ego functioning while reality-adaptive supportive (RAS) therapies were effective in reducing hospitalization and improving role performance. Kates and Rockland (1994) described the value of supportive psychodynamic therapy in fostering adaptive behaviour once symptoms had been stabilized by an effective drug regimen and psychoeducation. While the use of more classical psychoanalytic therapy may benefit a few selected clients, it is the less intensive and more supportive approach to therapy that carries the potential to contribute to the progress of clients in routine services in a way that complements other approaches. This application of psychodynamic theory takes account of fragility and enables theory to be used supportively to help improve adaptive functioning.

SUMMARY

The work with Tom described in this chapter was consistent with Kates and Rockland's (1994) approach, and drew directly on core aspects of psycho-dynamic theory in terms of the vulnerability of defence and the vulnerability of the self. It provided understanding and empathy alongside caution in avoiding anxiety and confrontation, but still offered different ways of making sense of disturbing experiences. It provided an overall opportunity for the development of a rather more securely established self with a greater capacity for less distorting defences – a person who was more able to accept and care for himself, and who was that bit more empowered to cope with the world around him.

REFERENCES

Alanen, Y. O. (1994). An attempt to integrate the individual-psychological interaction concept of the origins of schizophrenia. *British Journal of Psychiatry* 164 (suppl. 23): 56–61.

Bentall, R. P. *et al.* (1994). Cognitive behaviour therapy for persistent auditory hallucinations: From theory to therapy. *Behaviour Therapy* 25: 51–66.

Bleuler, E. (1950). *Dementia Praecox or the Group of Schizophrenias*. New York: International Universities Press.

Bullen, J. G. and Hemsley, D. (1987). Schizophrenia: A failure to control the contents of consciousness? *British Journal of Clinical Psychology* 26: 25–33.

Ciompi, L. (1994). Affect logic: An integrative model of the psyche and its relation to schizophrenia. *British Journal of Psychiatry* 164 (suppl. 23): 51–5.

Cramer, P. (1991). *Defence Mechanisms: Their Development and Measurement*. New York: Springer-Verlag.

Cullberg, J. (1991). Recovered versus non-recovered schizophrenic patients among those who have had intensive psychotherapy. *Acta Psychiatrica Scandinavica* 64: 242–5.

Cullberg, J. and Levander, S. (1991). Fully recovered patients who received intensive psychotherapy: A Swedish case-finding study. *Nordisk Psykiatrisk Tidsskrift* 45: 253–62.

Eissler, K. R. (1954). Notes upon defects of ego structure in schizophrenia. *International Journal of Psychoanalysis* 35: 141–6.

Federn, P. (1952). *Ego Psychology and the Psychoses*. New York: Basic Books.

Fowler, D. *et al.* (1995). *Cognitive Behaviour Therapy for Psychosis: Theory and Practice*. Chichester, UK: Wiley.

Freud, S. (1894). The neuropsychoses of defence. In *Standard Edition III*. London: Hogarth Press.

Freud, S. (1896). Further remarks on the neuropsychoses of defence. III: Analysis of a case of chronic paranoia. In *Standard Edition III*. London: Hogarth Press.

Freud, S. (1911) Psychoanalytic notes on an autobiographical account of a case of paranoia. In *Standard Edition XII*. London: Hogarth Press.

Frith, C. (1979). Consciousness, information processing and schizophrenia. *British Journal of Psychiatry* 134: 225–35.

Frith, C. (1992). *The Cognitive Neuropsychology of Schizophrenia*. Hove, UK: Erlbaum.

Garety, P. *et al.* (1994). Cognitive-behavioural therapy for drug resistant psychosis. *British Journal of Medical Psychology* 67: 259–71.

Gunderson, J. G. *et al.* (1984). Effects of psychotherapy in schizophrenia: II. Comparative outcomes of two forms of treatment. *Schizophrenia Bulletin* 10: 564–98.

Hartmann, H. (1953). Contribution to the metapsychology of schizophrenia. *Psychoanalytic Study of the Child* 8: 177–98.

Hartman, L. M. and Cashman, F. E. (1983). Cognitive-behavioural and psychopharmacological treatment of delusional symptoms: A preliminary report. *Behavioural Psychotherapy* 1: 50–61.

Hingley, S. M. (1992). Psychological theories of delusional thinking: In search of integration. *British Journal of Medical Psychology* 65: 347–56.

Hingley, S. M. (1997a). Psychodynamic perspectives on psychosis I: Theory. *British Journal of Medical Psychology* 70: 301–12.

Hingley, S. M. (1997b). Psychodynamic perspectives on psychosis II: Practice. *British Journal of Medical Psychology* 70: 313–24.

Jackson, M. (1993). Manic-depressive psychosis: Psychopathology and individual psychotherapy within a psychodynamic milieu. *Psychoanalytic Psychotherapy* 7: 103–33.

Jung, C. G. (1939). On the psychogenesis of schizophrenia. In *The Psychogenesis of Mental Diseases* (Collected Works 3). London: Routledge and Kegan Paul.

Kaney, S. and Bentall, R. P. (1989). Persecutory delusions and attributional style. *British Journal of Medical Psychology* 62: 191–8.

Kates, J. and Rockland, L. H. (1994). Supportive psychotherapy of the schizophrenic patient. *American Journal of Psychiatry* 48: 543–61.

Kernberg, O. (1972). Early ego integration and object relations. *Annals of the New York Academy of Sciences* 193: 233–47.

Kinderman, P. (1994). Attentional bias, persecutory delusions and the self-concept. *British Journal of Medical Psychology* 67: 53–66.

Kingdon, D. G. and Turkington, D. (1994). *Cognitive-Behavioural Therapy of Schizophrenia*. Hove, UK: Erlbaum.

Klein, M. (1986). Notes on some schizoid mechanisms. In J. Mitchell (ed.) *The Selected Melanie Klein*. Harmondsworth, UK: Penguin Books. (Original work published 1946.)

Kline, J. *et al.* (1992). Psychodynamic interventions revisited: Options for the treatment of schizophrenia. *Psychotherapy* 29: 366–77.

Kohut, H. (1977). *The Restoration of the Self*. New York: International Universities Press.

Kohut, H. (1984). *How Does Analysis Cure?* Chicago and London: University of Chicago Press.

Levander, S. and Cullberg, J. (1994). Psychotherapy in retrospect: Accounts of experiences in psychotherapy obtained from five former schizophrenic patients. *Nordic Journal of Psychiatry* 48: 263–9.

Mahler, M. S. (1968). *On Symbiosis and the Vicissitudes of Individuation, Vol. 1, Infantile Psychosis*. New York: International Universities Press.

McGlashan, T. H. (1984). The Chestnut Lodge follow-up study. II. *Archives of General Psychiatry* 41: 587–601.

Robbins, M. (1993a). Constitutional vulnerability and an epigenetic model. In *Experiences of Schizophrenia: An Integration of the Personal, Scientific and Therapeutic*. New York and London: Guilford Press.

Robbins, M. (1993b). The psychological system. In *Experiences of Schizophrenia: An Integration of the Personal, Scientific and Therapeutic*. New York and London: Guilford Press.

Rund, B. (1990). Fully recovered schizophrenics: A retrospective study of some premorbid and treatment factors. *Psychiatry* 53: 127–39.

Stone, M. (1983). Introductory comments on psychodynamically oriented treatment of schizophrenia. In M. H. Stone *et al.* (eds) *Treating Schizophrenic Patients*. New York: McGraw-Hill.

Tausk, V. (1988). On the origin of the influencing machine in schizophrenia. In P. Buckley (ed.) *Essential Papers in Psychosis*. New York: New York Universities Press. (Original work published 1933.)

Vaillant, G. E. (1971). Theoretical hierarchy of adaptive ego mechanisms. *Archives of General Psychiatry* 24: 107–18.

Varvin, S. (1991). A retrospective follow-up investigation of a group of schizophrenic patients treated in a psychotherapeutic unit. The Kastanjebakken study. *Psychopathology* 24: 336–44.

Part IV

The need for integration

Chapter 13

Neglected syndromes of schizophrenia – pervasiveness, profiles, and phenomenology

An overview of associated psychiatric syndromes

Paul C. Bermanzohn

INTRODUCTION: REDUCTIONISM OBSTRUCTS INQUIRY

Diagnostic reductionism, the tendency to attribute all of the symptoms and signs shown by those with schizophrenia to the schizophrenia alone, contributes to the widespread tendency to treat schizophrenia as if it were a single, unitary disorder (Bermanzohn *et al.* 2000, 2001). This tendency toward reductionism is greatly reinforced by hierarchical conceptions of diagnosis embedded in the *DSM* system (ibid.), which are still present in *DSM-IV* (APA 1994). The reductionist frame of mind causes psychiatry to neglect commonly occurring problems among schizophrenic patients.[1] This chapter will address depression, obsessive-compulsive disorder (OCD), and panic disorder. These three disorders are commonly found in schizophrenia and are often ignored or neglected.

In *DSM-IV*, psychopathological syndromes co-occurring with schizophrenia may only be diagnosed if they are 'not better accounted for' by the schizophrenia. We know of no guidelines to 'better account for' one syndrome in the presence of another. Nevertheless, it appears that these provisions in *DSM-IV* lead clinicians away from diagnosing other disorders, particularly anxiety disorders, in the presence of schizophrenia. This diagnostic rule has been traced to the traditional medical reluctance to give more than one diagnosis to a patient (Bermanzohn *et al.* 2001; Boyd *et al.* 1984). Studies show that anxiety and depressive disorders are not uncommon in patients with schizophrenia. The diagnostic system, in this way, may contribute to an underestimation of the frequency of these syndromes and to their clinical and scientific neglect.

The result is a common failure to treat or even to study these syndromes in the presence of schizophrenia, despite evidence that they appear to be not only common but a significant source of disability (Cheadle *et al.* 1978). While small preliminary studies suggest that both OCD (Sasson *et al.* 1997) and panic in schizophrenia (Kahn *et al.* 1988) are treatable, surprisingly few studies have been conducted to demonstrate this. The treatment of depression in schizophrenia has been relatively well studied and there are several authoritative studies of its treatability (see Siris 2001 for review).

These syndromes appear to be found in schizophrenic patients at rates higher than in the general population. This has led us to suggest that they are not comorbid disorders, the term most often used, but rather that they are associated with schizophrenia in some way not yet understood. Hence we refer to them as associated psychiatric syndromes (APS; Bermanzohn *et al.* 2001).

Thus, APS appear to present a tempting target for research: they are widespread, disabling disorders which appear to be treatable. The relative lack of such attention may be attributed in large part to the power of reductionism in psychiatric thought.

By treating schizophrenia in a reductionist way, clinically we often stop our inquiry into the patient's disorder prematurely, settling for an incomplete understanding. We settle for the idea that the schizophrenia alone is causing all the patient's signs, symptoms, and distress. Clinicians conclude, prematurely, that there is nothing else to look for. But many persons with chronic schizophrenia, perhaps even most of them, also suffer additional or associated forms of psychopathology, particularly depression, obsessive-compulsive disorder, and panic disorder, which may complicate the patient's course, diagnosis, and treatment.

APS may offer new insights into our patients and provide openings for developing innovative therapies for them, including psychological treatments. In this chapter I will focus on the frequencies with which APS are found in schizophrenia and the patterns of illness, or profiles, we have found in our clinical work and research. Finally, I will briefly review the debates on the significance of APS and the little that has been done to study their treatments in schizophrenia. Both pharmacological and psychological treatments will be touched upon.

STUDY DESIGN AND RESULTS

To study APS clinically, we conducted the following study (Bermanzohn *et al.* 2000).

Method

Patients who had a chart diagnosis of schizophrenia or schizoaffective disorder gave written informed consent for a Structured Clinical Interview for Diagnosis (SCID; First *et al.* 1994) for *DSM-IV* (APA 1994) with a specially-trained research rater. Evaluations were conducted in the order of each patient's most recent admission to the day program. The research team also reviewed each patient's clinical record and consulted clinical staff before and after each interview to minimize possible over-reporting of symptoms.

An effort was made to obtain conservative yet comprehensive diagnoses. Where there were diagnostic disagreements, consensus diagnoses were made in meetings between researchers and clinicians. Lifetime diagnoses were generated for each patient. In addition to the SCID, each patient was administered the Yale Brown Obsessive Compulsive Scale Symptom Checklist (YBOCS; Goodman *et al.* 1989a, 1989b) as a detailed probe for OC symptoms. Only patients with unequivocal *DSM-IV* SCID diagnoses of schizophrenia were included in the sample.

The *DSM-IV* diagnostic criteria were rigorously applied, but with several important modifications designed to highlight the role of hierarchy in diagnosis. Exclusion rules in the SCID (and *DSM-IV*) which prevent diagnosing APS were bypassed. In this way, if a diagnosis would have been blocked by an exclusion rule, the diagnosis was nevertheless made, but note was made that the diagnosis violated the usual exclusion rule.

For consistency, we operationalized 'substantial portion of the duration . . . of the (psychotic) illness,' a distinguishing feature for duration of mood disorder in the *DSM-IV* definition of schizoaffective disorder (APA 1994: 296), to mean at least one third of the time.

Treatments were not prescribed in this study but note was taken of treatments for APS which were used by the treating psychiatrists and of their clinical effects. All treatments reported on here were open and uncontrolled.

Results

In all, 42 patients with chart diagnoses of schizophrenia or schizoaffective disorder were examined; 37 patients met the *DSM-IV* criteria for schizophrenia, and data on these patients are presented here. The mean age of the patients was 38.7 years (SD ± 9.2); 15 (40.5%) were African-American, 21 (56.8%) were Caucasian, and one (2.7%) was Hispanic, of mixed racial descent; 15 were female (40.5%). The mean duration of schizophrenic illness was 18.5 years (SD ± 9.3).

Eighteen of the patients (48.6%) had one or more APS: 13 (35.1%) had one APS and five (13.5%) had two APS. None had all three syndromes.

Depressive disorders

Ten patients (27.0%) met the criteria for major depression. No patients met the 33% criterion which we set for duration of mood disorder to qualify for a diagnosis of schizoaffective disorder, so these depressive disorders were classed as 'superimposed on schizophrenia.' Four patients (10.8%) met the positive inclusion criteria for dysthymia. In two of these patients (5.4%), however, the dysthymia began after the onset of their schizophrenic disorder and so their dysthymic disorders would have been ruled out by the *DSM-IV* exclusion criterion (F). Two other patients (5.4%) had substantial depressive disorders but did not fulfill all criteria for major depressive disorder. Since they exhibited more than two but fewer than the five symptoms required for a diagnosis of major depression, they were diagnosed with minor depression (APA 1994: 719).

Obsessive-compulsive disorder

Eleven patients (29.7%) met the *DSM-IV* criteria for full obsessive-compulsive disorder (OCD). Eight patients in the sample (21.6%) exhibited an obsessive preoccupation with a delusional idea, but only six of them (16.2% of the total sample) qualified for a diagnosis of full OCD, since two were preoccupied exclusively with a delusional content. (See below, under 'obsessive delusions'.)

Panic

Four patients (10.8%) met the criteria for panic disorder (two with and two without agoraphobia). It is notable that three of the four patients with panic disorder also had OC symptoms and the fourth had major depression. We note a clinical association between panic and paranoia in several cases.

PATTERNS OF ILLNESS

Intriguing patterns of illness were noted among some of the patients with APS, especially those with OCD and panic.

Obsessive delusions

Eight patients (21.6%) exhibited complex intertwined symptoms which were psychotic in content and obsessive in form. We call these symptoms obsessive delusions. These patients had all been classed as neuroleptic refractory. They were considered refractory to treatment, at least in part, because of the failure of the obsessive delusions to respond to antipsychotic medicines (Bermanzohn *et al.* 1997a). Six of the patients (16.2% of the total sample) who had obsessive delusions also had full OCD with other nonpsychotic obsessions and compulsions. These nonpsychotic obsessions were of sufficient severity alone to diagnose OCD. Two patients who had only obsessive delusions could not be diagnosed with OCD. They had no 'ordinary' nonpsychotic obsessions, but were still counted among patients with OC-like symptoms. *DSM-IV* requires that an obsession's content cannot be limited to the content of another Axis I disorder (criterion D, APA 1994: 423). For this reason Eisen and colleagues (1997), unlike us, excluded from their study of obsessional phenomena in schizophrenia and schizoaffective disorder any patients who were preoccupied ('obsessed') with psychotic themes. It is very likely that this lowered their reported occurrence rates of OCD.

Five of the patients with obsessive delusions experienced obsessive symptoms as their first symptoms of psychiatric illness, in their teenage years or before. These symptoms endured throughout their lifetimes, causing them the most distress, and also causing clinicians the most diagnostic confusion. In all eight patients, the clinical overlap between obsessions and delusions, and the difficulty inherent in trying to separate such phenomena, contributed to their being called treatment-refractory. Four of these five were placed on clozapine as a result of being called refractory, possibly exacerbating the OCD.

I will now look at one case history in detail. (All eight cases histories are given in detail in the paper 'Are some neuroleptic-refractory symptoms of schizophrenia really obsessions?'; Bermanzohn *et al.* 1997a). Mr A's clinical history shows the difficulty of separating out psychotic from obsessive phenomena and also the persistence and intrusiveness of these phenomena. In his case 'the thoughts' led him to make repeated attempts at suicide over many years, attempts which were ultimately successful.

Case A

Mr A, from a strict Catholic home, was 43 years old when he died by his own hand. At 16 he had begun to be tormented by intrusive thoughts that people thought he was gay, and so were talking about him and making fun of him. He believed people wanted to hurt him and make his life miserable. He had to leave school because of these intrusive and distressing thoughts and became virtually housebound for about seven years, during which time he spent hours each day monitoring his walking in front of a mirror to be sure he did not walk in a way that was 'effeminate,' a way which might confirm what he believed others thought about him. He heard a voice do a running commentary on his thoughts and actions and two or more voices conversing with each other. He also heard laughter, his name being called and 'noises that didn't make sense.' He was depressed, but not suicidal.

From the ages of 17 to 20, Mr A would repeatedly comb his hair 'until I got the parting exactly right,' usually taking between 15 and 20 minutes daily, but sometimes hours. Preoccupations with violent, sexually aggressive, and homosexual thoughts led him to see his neighborhood priest daily to confess. For years these trips to confess were the only times he left his house. He had to synchronize his blinking with that of TV personalities. He said of these behaviors, 'I just couldn't stop', and recognized that they were excessive.

Despite recurrent depressions, he was about 37 years old before he clearly fulfilled *DSM-IV* criteria for a major depressive episode. At that time he was diagnosed and hospitalized with schizoaffective disorder and made several suicide attempts using an overdose of lorazepam. He also developed recurrent, intrusive thoughts of suicide. Hospitalizations followed other suicide attempts: he overdosed, crashed a car into a pole, tried to hang himself, and cut his wrists. He said, 'I keep trying to kill myself because I can't stand the thoughts.'

A variety of neuroleptics during his long illness had no effect on his preoccupation that others thought he was gay and were ridiculing him. He was on haloperidol decanoate, 150 mg IM Q 4 weeks for several years. Clomipramine (CMI), up to 250 mg per day, was added to his regimen. He remained on this regimen of injectable haloperidol and CMI for over a year with negligible improvement. After this trial failed, the CMI was tapered and discontinued and he was started on clozapine, which was slowly increased to 600 mg per day. On this dose for four weeks, he experienced a definite reduction in the intrusiveness of these thoughts and in the distress they caused him. However, his white blood cell count dropped below 2000/mm^3 and the clozapine had to be stopped. At this point his symptoms forcefully recurred and he hanged himself with a belt.

Discussion of obsessive delusions

Obsessive-compulsive symptoms have been reported in schizophrenia since the latter term was coined by Eugen Bleuler in 1911. Controversy over their prevalence in schizophrenia, their clinical significance (especially their impact on the course and outcome of schizophrenia), and whether obsessive-compulsive disorder could become schizophrenia has been almost constant since then. Difficulties with sorting out obsessions and delusions have been alluded to in earlier reports (Gordon 1950; Ingram 1961; Rosen 1957; Stengel 1945). Some of these reports grappled with whether the patients' symptoms were either delusions or obsessions – one or the other. We found many of these complex phenomena to be hybrids: obsessive in form and psychotic in content (Bermanzohn et al. 1997a, 1997b). The fact that over 20% of our patients exhibited these symptoms suggests that they are not unusual and should be considered when assessing complex patients for whom pathological repetitiveness appears to be a factor. The percentage of treatment-refractory cases that may be attributed wholly or in part to obsessive delusions is an empirical question not yet studied.

Rates reported for OC symptoms in schizophrenia have generally increased over the years, ranging from 1.1% (Jahrreiss 1926) to 59.2% (Bland et al. 1987). This may be in part due to the advent in recent years of treatments for OCD. A treatable disorder may be more readily diagnosed since there is something to be done for it. Untreatable diagnoses may be of academic but of less practical concern (Stoll et al. 1992). Another possible reason may be that atypical antipsychotics, which affect the serotonin system, may be increasing the frequency with which OC symptoms appear in schizophrenia (Bermanzohn *et al.* 1995).

Clozapine, risperidone, and other new, so-called 'atypical' antipsychotic agents have been implicated in creating or exacerbating OC symptoms (Baker *et al.* 1997). The basis for this claim is largely anecdotal and theoretical: case reports and the idea that the new generation of antipsychotics have serotonin-blocking activity which might be expected to exacerbate OCD. No prospective studies have been reported to test this effect. Four of our eight cases of obsessive delusions were receiving clozapine, but all four had OC symptoms before they got this medicine. So the clozapine did not cause their OC symptoms. Whether it played a role in exacerbating or sustaining the OC is not known.

Panic and paranoia

Panic and paranoia may be related to one another. Panic attacks may trigger paranoia; in other cases paranoia may trigger a panic attack. Three cases are presented here.

Case B

Mr B, a 42-year-old man with paranoid schizophrenia since the age of 22, was hospitalized five times for psychosis, depression, and suicidality.

Early in his illness voices threatened to cut off his genitals. He became convinced his neighbour wanted to shoot him, so he attempted suicide 'to die before they could torture me.' Voices which told him the Mafia was after him, and notions that he was being watched and would be tortured, continued episodically. He believed that others sent their thoughts to him telepathically. These symptoms were in good control on clozapine 200 mg/day and lorazepam 2 mg, except when he had panic attacks.

He had panic attacks with severe anxiety, shortness of breath, choking, racing heart, sweating, dizziness, light-headedness, chest pains, feelings he may lose control or 'blow up,' and, occasionally, numbness and tingling. These episodes were more likely to occur when he was in large groups. During these episodes he had a return of his paranoia, re-experiencing the thoughts that he would be kidnapped and his genitals would be cut off, and that others were talking about him behind his back. He referred to these episodes as 'paranoid attacks.'

Case C

Mr C, a 35-year-old man with paranoid schizophrenia, believed that his thoughts were responsible for major world events, like the tearing down of the Berlin Wall and the first Gulf War. He felt guilty and frightened by this, admitting: 'It's a big responsibility.' He had these symptoms for about a decade until they were well controlled by clozapine 450 mg/day. His paranoid thoughts would return whenever he went into a crowded room, which always made him nervous. This experience was especially intense when he went with his parents, with whom he lived, into a restaurant. He felt people were looking at him and that he would be humiliated by all this scrutiny. He felt embarrassed by people looking at him. He was sure they could tell he was a mental patient and would despise him for this.

Case D

Mr D was a 28-year-old man, diagnosed with paranoid schizophrenia. He was sure he was being pursued by the Mafia and that they wanted to kill him. While hospitalized on an inpatient unit, these beliefs became intense after dinner and were typically followed by episodes of anxiety similar to panic attacks, with great fear, heart palpitations, sweating, and a feeling that something terrible was about to happen.

Discussion of panic and paranoia

Panic and paranoia may be very similar to one another clinically, and may be especially difficult to distinguish in patients with schizophrenia. Both are states of fear not amenable to reason. Paranoia is, or should be, a delusion or a fixed false belief. But panic attacks may also be associated with a morbid conviction. For example, panic attacks are commonly experienced as heart attacks despite repeated normal ECGs. The conviction of a person with a panic attack that something horrible will happen to them is not alleviated by reassurance or by the repeated experience of panic attacks leading to no horrible consequences other than a transient terrible fear.

There are other similarities. In both panic and paranoia, the victims isolate themselves. This withdrawal and avoidance of social contact may be indistinguishable in panic and paranoia. People with schizophrenia may have difficulty communicating clearly and this may further complicate drawing a line between these two putatively different symptoms.

Penn et al. (1994) studied social anxiety in schizophrenia and noted that similarities exist between social anxiety and certain schizophrenic delusions, particularly paranoia. Argyle (1990) interviewed 20 consecutive patients with chronic schizophrenia in an outpatient clinic and found that seven (35%) had panic attacks. Four of these (20%) met DSM III-R (APA 1987) criteria for panic disorder. He noted that the relationship between panic and psychosis in his patients was complex. In some cases, the panic seemed to trigger the paranoia, as in Case B, while in others paranoia triggered panic, as in Case D.

Labbate and associates (1999) described 49 consecutively admitted VA (Veterans Administration Hospital) inpatients with schizophrenia or schizoaffective disorder: 21 patients (43%) had panic attacks and 16 (33%) had panic disorder. Patients with the paranoid subtype of schizophrenia were significantly more likely to have had panic attacks or disorder than patients with schizoaffective disorder or with the undifferentiated subtype of schizophrenia. Likewise, the three cases presented here all carried a diagnosis of paranoid schizophrenia.

In an unpublished re-analysis of the Epidemiologic Catchment Area (ECA) survey data (Regier *et al.* 1984), we found that among the 344 people diagnosed with schizophrenia, panic and paranoia were significantly more often associated with one another than would be expected by chance. The odds ratio for this association was 2.89 ($p < .001$).

Social phobia, or social anxiety, very common among those with panic attacks, may further complicate the problem of demarcating panic from paranoia. In Argyle's study (1990) 20% of the sample (four patients) exhibited social phobia, while in Zarate's study (1997) 30% exhibited social phobia.

From our clinical experience, in schizophrenia, symptoms of social phobia may merge into paranoia: We have seen several patients who cannot travel on public transportation because they feel they are being looked at, making them fear humiliation, like Mr C. For some, these feelings get stronger and they end up believing that they are being followed or will be killed, like in the paranoid attacks of Mr B. In such cases, panic appears to be on a continuum with paranoia – one gradually merging into or becoming the other.

Further complicating the distinction between social anxiety and paranoia is imprecision in the use of the word 'paranoia'. This word is used in the vernacular to refer to unease, uncertainty, or suspicion about the intentions of others, as when friends say to each other, 'Don't be paranoid.' In clinical psychiatry there is a similar lack of clarity. Paranoia may refer to nonpsychotic people with argumentative or litigious characters, as in paranoid personality disorder. The term has not been limited to denoting a fixed false belief (delusion) that one is in grave danger. Since the Greeks invented the term, paranoia has been used in this indefinite way across many generations and cultures (Berkowitz 1981; Lewis 1970; Ritzler & Smith 1976). It remains a serious, if unrecognized, problem in psychiatry (Kendler 1980).

RATES OF APS IN SCHIZOPHRENIA

Before *DSM-III*, 'neurotic' (anxiety and depressive) symptoms were found in over 65% (124 of 190) of schizophrenia patients living in the community, and the patients who had these disturbances were more disabled than the others (Cheadle *et al.* 1978). Soni and colleagues (1992) found that anxiety and depressive disorders were more common in schizophrenia patients living in the community than among hospitalized patients; they suggested this was because living in the community created more stress.

Table 13.1 Prevalence rates of co-occurring syndromes in schizophrenia

Authors	Sample/criteria employed	Findings		
		OCD	Depression	Panic

Studies of several APS all at once

Cheadle *et al.* (1978)	190 schizophrenic patients living in the community; pre-*DSM-III* categories used	65.3% (*n* = 124) had 'neurotic' (anxiety and depressive) symptoms; '[T]he neurotic problems are (almost exclusively) associated with . . . social handicaps, e.g., isolation, unemployment'		
Boyd *et al.* (1984)	Epidemiological study of a community sample in 5 US cities; *DIS/DSM-III*	12.3 28.5 37.9 (only odds ratios reported)		
Bland *et al.* (1987)	Random community sample in Edmonton, Alberta, Canada; *DIS/DSM-III*	59.2% < .01	54.2% < .001	29.5% < .001
Cosoff and Hafner (1998)	100 inpatients with psychosis (60 with schizophrenia) consecutively admitted to a public hospital in Adelaide, Australia; *DSM-III-R*	13.3% 16.6% social phobia	***	5%
Garvey *et al.* (1991)	95 psychiatric inpatients studied for coexisting anxiety disorders; 18 with schizophrenia/*DSM-III*	Comorbid anxiety in 44%, panic disorder in 17%, GAD in 22% of schizophrenia patients; results did not support validity of primary/ secondary distinction as it pertains to anxiety disorders; comorbid patients may have better prognosis		
Soni *et al.* (1992)	Compared hospitalized chronic schizophrenia patients (*n* = 201) to a matched sample living in the community (*n* = 142), all over age 40; RDC diagnoses*	Hospitalized patients were more disorganized and had more negative symptoms of schizophrenia (NSS); community patients had more anxiety and depression		
Strakowski *et al.* (1993)	102 acutely psychotic, hospitalized first-break patients, 10 in schizophrenia spectrum	13.7% Comorbidity in schizophrenia spectrum associated with longer hospitalization	**	6%
Zarate (1997)	60 randomly selected schizophrenic or schizoaffective outpatients; noncomorbid (*n* = 32) and comorbid (*n* = 28); *DSM-IV* criteria	6.67% 56.7% met criteria for lifetime anxiety disorders; 30% with social phobia; work and overall function were worse in the comorbid group	***	18.33%
Cassano *et al.* (1998)	96 consecutively hospitalized, currently psychotic patients, 31 with schizophrenia spectrum disorders, 10 with schizophrenia	58.1% comorbidity of schizophrenia spectrum 29%	**	19.4%

Bermanzohn et al. (2000)	37 consecutively admitted chronic schizophrenia patients in day program; mean duration of illness 18.5 years; *DSM-IV SCID*	29.7	27	10.8
Craig et al. (2002)	225 schizophrenia/schizoaffective disorder first-break patients from numerous mental health facilities in Suffolk County, NY, began study; 167–169 completed 24-month outcome assessments; *DSM-III-R SCID*	3.8% OCD; 11.2% panic; those with panic symptoms were more likely to have psychosis at 24-month assessment		

Studies of the prevalence of panic only

Boyd (1986)	5 large community samples (total n = 18,572) as part of Epidemiological Catchment Area (ECA) Survey; *DIS/DSM-III* criteria	28–63% of subjects with schizophrenia reported panic attacks, depending on the community
Argyle (1990)	20 consecutive patients attending an outpatient clinic for maintenance treatment of chronic schizophrenia; *DSM-III-R* criteria	7 patients (35%) had regularly occuring panic attacks; 4 of these 7 (20%) met full criteria for panic disorder; agoraphobia was present in 3 of those with panic attacks and in 1 patient without panic; among the 13 cases with significant social avoidance, 4 (20% of the total sample) had typical social phobia, with fears of appearing anxious and being humiliated
Cutler and Siris (1991)	45 patients, mostly outpatients with schizophrenia or schizoaffective disorder who also had operationally defined post-psychotic depression. *RDC* diagnoses*	11 patients (24.4%) had panic attacks; number of patients meeting full criteria for panic disorder not reported

Studies of prevalance rates for OCD and OC symptoms only

Jahrreiss (1926)	Chart review of 1000 hospitalized and clinic patients; strict criteria for OCD (similar to *DSM-IV*) but not for schizophrenia	1.1% OCD; n = 11
Rosen (1957)	Chart review of 848 hospitalized inpatients; criteria not specified for either OCD or schizophrenia	3.5% (n = 30) had OCD 'at some time'

Continued . . .

Continued . . .

Authors	Sample/criteria employed	Findings
		OCD Depression Panic
Fenton and McGlashan (1986)	After chart review, follow-up of 163 hospitalized inpatients an average of 15 years later; *DSM-III-R* criteria for schizophrenia and behavioral criteria for OC symptoms	21 patients (12.9%) met 2 of 8 behavioral criteria for OC symptoms
Berman *et al.* (1995a)	Structured interviews of 108 chronic schizophrenic patients' therapists at community mental health center; chart diagnoses for schizophrenia and criteria from Fenton and McGlashan (1986) for OC symptoms	27 patients exhibited OC symptoms at time of study = 26.5% point prevalence; 33 had OC symptoms at any time = 30.6% lifetime prevalence
Rae (unpublished)	Reanalysis of ECA survey; random community survey of 5 US communities; *DIS/DSM-III* criteria	23.7% OCD
Porto *et al.* (1997)	Interviews with 50 chronic schizophrenia patients in continuing day program for lifetime prevalences; *DSM-IV SCID* of schizophrenic and schizoaffective patients with OC symptoms and OCD	Lifetime prevalences 'clinically significant'; OC symptoms 60% (*n* = 30), full OCD 26%
Eisen *et al.* (1997)	Interviewed 77 schizophrenic and schizoaffective clinic outpatients using *SCID DSM-III-R* criteria	7.8% (*n* = 6) with OCD
Meghani *et al.* (1998)	All new admissions over 5 years to an outpatient psychiatry service in a large teaching hospital (*n* = 1458) were given structured diagnostic instrument and self report measures; criteria unspecified	31.7% (*n* = 61) of all schizophrenia patients (*n* = 192) met criteria for OCD; OCD-schizophrenia patients had 'less efficient psychosocial functioning . . . and lower self-satisfaction'; no treatment differences between the two groups noted except that OCD-schizophrenia patients were more likely to say that the meds they received 'made no difference'

For studies of prevalence rates of depression in schizophrenia, see Siris (2001).
* Spitzer *et al.* (1975), Siris (2001).
** Studied all psychotic disorders, including major depression, making this category redundant.
*** Data on depression not reported.

Many different rates of APS in schizophrenia have been found, but some modal rates have emerged. Depression has been found in 7–75% of patients with schizophrenia, with a modal rate of 25% (Siris 2001). OCD is reported in from 1.1% (Jahrreiss 1926) to 59.2% (Bland *et al.* 1987) of cases, with a modal rate of 30% (Bermanzohn *et al.* 1997a). Panic attacks were found in 10.8–63% (Boyd 1986) of cases, but no modal rate for panic is apparent.

Most of these studies have determined the prevalence rates either by epidemiological methods (Bland *et al.* 1987; Boyd *et al.* 1984; Soni *et al.* 1992), chart reviews (Fenton and McGlashan 1986), or by interviewing the patients' therapists (Berman *et al.* 1995a). The large-scale epidemiological studies have been criticized for using lay interviewers. Ours is the first wholly clinical study of APS of which we are aware; moreover, all our interviewers were highly trained mental health professionals.

Our study, like many in this area, has important methodological weaknesses. Based on a clinical sample at a single treatment facility, it may be of limited generalizability. Patients in a day centre like this one may be sicker and more chronically ill than other outpatient samples of schizophrenia patients. They may also be more compliant, since they attend programs for many years. This is hardly a universal practice among those with schizophrenia. The patients in this sample had a mean duration of illness of 18.5 years (±SD 9.3 years). So, because of sample bias, our findings may not represent the broad population of those with schizophrenia. A second weakness in our study method is the lack of a control group.

Patients with chronic schizophrenia have been the usual subjects in studies of APS. But chronic patients may have higher rates of APS than others. Craig and colleagues (2002) studied a sample of first-break psychosis patients. They criticize the reliance on samples made up of chronic patients and found a lower rate of OCD (3.8%) but not of panic symptoms (11.2%) in their schizophrenia patients. They suggest that rates of occurrence may increase with patients' age and duration of illness. High rates reported for APS in chronic schizophrenia have also led to speculation that APS might play some role in the development of chronicity in schizophrenia (Bermanzohn *et al.* 1995). The relationship between APS and the age of patients needs further attention.

WHAT IS THE RELATIONSHIP BETWEEN APS AND SCHIZOPHRENIA?

APS are commonly referred to as 'comorbid' disorders in schizophrenia (e.g. see *Management of Schizophrenia with Comorbid Disorders*, eds Hwang and Bermanzohn 2001). Yet it is unclear whether APS are separate and distinct co-occurring (or comorbid) syndromes, or whether they are a part of the patients' schizophrenic disorders – 'dimensions of schizophrenia' as proposed by Opler and Hwang (1994). Bland and associates (1987) suggest that this confusion may be in part resolved by studying the clinical validity of these syndromes using a three-part research strategy, to determine: whether the presence of APS is associated with a difference in the clinical course of patients when compared to the course of patients without these syndromes; whether corresponding syndromes occur in higher than expected rates among the family members of patients with APS as compared to the family members of schizophrenia patients without them; and whether these syndromes are treatable.

Comparing the rates of APS in schizophrenia to the rates of the corresponding syndromes in the general population may also shed light on this problem. If an APS occurs in schizophrenia at a rate much higher than in the general population, this would not support the idea that it is a comorbidity, or a randomly occurring convergence of two independent disorders. If a separate disorder co-occurs randomly with schizophrenia, its rate in schizophrenia should not exceed its rate in the general population (McGlashan 1997).

The three APS described here appear to be more common in schizophrenia than in the general population (see Table 13.2; Bland *et al.* 1987). Studies since then have supported this view (see Table 13.1; Craig *et al.* 2002 criticize methods used in this area). For example, two studies besides this one have reported lifetime diagnoses of OC among schizophrenia patients of about 30%. Berman and colleagues (1995a) found a lifetime rate of OC symptoms of 30.6%, while Meghani *et al.* (1998) reported a rate of 31.7%, making 30% the modal rate reported in the literature for OCD in schizophrenia. OCD occurs in about 2.5% of the general population.

EFFECTS ON COURSE AND PROGNOSIS

Like depression in schizophrenia (Harrow *et al.* 1998), anxiety disorders have been associated with a poor functional outcome (Zarate 1997). This has been found specifically when looking at OC symptoms (Berman *et al.* 1995a; Meghani *et al.* 1998; Samuels *et al.* 1993) and generally in studying anxiety levels (Huppert *et al.* 2001). Earlier reports (Rosen 1957; Stengel 1945),

Table 13.2 Lifetime prevalence rates of APS in schizophrenia and general population (from Bland *et al.* 1987)

	Panic	Major depressive episode	Obsessive-compulsive disorder
General population	7.3	7.3	4.0
Schizophrenia	29.5	54.2	59.2

largely based on case reports, maintained that schizophrenia patients with OC symptoms were less impaired than those without these symptoms. More recently, using the Global Assessment of Function scales, Tibbo and associates (1999) also reported that patients with OC symptoms had less impaired functioning. The effect of OC symptoms on schizophrenia remains controversial.

Panic disorder in schizophrenia has recently been examined by Goodwin and colleagues (2002, 2003). They found that such patients have a diminished quality of life and an increased likelihood of substance use disorders.

TREATMENTS OF APS

Depression

Depression in schizophrenia has been successfully treated in controlled trials using a variety of antidepressants added to the patients' antipsychotic medication (Siris 2001). In a particularly interesting study, Siris *et al.* (1994) found no exacerbation of psychosis while patients were on adjunctive imipramine and significantly more exacerbation of psychosis in the group on placebo. Treatment of depression in schizophrenia might provide some protection against relapse to psychosis, they concluded, suggesting that APS might work as 'endogenous stressors' in exacerbating psychosis (Siris 1988).

Treatments for OCD and panic disorder in schizophrenia have been studied less than those for depression.

OC symptoms

Five small case series and anecdotal reports using pharmacological treatment for OC-schizophrenia have been published (for a review see Sasson *et al.* 1997). All these case series added clomipramine to the patient's antipsychotic medication. Only one of these reports was controlled (Berman *et al.* 1995b). Several of these reports found that psychotic symptoms improved along with the OC symptoms. While promising, none of these reports is definitive. Recently, Poyurovsky and colleagues (2003) reported on two cases of OC-schizophrenia successfully treated with a combination of olanzapine and sertraline.

A single case in which cognitive behavioral therapy (CBT) helped a patient with OCD, hallucinations, and delusions has also been reported (Lelliott and Marks 1987). These psychotic symptoms were thought to be related to the OCD (I. Marks, personal communication, 19 September 1997).

Panic

No controlled treatment trials for panic in schizophrenia have been published. In one study, panic improved with addition and worsened with removal of alprazolam, which was openly administered then tapered and withdrawn, in a standardized treatment protocol given to seven chronic hospital patients with panic and schizophrenia (Kahn *et al.* 1988). In this study, both negative and positive symptoms of schizophrenia improved and worsened along with changes in panic symptomatology. Alprazolam and imipramine have been successfully used for panic in schizophrenia in several cases (Sandberg and Siris 1987; Siris *et al.* 1989). CBT has been used in several trials, including two in a group format (Arlow *et al.* 1997, 1999), and another in a series of individual cases (Hofmann 1999).

CONCLUSIONS

The percentages reported in our and many other studies of APS cannot be called 'prevalence rates' because they are findings from limited and non-random samples, so these rates should be called frequencies or occurrence rates. For this reason the rates we report here may not represent the broader universe of all those with schizophrenia. Our rates are similar, however, to those reported in many other studies of APS. Many studies of these phenomena, like ours, are done with 'samples of convenience,' such as clinic samples or admissions to a specific ward. Such samples of convenience must be viewed with caution. They may reflect unrecognized selection bias and not be representative.

Perhaps the most rigorous methods used in studying these syndromes in schizophrenia were those of Bland and colleagues (1987). Applying methods similar to those used by the Epidemiologic Catchment Area survey (Regier *et al.* 1984), Bland *et al.* conducted a randomized community survey of homes in Edmonton, Alberta, Canada. In their survey, 85% of the schizophrenia patients (17 out of 20) they identified had one or more of the three APS considered here. They used raters who were not mental health professionals, but laypersons trained for the survey. The use of laypersons as surveyors has been criticized. Nevertheless, the Bland paper seems to contain the best data currently available and, for this reason, we have used their numbers in Table 13.2 to compare the prevalence rates of APS in the general population with those with schizophrenia.

Survey methods, however rigorous statistically, are insensitive to individual clinical cases. They have a low resolution, like a map in which an entire city appears as a dot. But in a clinical science like psychiatry a more in-depth look at patients' patterns of illness is necessary to clarify phenomenology. In the last analysis it is phenomenology on which definitions of illness are based.

Well characterized individual cases may be instructive for phenomenology. Patterns discerned among specific cases may help define phenomenological types. To understand APS best we will need to shift back and forth between epidemiological approaches and case studies.

Our characterization of obsessive delusions as hybrid symptoms may help resolve inconsistencies and ambiguities in the literature on obsessions and delusions, especially where investigators have grappled with whether a symptom was an obsession or a delusion. Such ambiguities have bedeviled some reports. Finding obsessive delusions in 21.6% of our cases suggests these are not isolated or singular phenomena. Complex phenomena may be easier to ignore. More detailed study of obsessive delusions should be undertaken in order to characterize them more precisely and then to assess their frequency.

A combination of methods is needed to study these phenomena. Continuing with the map metaphor, if one wishes to get to know an area, a map is a good way to start and to use as needed. But the higher the altitude from which the map is drawn, the farther one is from the reality on the ground. On the other hand, one can more easily get lost without an overview. So with a clinical subject like the study of psychiatric patients, we should strive to combine the clinician's perspective, close to individual patients, on the ground, as it were, with a larger, broader perspective incorporating epidemiological and statistical studies of large numbers of cases and group effects to see how widespread phenomena are. To paraphrase the philosopher we might say: statistics without case studies are empty and case studies without statistics are blind.

Perhaps a preferable medical metaphor is provided by the microscope. When first looking at a slide, we look through a lower magnification to get a sense of the overall structure. Then we switch to a higher magnification (bringing us 'closer' to the object of study) to understand better its specific features. Like studying objects under a microscope, we can best understand APS, and other psychiatric phenomena, by shifting focus back and forth between the big picture and the fine detail.

When studying our patients, close up and in detail, intriguing clinical patterns of illness emerged. These patterns, which are often difficult to discern, may have clinical implications:

1   It appears likely that APS, which are associated with significant morbidity and dysfunction in schizophrenia, are treatable, using adjunctive agents appropriate to the particular APS (such as antidepressant, antiobsessional, or antipanic agents) added to the patient's antipsychotic therapy. Depression in schizophrenia has been effectively treated using a variety of agents. By analogy with depression, the evidence that OCD and panic disorder may be treatable is promising. But this is still just preliminary. Larger, randomized and controlled trials are needed. In

the meanwhile clinicians may wish to proceed cautiously when treating APS.

2   Difficulty recognizing OC symptoms in schizophrenia may lead to patients with these syndromes being considered as treatment-refractory, and no attempts made to treat the OC symptoms specifically (Bermanzohn *et al.* 1997a). Kane (1996) listed comorbid disorders among the factors making schizophrenia difficult to treat, but no studies have examined the frequency of OC symptoms among refractory schizophrenia patients.

3   Panic and social anxiety have been implicated in initiating psychosis, both as a trigger to psychosis in individual cases (Bermanzohn *et al.* 1997a) and as a sociodemographic risk factor in epidemiological studies (Tien and Eaton 1992). (OCD was also a significant predictor of the subsequent development of schizophrenia in the Tien and Eaton study.)

4   Treatment used for anxiety disorders without schizophrenia may be useful in treating anxiety disorders with schizophrenia. There are few studies to guide clinical practice on this point, so clinicians should exercise prudence in attempting to treat these complex cases.

NOTE

1   A related problem is that medical personnel may ignore physical complaints from those with schizophrenia. This arises from the dismissive attitude that mentally ill people are unreliable about reporting any aspect of their experience, a part of the stigma of mental illness. It can affect peoples' lives physically as well as socially.

REFERENCES

American Psychiatric Association (1987). *Diagnostic and Statistical Manual of Mental Disorders* (rev. 3rd ed.). Washington, DC: American Psychiatric Association.

American Psychiatric Association (1994). *Diagnostic and Statistical Manual of Mental Disorders* (4th ed.). Washington, DC: American Psychiatric Association.

Argyle, N. (1990). Panic attacks in chronic schizophrenia. *British Journal of Psychiatry* 157: 430–3.

Arlow, P. B. *et al.* (1997). Cognitive-behavioral therapy of panic attacks in chronic schizophrenia. *Journal of Psychotherapy Practice and Research* 6: 145–50.

Arlow, P. B. *et al.* (1999). A cognitive-behavioral approach for the treatment of panic in schizophrenia (Abstract). *Schizophrenia Research* 36: 160.

Baker, R. W. *et al.* (1992). Emergence of obsessive-compulsive symptoms during treatment with clozapine. *Journal of Clinical Psychiatry* 53: 439–41.

Berkowitz, R. (1981). The distinction between paranoid and non-paranoid forms of schizophrenia. *British Journal of Clinical Psychology* 20: 15–23.

Berman, I. *et al.* (1995a). Obsessive and compulsive symptoms in chronic schizophrenia. *Comprehensive Psychiatry* 36: 6–10.

Berman, I. *et al.* (1995b). Treatment of obsessive-compulsive symptoms in schizophrenic patients with clomipramine. *Journal of Clinical Psychopharmacology* 15: 206–10.

Bermanzohn, P. C. (1999). Prevalence and prognosis of obsessive-compulsive symptoms in schizophrenia: A critical view. *Psychiatric Annals* 29: 508–12.

Bermanzohn, P. C. *et al.* (1995, December). *Associated Psychiatric Syndromes (APS) in Chronic Schizophrenia.* Presentation at the 34th Annual Meeting of the American College of Neuropsychopharmacology (ACNP), San Juan, Puerto Rico.

Bermanzohn, P. C. *et al.* (1997a). Are some neuroleptic-refractory symptoms of schizophrenia really obsessions? *CNS Spectrums* 2(3): 51–7.

Bermanzohn, P. C. *et al.* (1997b). Obsessions and delusions: Separate and distinct, or overlapping? *CNS Spectrums* 2(3): 58–61.

Bermanzohn, P. C. *et al.* (2000). Hierarchical diagnosis in chronic schizophrenia: A clinical study of co-occurring syndromes. *Schizophrenia Bulletin* 26: 519–27.

Bermanzohn, P. C. *et al.* (2001). Hierarchy, reductionism and 'comorbidity' in the diagnosis of schizophrenia: Problems in the assessment of associated psychiatric syndromes (APS). In M. Hwang and P. C. Bermanzohn (eds) *Management of Schizophrenia with Comorbid Conditions.* Washington, DC: American Psychiatric Press, Inc.

Bland, R. C. *et al.* (1987). Schizophrenia: Lifetime comorbidity in a community sample. *Acta Psychiatrica Scandinavica* 75: 383–91.

Boyd, J. H. (1986). Use of mental health services for the treatment of panic disorder. *American Journal of Psychiatry* 143: 1569–74.

Boyd, J. H. *et al.* (1984). Exclusion criteria of DSM-III: A study of co-occurrence of hierarchy-free syndromes. *Archives of General Psychiatry* 41: 983–9.

Cassano, G. B. *et al.* (1998). Occurrence and clinical correlates of psychiatric comorbidity in patients with psychotic disorders. *Journal of Clinical Psychiatry* 59: 60–8.

Cheadle, A. J. *et al.* (1978). Chronic schizophrenic patients in the community. *British Journal of Psychiatry* 132: 221–7.

Cosoff, S. J. and Hafner, J. (1998). The prevalence of comorbid anxiety in schizophrenia, schizoaffective disorder and bipolar disorder. *Australian and New Zealand Journal of Psychiatry* 32: 67–72.

Craig, T. *et al.* (2002). Obsessive-compulsive and panic symptoms with first-admission psychosis. *American Journal of Psychiatry* 159: 592–8.

Cutler, J. and Siris, S. G. (1991). "Panic-like" symptomatology in schizophrenic and schizoaffective patients with postpsychotic depression: Observations and implications. *Comprehensive Psychiatry* 32: 465–73.

Eisen, J. L. *et al.* (1997). Obsessive-compulsive disorder in patients with schizophrenia or schizoaffective disorder. *American Journal of Psychiatry* 154: 271–3.

Fenton, W. S. and McGlashan, T. H. (1986). The prognostic significance of obsessive-compulsive symptoms in schizophrenia. *American Journal of Psychiatry* 143: 437–41.

First, M. B. *et al.* (1994). *Structured Clinical Interview for Axis I DSM-IV Disorders: Patient Edition (SCID – I/P, Version 2.0).* New York: Biometrics Research Department, New York State Psychiatric Institute.

Garvey, M. *et al.* (1991). Examination of comorbid anxiety in psychiatric inpatients. *Comprehensive Psychiatry* 32: 277–82.

Goodman, W. K. *et al.* (1989a). The Yale-Brown Obsessive Compulsive Scale (Y-BOCS). I: Development, use, and reliability. *Archives of General Psychiatry* 46: 1006–11.

Goodman, W. K. *et al.* (1989b). The Yale-Brown Obsessive Compulsive Scale (Y-BOCS). II: Validity. *Archives of General Psychiatry* 46: 1012–6.

Goodwin, R. *et al.* (2002). Panic attacks in schizophrenia. *Schizophrenia Research* 58: 213–20.

Goodwin, R. *et al.* (2003). Anxiety and substance use comorbidity among inpatients with schizophrenia. *Schizophrenia Research* 61: 89–95.

Gordon, A. (1950). Transition of obsessions into delusions. *American Journal of Psychiatry* 107: 455–8.

Harrow, M. *et al.* (1998, May). *How Vulnerable are Schizophrenic Patients to Depression?* Presentation at the 151st Annual Meeting of the American Psychiatric Association, Toronto, Canada.

Hofmann, S. G. (1999). Does cognitive-behavioral treatment of panic attacks improve schizophrenic symptoms? [Abstract] *Schizophrenia Research* 36: 326.

Huppert, J. D. *et al.* (2001). Quality of life in schizophrenia: Contributions of anxiety and depression. *Schizophrenia Research* 51: 171–80.

Hwang, M. Y. and Bermanzohn, P. C. (eds) (2001). *Management of Schizophrenia with Comorbid Conditions.* Washington, DC: American Psychiatric Press, Inc.

Ingram, I. M. (1961). Obsessional illness in mental hospital patients. *Journal Mental Science* 107: 382–402.

Jahrreiss, W. (1926). Obsessions during schizophrenia [in German]. *Archiv für Psychiatrie und Nervenkrankheiten* 77: 740–88.

Kahn, J. P. *et al.* (1988). Adjunctive alprazolam for schizophrenia with panic anxiety: Clinical observation and pathogenetic implications. *American Journal of Psychiatry* 145: 742–4.

Kane. J. M. (1996). Factors which can make patients difficult to treat. *British Journal of Psychiatry* 169(suppl. 31): 10–14.

Kendler, K. S. (1980). The nosologic validity of paranoia (simple delusional disorder). *Archives of General Psychiatry* 37: 699–706.

Labbate, L. A. *et al.* (1999). Comorbidity of panic disorder and schizophrenia. *Canadian Journal of Psychiatry* 44: 488–90.

Lelliott, P. and Marks, I. (1987). Management of obsessive compulsive rituals associated with delusions, hallucinations and depression: A case report. *Behavioral Psychotherapy* 15: 77–87.

Lewis, A. (1970). Paranoia and paranoid: A historical perspective. *Psychological Medicine* 1: 2–12.

McGlashan, T. H. (1997). Are schizophrenia and OCD related disorders? *CNS Spectrums* 2(4): 16–18.

Meghani, S. R. *et al.* (1998, May). *Schizophrenia Patients With and Without OCD.* Presentation at the 151st Annual Meeting of the American Psychiatric Association, Toronto, Canada.

Opler, L. and Hwang, M. Y. (1994). Schizophrenia: A multidimensional disorder. *Psychiatric Annals* 24: 491–5.

Penn, D. L. *et al.* (1994). Social anxiety in schizophrenia. *Schizophrenia Research* 11: 277–84.

Porto, L. *et al.* (1997). A profile of obsessive-compulsive symptoms in schizophrenia. *CNS Spectrums* 2(3): 21–5.

Poyurovsky, M. *et al.* (2003). Olanzapine-sertraline combination in schizophrenia with obsessive-compulsive disorder. Letter in *Journal of Clinical Psychiatry* 64: 611.

Regier, D. A. *et al.* (1984). The NIMH Epidemiologic Catchment Area: Historical context, major objectives, and study population characteristics. *Archives of General Psychiatry* 41: 934–41.

Ritzler, B. A. and Smith, M. (1976). The problem of diagnostic criteria in the study of the paranoid subclassification of schizophrenia. *Schizophrenia Bulletin* 2: 209–17.

Rosen, I. (1957). The clinical significance of obsessions in schizophrenia. *Journal Mental Science* 103: 773–88.

Samuels, J. *et al.* (1993). Obsessive-compulsive symptoms in schizophrenia. *Schizophrenia Research* 9: 139.

Sandberg, L. and Siris, S. G. (1987). 'Panic disorder' in schizophrenia: A case report. *Journal of Nervous and Mental Diseases* 175: 627–8.

Sasson, Y. *et al.* (1997). Treatment of obsessive-compulsive syndromes in schizophrenia. *CNS Spectrums* 2(4): 34–45.

Siris, S. G. (1988). Implications of normal brain development for pathogenesis of schizophrenia [Letter]. *Archives of General Psychiatry* 45: 1055.

Siris, S. G. (2001). Depression in the course of schizophrenia. In M. Hwang and P. C. Bermanzohn (eds) *Management of Schizophrenia with Comorbid Conditions*. Washington, DC: American Psychiatric Press, Inc.

Siris, S. G. *et al.* (1987). Adjunctive imipramine in the treatment of post-psychotic depression: A controlled trial. *Archives of General Psychiatry* 44: 533–9.

Siris, S. G. *et al.* (1989). Imipramine-responsive panic-like symptomatology in schizophrenia. *Biological Psychiatry* 25: 485–8.

Siris, S. G. *et al.* (1994). Maintenance imipramine for secondary depression in schizophrenia: A controlled trial. *Archives of General Psychiatry* 51: 109–15.

Soni, S. D. *et al.* (1992). Differences between chronic schizophrenic patients in the hospital and in the community. *Hospital and Community Psychiatry* 43: 1233–8.

Spitzer, R. R. *et al.* (1975). Research Diagnostic Criteria. Instrument No.58. New York: New York State Psychiatric Institute.

Stengel, E. (1945). A study on some clinical aspects of the relationship between obsessional neurosis and psychotic reaction types. *Journal of Mental Science* 91: 166–87.

Stoll, A. L. *et al.* (1992). Increasing frequency of the diagnosis of obsessive-compulsive disorder. *American Journal of Psychiatry* 149: 638–40.

Strakowski, S. M. *et al.* (1993). Comorbidity in psychosis at first hospitalisation. *American Journal of Psychiatry* 150: 752–7.

Tibbo, P. *et al.* (1999, April). *Obsessive-Compulsive Disorder in Schizophrenia*. Poster presented at the International Congress on Schizophrenia Research, Santa Fe, New Mexico.

Tien, A. Y. and Eaton, W. W. (1992). Psychopathologic precursors and sociodemographic risk factors for the schizophrenia syndrome. *Archives of General Psychiatry* 49: 37–46.

Zarate, R. (1997, November). *The Comorbidity Between Schizophrenia and Anxiety Disorders*. Presentation to the 31st Annual Meeting of the Association for Advancement of Behavior Therapy, Miami Beach, Florida.

Chapter 14

Dissociation and psychosis

The need for integration of theory and practice

Colin A. Ross

The most chronic and complex of the dissociative disorders, multiple personality disorder, was renamed 'dissociative identity disorder' in 1994 in *DSM-IV* (American Psychiatric Association). The rationale for the name change was, among other things, to clarify that there are not literally separate personalities in a person with dissociative identity disorder; 'personalities' was a historical term for the fragmented identity states that characterize the condition.

Almost a century earlier, 'dementia praecox' underwent a name change to 'schizophrenia'. Curiously, the term 'schizophrenia', derived from the Greek, means 'split mind disorder'. Schizophrenia is actually a more suitable name for the *DSM-IV-TR* entity of dissociative identity disorder than it is for the *DSM-IV-TR* disorder of schizophrenia, as these two diagnoses are described in their texts and diagnostic criteria (American Psychiatric Association 2000).

Bleuler (1950) chose the term 'schizophrenia' because he regarded a split between thought and emotion as central to the pathology of the disorder. His clinical description of schizophrenia, however, better matches the *DSM-IV-TR* text and criteria for dissociative identity disorder than that for schizophrenia, as pointed out by Gainer:

> I call dementia praecox 'schizophrenia' because (as I hope to demonstrate) the 'splitting' of the different psychic functions is one of its most important characteristics. . . . In every case we are confronted with a more or less clear-cut splitting of the psychic functions. If the disease is marked, the personality loses its unity; at different times, different psychic complexes seem to represent the personality. Integration of different complexes and strivings appears insufficient or even lacking . . . one set of complexes dominates the personality for a time, while the other groups of ideas or drives are 'split off' and seem either partly or completely impotent.
>
> (Gainer 1994: 265–67)

Nothing remotely resembling Bleuler's clinical description of schizophrenia is contained in the *DSM-IV-TR* text for schizophrenia. However, using different vocabulary, Bleuler's schizophrenia is described in the *DSM-IV-TR* text for dissociative identity disorder:

> Dissociative Identity Disorder reflects a failure to integrate various aspects of identity, memory, and consciousness. . . . Particular identities may emerge in specific circumstances. . . . Alternate identities are experienced as taking control in sequence, one at the expense of the other. . . . An identity that is not in control may nonetheless gain access to consciousness by producing auditory hallucinations (e.g., a voice giving instructions).
>
> (American Psychiatric Association 2000: 526)

The overlap and distinction between schizophrenia and multiple personality disorder have been unclear in the professional literature for almost a century. Likewise, in popular culture, the two disorders are often confused with each other or are thought to be synonymous (Ross 2004).

Currently, at least in North America, many if not most psychiatrists adhere to a conceptual system which makes a clear differentiation between the two disorders: schizophrenia is regarded as a major mental disorder with an endogenous biological aetiology based on a diagnostically specific genetic abnormality; it is treated primarily with medication and does not respond to individual psychotherapy. Dissociative identity disorder, on the other hand, is of peripheral interest. It is regarded as a variant of hysteria, represents a neurotic reaction to the environment, and is treated with either benign neglect or psychotherapy.

Dispute about the aetiology of dissociative identity disorder hinges on whether it is naturally occurring or an iatrogenic artifact. Adherents of both theories of aetiology agree that the disorder is a reaction to the environment and treated with psychological approaches. One would assume from this ideological system that the two disorders, schizophrenia and dissociative identity disorder, are clearly differentiated clinically.

The purpose of this chapter is to point out logical and scientific errors in the dominant conceptual system of psychosis and dissociation. The problem of the overlap and distinction between these two forms of psychopathology has numerous implications for theory, research and clinical practice. I will assume that schizophrenia and dissociative identity disorder are the major exemplars of the categories of psychosis and dissociation, and that arguments about each apply to the two general categories.

I will review evidence against the proposition that schizophrenia is primarily an inherited biological disorder treated with medication. I will then review evidence for there being an overlap and confusion between psychosis and dissociation, and go on to present evidence that the positive symptoms of schizophrenia are more characteristic of dissociative identity disorder than they are of schizophrenia. I will then review the evidence for the treatability of psychotic symptoms with psychotherapy in patients diagnosed with a dissociative disorder who also meet structured interview criteria for schizophrenia or schizoaffective disorder, and contrast this with the modest therapeutic impact of antipsychotic medications in schizophrenia. I will then argue for serious study of the conundrums and problems raised by my analysis, and will propose the existence of a dissociative subtype of schizophrenia.

My primary goal in this chapter is to dismantle the rigid, dichotomized categories of psychosis and dissociation, with reference to: genetic versus environmental causation; psychotic versus neurotic symptomatology; and treatability with medication versus psychotherapy. I will refer to dissociative identity disorder as multiple personality disorder when discussing data gathered before the name change in 1994.

EVIDENCE AGAINST THE GENETIC AETIOLOGY OF PSYCHOSIS

The major evidence against schizophrenia being predominantly an inherited disorder comes from the data on concordance rates in monozygotic twins. Kendler (1998), in accepting the Dean Award for lifetime research in schizophrenia from the American College of Psychiatrists, stated that, 'Most, if not all the reason that schizophrenia runs in families is due to shared genes and not shared environment.'

While making a concession to the possibility of an aetiological role for the environment, Kendler implied, by saying 'Most, if not all,' that this role was exceedingly minor.

In support of his conclusion, Kendler presented his own data from a study of 16,000 twin pairs in which concordance for schizophrenia in monozygotic twins was 31%. This finding is in fact conclusive proof that it is the role of inheritance that is minor in the aetiology of schizophrenia. The statement that most, if not all the aetiology of schizophrenia is genetic is clearly ideological in nature. It is contradicted by all the available evidence.

In a recent review, Sanders and Gejman (2001) stated that, overall, concordance rates for schizophrenia in monozygotic twins range from 30% to 45%. In a representative study, Cannon et al. (1998) concluded, from a concordance rate of 45% in a large sample of monozygotic twins, that 83% of the aetiology of schizophrenia is genetic. Their conclusion was based on a statistical model.

It is scientifically, biologically, genetically and medically impossible, based on a large body of data, that even half the aetiology of schizophrenia is genetic. The understanding of genetics required to make this analysis is contained in a ninth-grade biology text used in the state of Texas. A typical quotation from this text, illustrating the conceptual level expected of 14-year-old students, is: 'This means that two phenotypically normal people who are heterozygous carriers of a recessive mutation can produce children who are homozygous for the recessive gene. In such cases, the effects of the mutated genes cannot be avoided' (Johnson and Raven 1998: 154).

Other lines of evidence and arguments against the genetic basis of schizophrenia can be found in Ross (2004) and in Ross and Pam (1995). Since the concordance data are conclusive and irrefutable, other evidence will not be reviewed here. The scientific fact, based on the available evidence, is that schizophrenia is predominantly caused by the environment.

DATA ON THE EFFICACY OF ANTIPSYCHOTIC MEDICATION

Although psychiatrists commonly cite the efficacy of antipsychotic medications as evidence that schizophrenia is an endogenous 'chemical imbalance,' this conclusion is not warranted on either logical or empirical grounds. Medications can be effective for environmentally induced, genetically normal reactions to antigens, bacteria, viruses, physical trauma and numerous other forms of environmental input. The mechanisms of action of antihistamines, anti-inflammatories, antibiotics, painkillers and other medications used to treat these reactions have nothing to do with the genetic machinery controlling the reactions; the genome is normal in most of these medical problems, and there is no diagnostically specific 'genetic predisposition' involved in such normal responses to the environment. We do not search for the gene for fractured tibias in alpine skiers, although we do treat some of the symptoms with medication. Nor do we search for genes for streptococcal pneumonia, myocardial infarction or numerous other medical disorders.

It is clear, medically, that only a tiny subset of myocardial infarctions are caused by specific genetic defects such as familial hyperlipidoses. From a public health perspective, specific genetic treatment strategies aimed directly at diagnostically specific sections of abnormal genome, or their immediate products, can potentially help only a tiny subset of affected individuals. Behaviours are the primary target of treatment both before and after myocardial infarction. The relevant variables are diet, exercise, smoking, drinking, compliance with medications (for blood pressure and cholesterol) and stress management.

The conclusion that an endogenous biomedical aetiology can be inferred from response of symptoms to medication is unscientific. Such thinking is not medical.

An additional argument must be considered: if one accepts that the efficacy of antipsychotic medications can provide evidence that schizophrenia is an endogenous biomedical disorder, presumably this is true only if the medications are in fact effective, and only to the degree to which they are effective. If one accepts the erroneous logic of the 'medication response – chemical imbalance – endogenous biomedical aetiology' equation, then one is locked into a conclusion that schizophrenia is an endogenous biomedical disorder only to a modest degree, if at all.

Why is this so? The data on the efficacy of antipsychotic medications are conclusive: they reduce symptoms to a minor degree in most patients and are only marginally more effective than placebo.

These facts are illustrated by multi-center trials of the atypical antipsychotic, quetiapine (Seroquel). Arvantis and Miller (1997) describe a study in which 361 patients with schizophrenia from 26 centers in North America participated in a randomized, prospective, double-blind, placebo-controlled trial of Seroquel versus placebo. Data from this study are also summarized in Kasper and Muller-Spahn (2000), who present a bar graph of the principal findings. On the Brief Psychiatric Rating Scale (BPRS), subjects on 150 mg of Seroquel experienced an average score reduction of 8.67, while the subjects receiving placebo experienced an average increase in score of 1.71. It was found that 150 mg was the most effective dose of Seroquel. These data look quite impressive on a bar graph.

However, the average reduction in BPRS score per subject looks different when one examines the actual numbers rather than the bar graph. The baseline BPRS score for the subjects receiving 150 mg of Seroquel was 47.2; the scores fell to 38.2 on average, which is a reduction of only 19.1%. Scores of 38.2 on the BPRS are in the range for severe psychosis, and well above the cutoff score of 27 required for entry into the study.

At its most effective dose, Seroquel only reduces symptoms by 19.1%. Imagine an antipyretic which reduced fever by 19.1%. Assume that a temperature of 98.6° was set as zero on a 'Brief Fever Rating Scale.' Assume further that the average temperature of subjects randomized to the antipyretic was 102.6. If the average subject recruited into a multi-center, randomized, prospective, double-blind, placebo-controlled trial of the antipyretic experienced a symptom reduction of 19.1% in response to the most effective dose of antipyretic, the average temperature at the end-point of the study would be 101.6.

Mothers would not purchase this medication and it would fail in the marketplace. However, if paediatricians thought like psychiatrists, they would hail the efficacy of the drug as evidence that fever is a specific genetic syndrome. This conclusion would exactly parallel the rules of the *DSM-IV-TR* (American Psychiatric Association 2000) and the logic of the 'medication response – chemical imbalance – endogenous biomedical aetiology' equation. According to *DSM-IV-TR*, schizophrenia can be diagnosed based on the presence of a single Criterion A symptom, auditory hallucinations. Schizophrenia is the psychiatric equivalent of 'fever disorder,' and could be called 'auditory hallucination disorder.'

Kasper and Muller-Spahn (2000) go on to describe the percentage of responders to drug and placebo, defined as those with a 40% or greater reduction in BPRS scores. Again, they construct a visually impressive bar graph. However, the percentage of subjects who responded to Seroquel, using the 40% score reduction criterion, was only 29.2%, while the percentage responding to placebo was 5.9%.

This is not a big difference between drug and placebo. Nor is it a very impressive response to medication: under one third of subjects responded to the Seroquel.

Further, the term 'responder' disguises the fact that the average patient with an entry BPRS score of 47.2 can experience a 40% score reduction yet, with an end-point score of 28.3, still be psychotic enough to qualify for entry into the study. Only about 25% of subjects on 150 mg of Seroquel experienced a score reduction large enough to drop them below the BPRS entry cutoff score of 27.

The scientific facts are that Seroquel is effective in less than one quarter of patients and, overall, causes a minor reduction in symptom scores within the severely ill range on the BPRS.

The strangest Seroquel bar graph of all appears in Kasper and Muller-Spahn (2000). They provide evidence demonstrating that Seroquel is as effective as olanzapine (Zyprexa). They compare Arvantis and Miller's (1997) data to a study of Zyprexa by Beasley *et al.* (1996). Kasper and Muller-Spahn fail to comment on the fact that the response rate to placebo in the Zyprexa study was higher than the response rate to any dosage of Seroquel in the Seroquel study.

The existing data prove that in some groups of schizophrenics, placebo works better than Seroquel does in other groups. This is so even when both groups meet the criteria required by the Food and Drug Administration for entry into a clinical trial. This is not an anomalous or unusual finding. In fact it is the way the data look for all antipsychotic medications. This information has been readily available in the psychiatric literature for over twenty years.

Davis (1980), for example, described the results of 122 separate studies comparing 19 other neuroleptics to chlorpromazine. In none of these studies was the other medication found to be more effective than chlorpromazine. It is accepted that the different neuroleptics are equally effective if given in equivalent doses. Technically speaking, the neuroleptics are equi-effective if given in equi-potent doses. Therefore one can generalize from a comparison of chlorpromazine versus placebo to all neuroleptics.

Davis (1980) describes 66 studies in which chlorpromazine was compared to placebo for treatment of psychosis; there was no difference between the two in 11 of the 66 studies (17%). The superiority of neuroleptic over placebo is non-existent in almost one out of every five populations studied.

What about the studies in which there was a finding in favour of active medication? Typically, in such studies, there is a response to placebo, in terms of average score reduction, but the reduction is somewhat greater in the subjects randomized to a neuroleptic. The literature is conclusive that psychosis responds to placebo, and it is conclusive that the symptom reduction caused by neuroleptics is marginally superior to that caused by placebo. Subjects treated with neuroleptics in randomized trials, on average, still have significant residual symptoms of psychosis. Only a tiny minority experience a symptom reduction of 80%, that is, sufficient to classify them as 'normal' or 'in full remission.' This is such a small percentage that it is almost impossible for it to be clinically different from placebo.

The usual statistical analyses of antipsychotic medication versus placebo disguise the fact that the absolute magnitude of the treatment response is modest, and minimally superior to placebo. The pharmaceutical industry and 'biological psychiatry' have promoted a picture of the biological nature of major mental illness and the efficacy of psychotropic medication that is far out of proportion to the data. The statistically significant difference between medication and placebo seen in most, but not all, drug trials is of marginal clinical and conceptual significance.

EVIDENCE FOR AN OVERLAP BETWEEN DISSOCIATION AND PSYCHOSIS

Rosenbaum (1980), Bliss (1980) and Kluft (1987) were the first to point out that there is an overlap and confusion between dissociation and psychosis. My own study of this problem was inspired by and follows on from Kluft. In my Trauma Program in Dallas over the past ten years, several thousand individuals with dissociative disorders have received treatment. It is common for them to have received diagnoses of bipolar mood disorder, schizoaffective disorder, schizophrenia or psychotic disorder not otherwise specified from previous clinicians who did not make dissociative diagnoses.

In two large series of multiple personality cases summarized by Ross *et al.* (1990) ($n = 236$; $n = 102$), 40.8% and 26.5% had received previous diagnoses of schizophrenia, 54.5% and 57.0% had received antipsychotic medications, and 12.1% and 16.7% had been treated with electroconvulsive therapy (ECT). These figures provide clear evidence that these individuals were perceived by prior psychiatrists as suffering from major mental disorders with prominent psychotic symptoms.

Diagnoses justifying ECT and neuroleptics would have included schizophrenia, bipolar mood disorder, psychotic depression and schizoaffective disorder. Individuals in treatment for a dissociative disorder are consigned to the category of 'hysteria' by psychiatrists who do not believe in dissociative identity disorder. If they enter treatment with a non-believer psychiatrist prior to the dissociative diagnosis, however, they are regarded as suffering from a major endogenous biomedical brain disorder.

Ross *et al.* (unpublished data) interviewed 83 subjects with stable, long-term clinical diagnoses of schizophrenia and 166 subjects with multiple personality disorder (MPD) with the Dissociative Disorders Interview Schedule (Ross 1997). The two groups differed at $p < .05$ on all demographic variables using t tests or chi squares: average age, MPD 31.8 years, schizophrenia 41.9 years; average number of children, MPD 1.0, schizophrenia 0.6; per cent female, MPD 89.2, schizophrenia 30.9; per cent married, MPD 30.1, schizophrenia 13.3; and per cent employed, MPD 45.5, schizophrenia 9.9.

The MPD subjects reported higher rates of childhood physical and/or sexual abuse than those with schizophrenia: MPD 91.0%, schizophrenia 44.6% (χ^2, 65.544, $p < .001$). However, the difference was a matter of degree, since the schizophrenic subjects reported high rates of trauma compared to the base rate of 12.6% in the general population of the same city using the same structured interview (Ross 1991).

The MPD subjects more often met *DSM-III-R* criteria for: somatization disorder, MPD 39.8%, schizophrenia 4.8%; major depressive disorder, MPD 89.8%, schizophrenia 53.0%; and borderline personality disorder, MPD 61.4%, schizophrenia 21.7%. These differences were all significant at $p < .00001$ using chi-square tests. The two groups did not differ on rates of substance abuse: MPD 51.2%, schizophrenia 43.4%.

The MPD subjects also scored higher on the Dissociative Experiences Scale (DES; Bernstein and Putnam 1986) and symptom clusters of the Dissociative Disorders Interview Schedule: DES score, MPD 39.7, schizophrenia 14.2; somatic symptoms, MPD 14.1, schizophrenia 2.8; and borderline personality disorder criteria, MPD 5.1, schizophrenia 2.6. All these differences were significant at $p < .00001$.

The sensitivity of the structured interview in the MPD group was 94.6%, which is the percentage of subjects diagnosed as having MPD using the interview schedule. The remaining subjects all had numerous chronic dissociative symptoms on the interview schedule.

Most important for the present discussion, however, 25.3% of the schizophrenic subjects also met criteria for MPD, while others met criteria for other dissociative disorders.

Conversely, when 107 subjects with stable clinical diagnoses of dissociative identity disorder were interviewed with the Structured Clinical Interview for *DSM-III-R* (Ellason *et al.* 1996), 49.5% met criteria for schizoaffective disorder, 18.7% for schizophrenia, 2.8% for psychotic disorder not otherwise specified and 1.9% for delusional disorder.

The conceptual system of modern psychiatry, clinical diagnostic practices and the most valid and reliable structured interviews for making dissociative and psychotic diagnoses clearly yield substantial rates of false positive diagnoses in one or both directions. The data clearly demonstrate significant overlap and confusion between the two categories. This confusion and overlap is seen routinely in the diagnoses previously given to patients entering my hospital trauma programs.

EVIDENCE THAT THE POSITIVE SYMPTOMS OF SCHIZOPHRENIA ARE MORE COMMON IN DISSOCIATIVE IDENTITY DISORDER THAN IN SCHIZOPHRENIA, AND ARE RELATED TO CHILDHOOD TRAUMA

Individuals with dissociative identity disorder score highly on psychotic symptom measures, as well as meeting *DSM-IV-TR* and structured interview criteria for psychotic disorders. In my own research, these measures include the Dissociative Disorders Interview Schedule, the Symptom Checklist-90 (SCL-90), the Multidimensional Inventory of Dissociation, the Millon Clinical Multiaxial Inventory-II, the Positive and Negative Syndrome Scale and the Diagnostic Interview Schedule. Dissociative identity disorder subjects also characteristically have highly elevated scores on the schizophrenia scale of the Minnesota Multiphasic Personality Inventory (Coons and Fine 1988).

In fact, the positive symptoms of schizophrenia are more characteristic of multiple personality disorder than they are of schizophrenia. Ross *et al.* (1990) compared 12 published series of schizophrenia cases ($n = 2576$) to three series of MPD cases ($n = 368$) and found that the prevalence of one or more Schneiderian first rank symptoms was 87.0% among the MPD subjects but only 55.5% among the schizophrenic subjects. Similarly, the average number of Schneiderian symptoms was 4.9 in MPD but only 1.3 in schizophrenia.

When the authors compared the frequency distribution of Schneiderian symptoms in one series of MPD cases ($n = 102$) to that in three series of schizophrenia cases, the differences were even more striking. In the three series of schizophrenia cases ($n = 361$), only 16 subjects (4.4%) reported six or more of the 11 Schneiderian first rank symptoms, compared to 54 (52.9%) of the MPD subjects; only three of the schizophrenic subjects (0.8%) reported nine or more symptoms, compared to 27 (26.5%) of the MPD cases.

Ellason and Ross (1995) compared 108 subjects with dissociative identity disorder (DID) to norms for schizophrenia ($n = 240$) in the manual for the Positive and Negative Syndrome Scale. The average score on the positive symptom scale was 23.80 for the DID subjects and 19.86 for the schizophrenia subjects ($t = 5.80$, $p < .00001$). The average score on the negative symptom scale was 17.06 for the DID subjects and 21.75 for the schizophrenia subjects ($t = 7.19$, $p < .00001$).

The available data indicate that the positive symptoms of schizophrenia are more characteristic of dissociative identity disorder than they are of schizophrenia.

Ross *et al.* (unpublished data) interviewed 83 subjects with stable, long-term clinical diagnoses of schizophrenia with the Dissociative Disorders Interview Schedule. They divided the subjects into those who reported childhood physical and/or sexual abuse ($n = 37$) and those who did not

($n = 46$). The abused schizophrenics reported higher scores on the Dissociative Experiences Scale, and on six symptom scales of the Dissociative Disorders Interview Schedule.

Most important, the abused schizophrenics endorsed an average of 6.3 Schneiderian symptoms compared to 3.3 for the non-abused subjects ($t = 3.9$, $p < .001$). On the Positive and Negative Syndrome Scale, the abused schizophrenics had an average positive symptom score of 20.4 compared to 15.7 for the non-abused ($t = 3.2$, $p < .002$). The abused subjects had an average negative symptom score of -17.7, compared to -21.0 for the non-abused ($t = 1.9$, $p < .06$).

Laddis *et al.* (2001) compared subjects with dissociative identity disorder ($n = 35$) to those with schizophrenia ($n = 20$) on the Multidimensional Inventory of Dissociation. On this measure, the dissociative subjects more frequently endorsed all eight Schneiderian symptoms inquired about in the inventory. A typical finding was for voices arguing: dissociative subjects 71.5%, schizophrenic subjects 27.0%, a difference significant at $p < .05$.

Ellason and Ross (1996) noted high scores on the psychotic subscales of the Millon Clinical Multiaxial Inventory in a sample of 96 subjects with dissociative identity disorder. These included mean base rate scores on the different subscales of 77.7 for schizoid, 81.1 for schizotypal, 67.5 for paranoid and 77.6 for thought disorder. A base rate of 60 for a given scale was the mean for clinical subjects in the original development of the Millon Clinical Multiaxial Inventory: the higher the score above 60, the more disturbed the individual. In comparison, the highest scale score for the 96 subjects was 96.5 for avoidant and the lowest was 57.5 for bipolar:manic.

In a sample of 144 psychiatric inpatients, of whom 92 had dissociative identity disorder (Ross *et al.* 1996), scores on the psychoticism subscale of the SCL-90 correlated at $r = .40$ with the number of perpetrators of physical abuse ($p < .0001$) at $r = .31$ with the number of perpetrators of sexual abuse ($p < .0001$) and at $r = .27$ with the number of types of sexual abuse perpetrated ($p < .01$). The childhood abuse histories were gathered using the Dissociative Disorders Interview Schedule.

In this study, a regression analysis revealed that the number of perpetrators of physical abuse was an especially powerful predictor of scores on the psychoticism subscale of the SCL-90 ($R = .17$, $\beta = .34$, $F = 10.72$, $p < .001$) and the Schneiderian symptoms section of the Dissociative Disorders Interview Schedule ($R = .65$, $\beta = .36$, $F = 18.81$, $p < .00001$). The average score on the Global Severity Index of the SCL-90 is 2.11 (SD 0.68) for dissociative identity disorder, and the psychoticism subscale is one of the most elevated scales (Ross *et al.* 1996).

In a stratified cluster sample of the general population ($n = 502$) in the city of Winnipeg, Canada, subjects were divided into those who reported no Schneiderian first rank symptoms on the Dissociative Disorders Interview Schedule and those who reported three or more (Ross and Joshi 1992). The subjects with psychotic symptoms reported a rate of childhood physical and/ or sexual abuse of 45.7% compared to 8.1% for those without psychotic symptoms. The psychotic subjects also scored higher on the Dissociative Experiences Scale and five symptom scales of the Dissociative Disorders Interview Schedule.

In a regression analysis of this general population data, with the number of Schneiderian symptoms as the criterion variable, a history of physical and/or sexual abuse was a powerful predictor variable (β = .51, F = 22.337, p < .00001).

All the available data, then, which involve a wide range of self-report, computer-scored and structured interview measures, demonstrate that positive symptoms of psychosis are strongly related to and predicted by childhood physical and/or sexual abuse, and are more characteristic of dissociative identity disorder than of schizophrenia. This is true in both the general population and clinical populations: the more traumatized a sample, the more dissociative and psychotic it will be.

EVIDENCE FOR THE TREATABILITY OF PSYCHOTIC SYMPTOMS WITH PSYCHOTHERAPY IN DISSOCIATIVE IDENTITY DISORDER

The clinical literature on the treatment of dissociative identity disorder repeatedly describes the stable, long-term remission of Schneiderian symptoms on integration, in the absence of antipsychotic medication (Ross 1997). There is only a limited amount of more systematic, prospective treatment outcome data for the disorder, and none of it involves randomization of subjects or control groups. Randomization to waiting list or treatments assumed to be ineffective would be difficult for several reasons. First, there would be ethical problems randomizing subjects to a waiting list when the disorder carries such a high burden of hopelessness, depression and suicidal ideation, and when these symptoms respond so effectively to acute inpatient treatment (Ross and Ellason 2001; Ross and Haley 2004).

Typical reductions in scores after three to four weeks of acute inpatient and day hospital treatment for a sample of 30 subjects are: Beck Depression Inventory, admission 40.5, discharge 25.0; Beck Suicide Scale, admission 17.4, discharge 11.1; and Beck Hopelessness Scale, admission 13.9, discharge 8.7 (Ross and Ellason 2001). All these differences were significant at p < .0001 using t tests.

It would be almost impossible to convince subjects to participate in a waiting list or placebo treatment, even if it was deemed necessary to do so. The logistical problems of maintaining sufficient numbers of control subjects in the trial without almost 100% dropout rates would be insurmountable. Finally, the likelihood of obtaining grant money for a large prospective treatment outcome study for dissociative identity disorder is almost nil in the current ideological climate.

Despite these difficulties, the existing data indicate that treatment of dissociative identity disorder has a profound impact on a wide range of comorbid symptoms including psychosis. In reviewing these data, one must keep in mind that the standard of comparison is a 19.2% reduction of psychotic symptoms on 150 mg of Seroquel.

Ellason and Ross (1995) described a single case of dissociative identity disorder in which the Millon Clinical Multiaxial Inventory-II was administered pre-integration and two years later at post-integration. Base rate score reductions were similar to those observed in a larger sample of eight subjects treated to integration (Ellason and Ross 1996). In the larger sample, pre-integration base rate scores and post-integration base rate scores two years later were: schizoid, pre 64.3, post 54.0; schizotypal, pre 71.9, post 51.1; paranoid, pre 59.0, post 54.4; and thought disorder, pre 72.3, post 43.6. The percentage reduction in scale scores was: schizoid, 16.0%; schizotypal, 28.9%; paranoid, 7.8%; and thought disorder, 39.7%.

A base rate score of 60.0 is the cutoff for clinical significance on the Millon Clinical Multiaxial Inventory.

Ellason and Ross (1997) reported data on a variety of other measures for 54 dissociative identity disorder subjects interviewed in 1993 and again in 1995. The average number of Schneiderian symptoms endorsed for the previous year on the Dissociative Disorders Interview Schedule dropped from 6.8 to 4.2, a reduction of 38.2%. Among 12 subjects who reached integration during this time period, however, the reduction in Schneiderian symptoms was from an average of 6.2 to 1.4, which is 77.4%.

The end-point average of 1.4 Schneiderian symptoms is artificially high because in order to be classified as integrated, subjects must have experienced three months of integration. Symptoms were reported for the previous year, during which time some of the 12 subjects were not yet integrated.

For this chapter, I conducted an additional analysis on 36 subjects from Ellason and Ross (1997) who met Structured Clinical Interview for DSM-III-R (American Psychiatric Association 2000) criteria for schizophrenia or schizoaffective disorder at baseline in 1993. Reductions in scores on various measures between 1993 and 1995 are shown in Table 14.1. All the symptom reductions were significant at $p < .00001$ using t tests, except for the thought disorder scale of the Millon Clinical Multiaxial Inventory, which was significant at $p < .007$.

Overall, my clinical experience with this population indicates that no integrated individuals who formerly had dissociative identity disorder receive long-term neuroleptics post-integration. A few are prescribed selective serotonin re-uptake inhibitors on a long-term basis and none receive mood stabilizers long-term. No integrated subjects continue to experience any positive symptoms of psychosis.

Table 14.1 Two-year prospective follow-up on subjects with schizophrenia and schizo-affective disorder (*n* = 36)

Measure	1993	1995	% Reduction
PANNS positive symptoms	24.4	16.4	32.8
PANNS negative symptoms	-17.2	-13.4	22.1
SCL-90 psychoticism subscale	2.3	1.4	39.1
DDIS Schneiderian symptoms	6.7	3.9	41.8
MCMI-II thought disorder	74.9	69.1	7.7
	1993	1995	% Reduction
SCID schizophrenia or SCID schizoaffective disorder	100%	26.5%	73.5%

PANNS = Positive and Negative Syndrome Scale; SCL-90 = Symptom Checklist-90; DDIS = Dissociative Disorders Interview Schedule; SCID = Structured Clinical Interview for DSM-III-R

No professional with direct clinical experience of the minutely described sequence of therapeutic tasks and strategies for dissociative identity disorder (Ross 1997) would conclude that the remission of psychotic symptoms is anything but a treatment effect, although this cannot be proven scientifically with the available data.

CONUNDRUMS AND PROBLEMS CONCERNING DISSOCIATION AND PSYCHOSIS – THE CONTRAST BETWEEN NORTH AMERICA AND NORWAY

When I first went to Stavanger, Norway, in 1999 to talk about dissociation, I was completely unprepared for the conversations I experienced concerning dissociation and psychosis. In North America, at professional meetings, I had encountered only rigid, dichotomized thinking about these two categories. I had never met a person with a serious research or clinical interest in schizophrenia who took dissociative identity disorder seriously.

I presented an argument that some individuals in treatment for schizophrenia actually have dissociative identity disorder, and can be treated effectively with psychotherapy. This argument was well received by the clinicians already treating dissociative disorders, as I anticipated it would be.

An alternative and previously unconsidered viewpoint was presented to me by Jan Olav Johannessen. He proposed that rather than defining patients as having a dissociative disorder, I diagnose them as having schizophrenia. This is warranted because of their high scores on all measures of psychosis administered to date. Dr Johannessen's argument in favour of defining these people as psychotic was that doing so would improve the prognosis for schizophrenia.

I also learned that in Norway it is standard practice to provide long-term psychotherapy for individuals with schizophrenia. The therapy is active and directed at symptoms of the disorder. It is not merely educational or support-ive. Norwegian psychiatrists who do not adhere to the trauma model of psychosis (Ross 2000, 2004) nevertheless consider it standard practice to provide psychotherapy for their schizophrenic patients.

In North America, if I diagnosed someone as having schizophrenia, and treated them as described in my 1997 text on dissociative identity disorder, I would be liable for a seven-figure judgment in a medical malpractice lawsuit. I would be scoffed at as unscientific by virtually the entire community of researchers and clinicians dealing with schizophrenia. I could not get an academic appointment at a medical school in North America to conduct such treatment and I could not get a research grant to do so. Nor could I publish my description of the treatment in a biologically-oriented psychiatry journal. There is very little chance that the present chapter would be published by a North American editor with an academic track record in schizophrenia treatment or research.

My experience in Norway brought home to me the extreme ethnocentric nature of North American psychiatry. In more intellectually fluid, open and inquiring cultures, one is allowed to consider the possibility that some forms of schizophrenia could occur in genetically normal individuals in reaction to toxic input from the psychosocial environment, and be treatable with psychotherapy.

These possibilities, in my opinion, are worthy of serious academic, clinical and research attention.

A DISSOCIATIVE SUBTYPE OF SCHIZOPHRENIA

I propose the existence of a dissociative subtype of schizophrenia. According to this model, there is a spectrum of psychopathology as shown in Figure 14.1.

According to the Johannessen argument, one could include all cases to the right of the dissociative subtype of schizophrenia within the category of dissociative schizophrenia. I do not have a fixed position on this aspect of the model, and would be open to reclassifying all cases of dissociative identity disorder as dissociative subtype of schizophrenia. I am against this solution to the problem in North America solely because of the ideological climate in

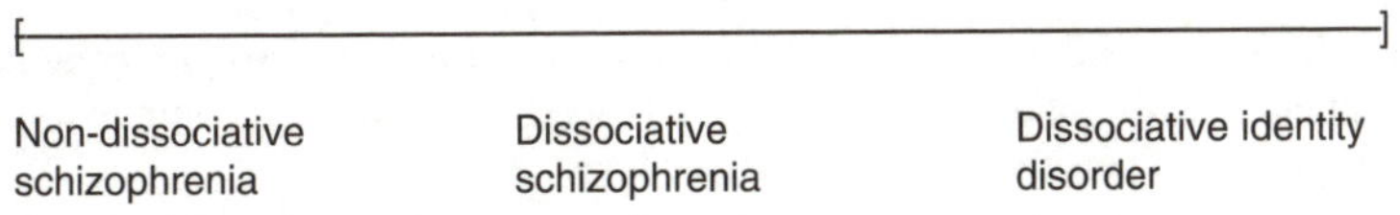

Non-dissociative   Dissociative   Dissociative identity
schizophrenia   schizophrenia   disorder

Figure 14.1 A dissociative subtype of schizophrenia.

North American psychiatry. In North America, that reclassification would eliminate the possibility of active psychotherapy for the psychosis.

If individuals with the dissociative subtype of schizophrenia could be treated according to the principles and strategies of the Trauma Model (Ross 2000, 2004) and treatment for dissociative identity disorder (Ross 1997), then I would have no objection to classifying them as suffering from schizophrenia.

According to the Trauma Model, the dissociative subtype of schizophrenia, compared to other subtypes, is characterized by more positive symptoms of psychosis, fewer negative symptoms, more comorbidity on both Axis I and Axis II, higher scores on measures of dissociation, a greater amount of psychological trauma, more of the psychobiology of trauma, less of the psychobiology of endogenous biomedical forms of schizophrenia, greater response to trauma therapy, more clearly defined, structured and dissociated identity states, and greater capacity for the voices to engage in psychotherapy. The dissociative subtype of schizophrenia may also have a differential response to antipsychotic medication; for instance non-responders to conventional D2 neuroleptics who then respond to clozapine may be more likely to have the dissociative subtype of schizophrenia.

If dissociative identity disorder was redefined as a dissociative subtype of schizophrenia, then the prognosis for schizophrenia would improve and it would be treatable, in some forms, with psychotherapy. The environmental aetiology of the dissociative subtype of schizophrenia could be demonstrated with adoption and twin studies. The prediction of the Trauma Model is that this subtype rarely if ever occurs in the absence of severe, chronic childhood trauma and that monozygotic twins discordant for severe trauma are almost never concordant for dissociative schizophrenia.

The current rigid categories concerning the aetiology, classification and treatment of dissociation and psychosis should be dismantled, to the potential benefit of many patients with psychoses. Unfortunately, these categories will probably continue to dominate North American psychiatry for years if not decades. They are not supported by the data and are not scientific in nature.

REFERENCES

American Psychiatric Association (1994) *Diagnostic and Statistical Manual of Mental Disorders* (4th ed.). Washington, DC: APA.

American Psychiatric Association (2000). *Diagnostic and Statistical Manual of Mental Disorders* (4th ed., text revision). Washington, DC: APA.

Arvantis, L. A. and Miller, B. G. (1997). Multiple fixed doses of 'Seroquel' (quetiapine) in patients with acute exacerbation of schizophrenia: A comparison with haloperidol and placebo. *Biological Psychiatry* 42: 233–46.

Beasley, C. M. *et al.* (1996). Olanzapine versus placebo and haloperidol. Acute phase results of the North American double-blind olanzapine trial. *Neuropsychopharmacology* 14: 111–23.

Bernstein, E. M. and Putnam, F. W. (1986). Development, reliability, and validity of a dissociation scale. *Journal of Nervous and Mental Disease* 174: 727–33.

Bleuler, E. (1950). *Dementia Praecox or the Group of Schizophrenias*. New York: International Universities Press.

Bliss, E. L. (1980). Multiple personalities. A report of four cases with implications for schizophrenia. *Archives of General Psychiatry* 37: 1388–97.

Cannon, T. D. *et al.* (1998). The genetic epidemiology of schizophrenia in a Finnish twin cohort. *Archives of General Psychiatry* 55: 67–74.

Coons, P. M. and Fine, C. (1988). Accuracy of the MMPI in identifying multiple personality disorder. In B. G. Braun (ed.) *Proceedings of the Fifth International Conference on Multiple Personality/Dissociative States*. Chicago: Rush-Presbyterian-St. Luke's Medical Center.

Davis, J. M. (1980). Antipsychotic drugs. In H. I. Kaplan *et al.* (eds) *Comprehensive Textbook of Psychiatry/III*. Baltimore: Williams and Wilkins.

Ellason, J. W. and Ross, C. A. (1995). Positive and negative symptoms in dissociative identity disorder and schizophrenia: A comparative analysis. *Journal of Nervous and Mental Disease* 183: 236–41.

Ellason, J. W. and Ross, C. A. (1996). Millon Clinical Multiaxial Inventory-II follow-up of patients with dissociative identity disorder. *Psychological Reports* 78: 707–16.

Ellason, J. W. and Ross, C. A. (1997). Two-year follow-up of inpatients with dissociative identity disorder. *American Journal of Psychiatry* 154: 832–9.

Ellason, J. W. *et al.* (1996). Lifetime Axis I and II comorbidity and childhood trauma history in dissociation identity disorder. *Psychiatry* 59: 255–66.

Gainer, K. (1994). Dissociation and schizophrenia: An historical review of conceptual development and relevant treatment approaches. *Dissociation* 7: 261–8.

Johnson, G. B. and Raven, P. H. (1998). *Biology: Principles and Explorations*. New York: Holt, Rhinehart and Winston.

Kasper, S. and Muller-Spahn, F. (2000). Review of quetiapine and its clinical applications in schizophrenia. *Expert Opinions in Pharmacotherapy* 1: 783–801.

Kendler, K. S. (1998, February). *The Genetics of Schizophrenia: Toward the Identification of Individual Susceptibility Loci*. Dean Award Lecture, Annual Meeting of the American College of Psychiatrists, San Juan, Puerto Rico.

Kluft, R. P. (1987). First-rank symptoms as a diagnostic clue to multiple personality disorder. *American Journal of Psychiatry* 144: 293–8.

Laddis, A. *et al.* (2001, December). *A Comparison of the Dissociative Experiences of Patients with Schizophrenia and Patients with DID*. Paper presented at the 18th International Fall Conference of the International Society for the Study of Dissociation, New Orleans.

Rosenbaum, M. (1980). The role of the term schizophrenia in the decline of diagnoses of multiple personality. *Archives of General Psychiatry* 37: 1383–5.

Ross, C. A. (1991). Epidemiology of multiple personality and dissociation. *Psychiatric Clinics of North America* 14: 503–17.

Ross, C. A. (1997). *Dissociative Identity Disorder: Diagnosis, Clinical Features and Treatment of Multiple Personality* (2nd ed.). New York: John Wiley and Sons.

Ross, C. A. (2000). *The Trauma Model: A Solution to the Problem of Comorbidity in Psychiatry*. Richardson, TX: Manitou Communications.

Ross, C. A. (2004). *Schizophrenia: Innovations In Diagnosis and Treatment.* Binghamton, NY: Haworth Press.

Ross, C. A. and Ellason, J. W. (2001). Acute stabilization in an inpatient trauma program. *Journal of Trauma and Dissociation* 2: 83–7.

Ross, C. A. and Haley, C. (2004). Acute stabilization and three month follow-up of inpatients in trauma program. *Journal of Trauma and Dissociation* 5: 103–12.

Ross, C. A. and Joshi, S. (1992). Schneiderian symptoms and childhood trauma in the general population. *Comprehensive Psychiatry* 33: 269–73.

Ross, C. A. and Pam, A. (1995). *Pseudoscience in Biological Psychiatry.* New York: Wiley and Sons.

Ross, C. A. *et al.* (1990). Schneiderian symptoms in multiple personality disorder and schizophrenia. *Comprehensive Psychiatry* 31: 111–8.

Ross, C. A. *et al.* (1996). Lifetime Axis I and II comorbidity and childhood trauma history in dissociative identity disorder. *Psychiatry* 59: 255–66.

Sanders A. R. and Gejman P. V. (2001). Influential ideas and experimental progress in schizophrenia genetics research. *Journal of the American Medical Association* 285 (22): 2831–3.

Chapter 15

Classic literary categories as a measure of progress in the psychotherapy of schizophrenia

Ann-Louise S. Silver

INTRODUCTION

The stages of treatment of schizophrenia take place within a cultural matrix, in a particular political climate, in treatment settings whose stability changes, and within evolving family matrices (both our patients' and our own). In reviewing my 25 years at the now-closed sanatorium, Chestnut Lodge, which specialized in the psychoanalytically-oriented treatment of chronically schizophrenic patients, I sought trends and generalizations about my colleagues' and my own work, and concluded that each of us brought a uniquely personal and evolving perspective to each individual enterprise (Fromm-Reichmann 1990; Greenberg 1967; Silver 1989, 1996, 1997). Jay Greenberg's comments help set realistic limitations to theorizing:

> Few issues in psychoanalysis are quite so muddled . . . as the relationship between theory and technique . . . [due to] the poor match between the kind of work that theory-making is, and the kind of work that clinical practice is. . . . Theorizing, necessarily, is done publicly. . . . [A]ll participants have access to what is said, if not necessarily to what is meant. Technique, on the other hand, is obviously private. There exists no record of all the transactions constituting an analysis, nor could such a record exist, even in principle. . . . By the time it is run through the analyst's particular vision of human life, not to mention his personality, the impact of theory is difficult to trace.
>
> (Greenberg 1986: 87)

Gertrude Stein made this same point, in her own unique style:

> Repeating then is in every one, in every one their being and their feeling and their way of realizing everything and every one comes out of them in repeating. More and more then every one comes to be clear to some one. Slowly every one in continuous repeating, to their minutest variation, comes to be clearer to some one. Every one who ever was or is or will be

living sometimes will be clearly realised by someone. Sometime there will be an ordered history of every one. Slowly every kind of one comes into ordered recognition.

(Stein 1934: 206)

Freud's famous comments on the stages of analytic treatment are similarly humble:

Anyone who hopes to learn the noble game of chess from books will soon discover that only the openings and end-games admit of an exhaustive systematic presentation and that the infinite variety of moves which develop after the opening defy any such description. This gap in instruction can only be filled by a diligent study of games fought out by masters. . . . The extraordinary diversity of the psychical constellations concerned, the plasticity of all mental processes and the wealth of determining factors oppose any mechanization of the technique.

(Freud 1913: 123)

The stages of treatment are often connected with the game of chess. Ernest Jones's paper 'The Problem of Paul Morphy' (1931) discusses the man said to be the best chess player ever. Jones describes chess as the ultimate game of war, and relates it to paranoia and to dread and denial of death. The first reported dream of my first analysand, a man suffering from non-psychotic obsessive doubts, illustrates this. In his recurring nightmare dating back perhaps to high school, he is playing chess, possibly against himself. The chessmen are beautiful but extremely fragile and valuable cut-glass crystal. The game is agonizing not only because of its strategic intricacy, but because he knows that if he accidentally breaks a glass, he will destroy the entire universe. The dream includes terror over waking up. What if in awakening he knocks over the board? This 'getting up' would later connect both to his severe ambivalence about moving up in the world, far beyond his explosive father, and his dread of 'getting up' into his wife and impregnating her; she was sometimes linked with his sexy mother of his childhood. Were he to father a child, his hopes of achieving personal ambitions would be shattered, and he would rage impotently as had his father.

This dream, with its immediate grandiose destructiveness, illustrates the core of the waking terror of patients suffering from psychoses, as Frieda Fromm-Reichmann and others have stressed (Fromm-Reichmann 1950, 1959). Regarding the rules of the game of psychotherapy in psychosis, Fromm-Reichmann's *Principles of Intensive Psychotherapy* (1950) is probably our profession's fundamental text, most of which remains currently relevant. She emphasized the patient's exaggerated dread of his or her destructive potential.

I will use Roy Schafer's 1970 article, 'The Psychoanalytic Vision of Reality,' to organize my thesis that the four categories of visions of reality – comic, romantic, tragic and ironic – correlate with the steps in successful psychotherapy of schizophrenia. They also apply to the developmental stages of therapists specializing in treating schizophrenia, and to the historical phases of our psychodynamically-oriented asylums. Like all categorizations, my thesis over-generalizes. It is susceptible to effective challenges and disagreement. Philosopher Wilfried Ver Eecke, on reading a draft of this chapter, highlighted Hegel's ranking of the aesthetic values in ascending order in 'Lectures on Aesthetics': architecture, sculpture, painting, music, poetry and, at the top, tragedy, comedy and drama (Hegel 1835). I believe that were we to evaluate the aesthetics of the drama of psychotherapy, work with sufferers of psychosis would rank far above treatment of the neuroses.

Schafer stresses that psychoanalysis has its roots in the humanities. He says, 'These roots have been all but lost sight of in this, the heyday of the medical-scientific programme for psychoanalysis' (Schafer 1970: 280). Schafer explains that the four categories referred to above are those which 'scholars have discerned in the mythic and artistic products of this imaginative mind confronting reality' (ibid.). I will relate each vision to the evolution of our institutional philosophies and to the individual therapist's maturational process; some illustrative clinical vignettes are included.

THE COMIC VISION

> The comic vision seeks evidence to support unqualified hopefulness regarding man's situation in the world. It serves to affirm that no dilemma is too great to be resolved, no obstacle too firm to stand against effort and good intentions . . . no suffering so intense that it cannot be relieved, and no loss so final that it cannot be undone or made up for. The programme is reform, progress and tidings of joy.
>
> (Schafer 1970: 281)

Gail Hornstein's biography of Fromm-Reichmann, published in 2000, is entitled *To Redeem One Person is to Redeem the World*. Before it was available, Joanne Greenberg, author of *I Never Promised You a Rose Garden* (1964), wrote to me,

> WAIT until you read Gail Hornstein's book!! It is just about everything we all wanted to say about what happened and what has been happening in psychiatry recently – it seems to me she got it all right. Like any really good biography, she does the milieu, but also the writing is good, and the conclusions she comes to are what we all would have wanted.
>
> (Greenberg, personal communication)

Fromm-Reichmann illustrated the comic vision in a lecture delivered at the 1954 annual meeting of the American Psychiatric Association in St. Louis, USA:

> My experience during the last twenty years has been mainly with schizo-phrenic patients who came to our hospital in a state of severe psychotic disturbance, from which the majority emerged sooner or later under intensive dynamic psychotherapy. . . . Sometimes relapses occurred. Such relapses were due to failure in therapeutic skill and evaluation of the extent of the patient's endurance for psychotherapy, to unrecognized difficulties in the doctor–patient relationship, or to responses to intercur-rent events beyond the psychiatrist's control. As a rule, these relapses could be handled successfully if the psychiatrist himself did not become too frightened, too discouraged, or too narcissistically hurt by their occurrence.
>
> (Fromm-Reichmann 1959: 196)

This certainly gave members of the audience a sense that patients they referred to Chestnut Lodge would recover or improve markedly, or that if they themselves worked at the Lodge, their therapeutic prowess would be transformed. Robert Cohen served as Chestnut Lodge's Clinical Director, then was head of intramural research at the National Institute of Mental Health before returning to the Lodge as Director of Psychotherapy. This was the post his analyst, Fromm-Reichmann, had held. He often said that those working at the Lodge in those years were chronically discouraged by the obdurate nature of schizophrenia. They needed the small group meetings, and the system wherein everyone was in ongoing supervision, to keep their spirits up.

Schafer continues:

> Thus, the protagonist in difficulty is regarded as being blocked in the pursuit of his goals by representatives of an obstructive society and as ultimately triumphing over these representatives and becoming the centre of a new and better one. As he makes his way to the influential centre of affairs, his attitude toward the blocking figures changes for the most part from opposition to their exclusiveness to acceptance and inclusiveness.
>
> (Schafer 1970: 281)

For me, this resonates with Fromm-Reichmann's and others' tendency to view family dynamics as the crucial factor in the development of schizo-phrenia. It also resonates with a contradictory but very intriguing statement made by Fromm-Reichmann at a Lodge Wednesday Conference:

It is our experience that whenever a patient gets well, it has the power to change the relatives. Now, if she breaks out of all the hostile interplay and resentment by virtue of her insight, the mother and father will change too. If she learns how to get along with the parents, the parents will get along with her. You are the [inter]mediary for that.

(Silver and Feuer 1989: 30)

Schafer emphasizes that 'Laughter and gaiety are not considered essential to the comic. Worldly gratification and security are' (Schafer 1970: 281). The comic vision emphasizes ideas of rebirth, springtime and 'the world view of cyclic return, another chance: the view of cyclic return implies that the past can be redone, if not undone. Thereby it implicitly denies the passage of time. It cancels out pastness' (ibid.: 283). For me, this resonates with my sense, mid-treatment, of re-parenting my patient. Parental outrage against such professional strivings and hubris has largely forced discussion of this quandary into the silent and therefore dangerous realm of political incorrectness. Schafer concludes, 'A legitimate comic element is preserved . . . in the acknowledged possibility of accomplishing some revision of [the patient's] inner world – of developing a fresh view of it, and, through that, a healthier narcissism and social existence' (ibid.: 283).

THE ROMANTIC VISION

In the romantic vision . . . life is a quest or a series of quests. The quest is a perilous, heroic, individualistic journey. Its destination or goal combines some or all of the qualities of mystery, grandeur, sacredness, love, and possession by or fusion with some higher power or principle.

(Schafer 1970: 283)

The romantic vision develops out of the comic vision, as the following point by Barbro Sandin, at the International Society for the Psychological Treatments of the Schizophrenias and Other Psychoses at Turin in 1988, illustrated:

By what right do we reject our patients and see their life and death struggle only as an illness, thus making impossible their chances of finding a way? In daily life together with my patients, I am helped by the thoughts underlying the concept 'being-with-the-other.' It means to be *with* – NOW – in time and space and in myself. . . . This is the beginning of the solution to the mystery or the illumination of the paradox: I do not exist now, but I have existed. I know something about existing. I was then, and I can begin to exist again, now, in a new experience, different from then.

(Sandin 1993: 26–7)

Gaetano Benedetti, in *Psychotherapy of Schizophrenia*, quotes a metaphoric passage written by his patient because, 'Such a report shows us how it is possible, in psychotherapy, for suffering and participation to become the *power of liberation*' (Benedetti 1987: 221). The patient writes:

> Gaetano Benedetti was called, one day, by an unknown voice, and told to set on the way to Hades . . . to look for a certain corpse. . . . He had only himself to depend upon, as he was alone, or rather not quite, but his companionship consisted only of a lifeless doll that he had found on a compost heap. . . . He prepared a comfortable resting place for the puppet one night, and lovingly covered her, and hid his tears from her. . . . The doll knew very well that it was her own soul for which he had gone wandering.
>
> (Benedetti 1987: 220–1)

The patient describes terrifying near-catastrophes, and concludes, 'Even the sight of the castle at a distance created such fear in the doll such as the living do not know, but the man pulled her ever onward' (ibid.).

Schafer explains 'The romantic vision is, implicitly if not explicitly, regressive and childlike, particularly in its persistent nostalgia for a golden age in time or space that is the essential destination of the quest, the prize for the counterphobic victor in the central conflict' (Schafer 1970: 284). My persistent nostalgia for the old Lodge, which I've called my perpetual residency, my marvelling at the intensity of supportive review, at the uniqueness of each treatment pair and trios of patient, therapist and supervisor, and at the kaleidoscopic effect of working among so many such trios, I am sure leads readers to think, 'Grow up already. Face reality. Rose gardens have their season.' Again Schafer: 'Sooner or later experience becomes a failed quest as "nature" and "triumph" remain ambiguous, elusive and costly' (ibid.: 284).

> [Y]et fundamental changes take place . . . the quest continues, but, for the patient, the dragons change, the modes of combat change, and the concepts of heroism and victory change. . . . Gaining insight into this world replaces much interpersonal and intrapersonal aggressive and libidinal manipulation as the way to fight it all out. . . . Analysis as investigation is the quest.
>
> (ibid.: 284–5)

While the McGlashan follow-up study (McGlashan 1984, 1986a, 1986b) reported moderate to marked improvement among only one third of the Lodge's patients diagnosed with schizophrenia, it found an astounding rate of significant improvement or recovery in 80% of patients diagnosed as borderline. And in a study by Fenton and McGlashan (1987) into sustained remission in drug-free schizophrenia, the course of 163 patients was reviewed, averaging 15 years post-discharge from the Lodge. The authors defined a good outcome as including no further hospitalizations and no exposure to psychotropic medication, while having a moderate-or-better outcome. There were 23 patients, or 14% of the total: 8 men (10%) and 15 women (19%). Of these, 80% were working and 70% had married. Most stayed in outpatient therapy for two years after leaving the hospital and then had no therapy, and only 13% were in treatment at follow-up. As in other studies, they were more likely to have left the hospital against medical advice. Thus, the quest reached its goal more often, it seems to me, than it does currently.

Within the romantic vision, each therapist and each patient struggles to assert the constructive aspects of his/her personality, often at the expense of the other. Mutual therapeutic zeal and mutual resistance lead to a sometimes exciting but more often an exasperating and boring redundancy. Each party tries to inculcate and indoctrinate the other into his or her world view. Each says, 'What works for me might work for you.' For example, an analytically trained researcher at the Lodge presented his work with a chronically depressed and psychotic woman. He quoted her ruefully complaining that she was alone in the world – she had no-one and never would have anyone in her life. 'But look how many friends you have,' he said, and then told the listeners how he had counted out the number of her friends – the fellow patients with whom she walked into town for dinners. He felt confident that he was working well with her, and yet many of us groaned and then commented that he was denying the patient her reality, and forcing his perceptions of reality onto her. How do we differentiate this from my repeatedly highlighting my patients' ambivalences or transferences? Am I pushing my perspective onto their accounts? Ver Eecke comments here that dialogue must be distinguished from imposing. There might be a danger in pushing our perspectives, but this is bad psychoanalysis – the sort of problem Freud had with Dora.

During a session with a chronically psychotic woman, I spun out a metaphor of our work. The patient has created a balloon with its own light atmosphere in which she floats above the earth; however, the balloon has a string. The string grows finer as its distance from the balloon increases. At the start of the work it is spider-web-thin. I catch hold and pull very gently, winding it into a skein. Sometimes or many times it breaks when I or the patient tug. But as the process continues, the thread grows stronger and can endure more tugs and jerks without disruptions that feel final. At last, we are really looking at each other. The balloon's wall grows thinner – even permeable – and disappears, as the patient stands firmly on the ground of our vulnerability, fallibility and mortality.

Harold Searles's observations on the stages of treatment, definitive during the non-medication era, delineate the stages of this romantic quest. But are they still applicable from a psycho-bio-social, psycho-pharmacologically influenced perspective?

The 'technique' of psychotherapy of schizophrenia is best spelled out in terms of an evolutionary sequence of specific, and very deep, feeling involvements in which the therapist as well as the patient becomes caught up, over the course of what has emerged. . . . That is, both the therapist and the patient bring the full range of their humanities to the new relationship, and this involves their emotional histories as individuals, and the ways they have learned to process these emotions. The most important skill in reaching successful maturity is the ability to recognize one's ambivalences and to accept them, to know that one both loves and hates each of one's parents, one's spouse, children, patients, co-workers, etc. When this state of inner contradiction has not been accepted emotionally and intellectually, a person is at risk for psychotic regression, having relied too long on symbiosis, or psychological merge, or lack of boundaries, with the mother. The therapist of such a person will resonate with the patient; the therapist's own primitive states of mind which preceded the owning of ambivalence will be heightened, analogous to harmonic vibration. The therapist needs to be open to these states of mind: to be mother to her new baby, or baby to his or her new mother, in a wordless mix-up which can later develop towards mutual autonomy.

(Searles 1961: 521)

Searles, quoting Mabel Blake Cohen, emphasizes the patient's efforts to manipulate 'the relationship in such a way as to elicit the same kind of behaviour from the analyst' that the patient experienced from the parents (ibid.: 522). He then maps out:

The successive phases which in my experience best characterize the psychotherapy of chronic schizophrenia: . . . the 'out-of-contact' phase, the phase of ambivalent symbiosis, the phase of pre-ambivalent symbiosis, the phase of resolution of the symbiosis, and the late phase – that of establishment, and elaboration, of the newly won individuation through selective new identifications and repudiation of outmoded identifications. The first three of these phases retrace, in reverse, the phases by which the schizophrenic illness was originally formed.

(ibid.: 523)

Is such work possible when the patient is receiving a complex and changing psychopharmacologic regimen? Do we now work through these phases, but on a new level of mental organization, or if we now trace such phases, is it in an 'as if' mode, as we pretend such working through is still possible? Perhaps anti-psychotic medications preclude the formation of a transference psychosis. And how many of us are left who still say that such a transference psychosis is necessary for ultimate recovery?

THE TRAGIC VISION

The tragic vision is expressed in a keen responsiveness to the great dilemmas, paradoxes, ambiguities, and uncertainties pervading human action and subjective experience. It manifests itself in alertness to the inescapable dangers, terrors, mysteries, and absurdities of existence. It requires one to recognize the elements of defeat in victory and of victory in defeat. . . . Of all the perspectives on human affairs, the tragic is by far the most remorselessly searching, deeply involved, and, along with the ironic, impartial. . . . The tragic sense of time is linear rather than cyclic . . . a second chance cannot be the same as the first; life is progression towards death without rebirth. . . . [I]nternal split or opposition is essential to the tragic vision, according to which the protagonist is inevitably divided within himself, some of his rights, values, duties, and opportunities necessarily clashing with others, and his choices consequently always entailing sacrifice, ambivalence, and remorse, if not guilt. Scheler (1954) extending Hegel's (Abel 1967: 367–416) line of thought, speaks of the 'tragic knot', which expresses 'the entanglement between the creation and destruction of a value'; by this he refers to the coinciding in an event, person or thing, and, above all, in one quality, power or ability, of the influences that both champion the value and destroy it. Much of analysis is concerned with tragic knots.

(Schafer 1970: 285–6)

Treatment terminations highlight the tragic vision. While some are agreed upon, far more often the duo is disrupted. The therapist moves away geographically or moves away from this grueling work, or becomes sick or dies. The patient's family runs out of money or patience or both, and pushes for less costly treatment, or they or the patient suffer a disaster – an accident or a suicide. Or, as was the case for Chestnut Lodge, the hospital itself may metaphorically move away or die.

Meanwhile, I regret how my current clinical efforts have a cheer-leading quality, like those of the researcher-clinician I mentioned earlier. I promote unknown risk-taking for the sake of seeming progress. I cannot be simultaneously playful and in authority, and too often find my work stultifying, depressing, frustrating and almost inauthentic. But I have the rare luxury of meeting frequently with my patients, without the intrusion of managed care pressures which have generally demolished confidentiality and forced clinicians into a behaviourally-based system of specific short- and long-term goals. Bertram Karon (2003; Karon and Vandenbos 1981) has spoken eloquently and forcefully about the current tragedy – that people suffering from schizophrenia are almost always blocked from the opportunity for insight-oriented psychotherapy.

Clinical case

The treatment termination that I experienced as the most tragic involved the end of five years of work with a man who was 22 when we met. He typifies the Holocaust second generation, as described by Grubrich-Simitis (1981, 1984) and others. He had broken down at age 18, in his freshman year at a prestigious university. He was hospitalized, tried to return to college, but then needed increasingly long hospitalizations.

When his father was 18, he and his family were deported to Auschwitz, where father's mother was killed immediately, and father's father survived until the final months of the war. My patient's father and uncle escaped in its final chaotic weeks. Father became a prominent physicist in the USA, but terrorized his family with huge outbursts, followed by enormous contrition. He wolfed down each meal as if to eat slowly risked starvation.

My patient was brilliant. He trounced me at chess in the midst of florid delusions. He had been a successful actor, and dramatic displays remained his specialty. In a session when he was in a cold wet sheet pack, he 'became' Hitler and raged at me, describing the tortures he had in store for me. He frothed at the mouth. I gagged and almost vomited. At other times he was Christ. Once he 'was' a comet, a cluster of ice crystals hurtling through space, held together by their shared gravitational field. He warned me not to get too close, since I might become another such comet.

He sometimes commanded my absolute silence because he was watching hallucinated cartoons, in the style of Art Spiegelman's *Maus* (1986). My patient had actually won a national cartooning contest, and I really wanted to see these hallucinations. In one session, he asked me to take dictation of his poetry in the steno pad where I kept my process notes. I was pleased to do this, but got irritated as he scornfully insisted on my adding a comma, 'No! Not there, you idiot! On the line above!' We filled one side of a page. I turned the page and began on the back of the just-completed page, as is my routine. 'Don't write on both sides of the page. I want my poetry written on just one side.' 'I don't feel like it,' I said. We got into a stubborn stand-off, and he spat at me. I have no justification for not complying with his simple request.

His outbursts continued, and the staff all agreed to resume phenothiazine prescription. He progressed and moved to supervised living and had a job. But he knew his treatment was diminishing his parents' retirement fund. He announced to me his decision to make the hospital fire him. He was determined to 'win' this one. He took a hated housemate's record collection out to the pavement on the day the dustbin men were due. The collection was removed. About a month later, the housemate (who had been, before his breakdown, a promising physicist) committed suicide. A few days after trashing those records, at a hospital talent show, my patient sang hard rock songs and then, in the Pete Townsend tradition, hurled the microphone and speakers at the wall. He was re-admitted to the hospital while his parents arranged a transfer to a distant state.

In our final session, he paced back and forth expressing intense ambivalence – gratitude and disappointment, hope and despair. Sometimes he paced behind me. He took off the bandanna he wore as a head band, and whipped it around my neck. As quickly as he tightened it around my neck he released it and rushed out of the room. I found a staff member to stay with us. My patient claimed he was only joking. He never intended to harm me. I think he meant it as a dramatic communication, an enactment of the tragedy of his father's life and of his own, the experience of chronic dread of murder, being killed or doing the killing. With his 'joke' he was depositing this dread-filled tension in me. I would remember both of us as terrified and terrifying, trusting and paranoid, creative and destructive, all in ways too complex to elaborate fully. He still resides in that distant community, holding intermittent jobs, and avoiding ambitions and creative challenges. I was sad to hear from his parents that he burned his often evocative poetry, some of which has survived in my note pads.

I experienced each of my patients who required reinstatement of medications as slipping away as their formerly 'real' issues became obscured. They seemed both more coherent and less authentic; I have felt more muddled, more cheer-leading and less authentic.

When I was in psychiatric residency in the early 1970s, I participated in a teaching seminar given by a distinguished analytic teacher who had begun his career at Chestnut Lodge. He shared process material from his work with a young psychotic woman who, when the seminar began, was his outpatient. I was awed by his skill and very appreciative of his ability to let us in on how he formulated his comments to her. However, she became increasingly depressed and frightened, and was hospitalized on one of our wards. There, she did some extraordinary painting in the occupational therapy programme. I still recall my deep disappointment when, having begun on phenothiazines, she covered my favourite painting, a self-portrait, with a whitewash that obscured her in a fog, muted the work and robbed it of its evocative power. Some weeks later she was discharged from the hospital and, rather soon after, died by suicide. Our seminar became a memorable group experience as we agonized over our limited therapeutic power. We knew that no matter how much expertise we might gain, and no matter what our empathic capabilities and real fondness and admiration for our patients, this might not suffice to prevent the disaster that ends all possibility of hopeful resolution. This conclusion is a too-common final stage of treatment in schizophrenia; approximately 10% of patients end their own lives. This statistic has remained constant in both the pre- and post-medication eras.

THE IRONIC VISION

Schafer writes:

> The ironic vision I shall characterize chiefly as a readiness to seek out
> internal contradictions, ambiguities and paradoxes. In this respect it
> overlaps the tragic vision. The difference between the two lies in their
> aims. The tragic vision aims at seeing the momentous aspects and
> implications of events and people; it values total involvement and great
> crises. . . . The ironic vision considers the same subject matter as the
> tragic but aims at detachment, keeping things in perspective, taking noth-
> ing for granted, and readily spotting the antithesis to any thesis so as to
> reduce the claim of that thesis upon us. . . . Applied to oneself, irony is
> self-deprecatory.
>
> (Schafer 1970: 293)

He adds, 'A useful capacity for irony is not reliably available to psychotic
patients undergoing treatment' (ibid.: 294). This is Schafer's only single-
sentence paragraph. It calls out for an intensive study of the development of
increasingly reliable capability for irony as a marker for progress in psychodynamic treatment of the psychoses. Such study might be approached by
tracking the use of humor in a given treatment. As observed by Ver Eecke, if
both parties have enjoyed a particular joke, they have each been able to see two
points of view simultaneously, this reinforcing an inner dialogue for both.

My vision of irony is most intense as I consider my work with one of my
first Lodge patients, who was called the sickest patient to have been admitted
to the adolescent unit. I worked with her for seven years, with no meds, and
she went on to college and graduate school, marriage and kids. We had
succeeded after seven intensive years. But then, following an accident that left
her in chronic severe pelvic pain, her psychosis and suicidality returned. She
had since moved far away. We began weekly phone sessions. She revealed
that she had been chronically molested from the age of eight until coming
to the hospital. None of us at the Lodge had known or really suspected as
the treatment occurred in the 1970s before incest became clearly thinkable.
She has many explanations for keeping her secret, including her having
wished her abuser might come to rescue her. If she told, it would have made it
harder for him to do so. I am left humbled by my inability to imagine the
unthinkable.

CONCLUSION

We need, I believe, to re-examine the roots of our interest in this work. Are
we in error when we keep private our personal histories as an extension of

analytic anonymity? This professionalistic isolation, this privacy or aloofness, distances us from other mental health workers, and from our patients' families and our patients themselves. About fifteen years ago, a group of women psychiatrists at the Lodge formed a study group, at first reading and discussing some classic papers. We then focused on our work with violent patients. Talking about our countertransferences led to our sharing aspects of own life stories. We gave as much or as little intimate detail as we chose in the 45 minutes we allotted. We organized our remarks around the question, 'What's a nice girl like you doing in a place like this?' We went through three cycles of autobiography among the five of us, and were astounded by the lack of much coincidence. But this variety only highlighted the powerful point of consensus: we all emphasized our mothers' depressions. One had made a suicide attempt. One suffered a vegetative, another an agitated depression, and another was intermittently raging, with insomnia and persecutory delusions (LaVia *et al.* 1986).

Our study group also discussed our siblings' emotional difficulties, and our yearnings to help them. Wally Lamb's novel (1998) and Jay Neugeboren's (1997) and Robin Hemley's (1998) memoirs exemplify the siblings' ambivalent therapeutic strivings. Just as Fromm-Reichmann had said that she was a therapist from the age of three, managing her parents' interpersonal tensions (Fromm-Reichmann 1956), we too felt we had been attempting to be family therapists, and therapists to each of our parents, mainly our mothers. We began our professional training before we were enrolled in nursery school. We all acknowledged that our patients had striven similarly. We could see this in the transference, our patients as our therapists, as first recognized by Georg Groddeck and as elaborated by Sándor Ferenczi and Harold Searles (see Silver 1993). I now think of our professional training as advancing a life's work. It provides us with professional orientation and jargon, guild affiliations and guild agendas. It strengthens elitism as we compete for earnings and market share. But as we see our asylums downsizing or closing, we no longer hold court in our ivory towers. Those of us who have reached the life stage characterized by an ironic orientation have an obligation to be with the younger generations of mental health workers, who are still energetically in the comic and romantic phases of their careers. Their youthful optimism, their quest to slay the dragon of psychosis, can help us as we labour along, maturely and depressively ironic. Perhaps they can continue their quest to help their depressed parents in their transferences with us. While our orientation can help them master their anxieties, so that the treatment of psychosis may still proceed with humanism and dignity, they can help us stay connected to the rapidly evolving scene.

Mental health services in the USA have been enduring a long and complex siege, and we are often left impotently battling each other and working at cross purposes. The frequency of psychoanalytic work in the USA has plummeted, and analytically-oriented work with people with psychotic illness is even rarer. For me, in these challenging times, the International Society for the Psychological Treatment of the Schizophrenias and Other Psychoses has become an increasingly cherished container and support, as I struggle to develop an ironic vision of reality that allows me to continue questing. But the dragons won't stay slayed. They refuse even to be defined, and I notice that I myself am often shooting flames.

REFERENCES

Benedetti, G. (1987). *Psychotherapy of Schizophrenia*. New York: New York University Press.

Fenton, W. S. and McGlashan, T. (1987). Sustained remission in drug free schizophrenia. *American Journal of Psychiatry* 144: 1306–9.

Freud, S. (1913). On beginning the treatment: Further recommendations on the technique of psychoanalysis. *Standard Edition* 12: 121–44. London: The Hogarth Press and the Institute of Psychoanalysis.

Fromm-Reichmann, F. (1950). *Principles of Intensive Psychotherapy*. Chicago: University of Chicago Press.

Fromm-Reichmann, F. (1956/1989). Reminiscences of Europe. In A.-L. Silver (ed.) *Psychoanalysis and Psychosis*. Madison, CT: International Universities Press.

Fromm-Reichmann, F. (1959). *Psychoanalysis and Psychotherapy* (edited by D. M. Bullard). Chicago: University of Chicago Press.

Fromm-Reichmann, F. (1990). The assets of the mentally handicapped: The interplay of mental illness and creativity. *Journal of the American Academy of Psychoanalysis* 18: 47–72.

Greenberg, J. (1964). *I Never Promised You a Rose Garden*. New York: Holt, Rinehart and Winston. (Early editions published under pseudonym of Hannah Green.)

Greenberg, J. (1967). In praise of my doctor – Frieda Fromm-Reichmann. *Contemporary Psychoanalysis* 4: 73–5.

Greenberg, J. R. (1986). Theoretical models and the analyst's neutrality. *Contemporary Psychoanalysis* 22: 87–106.

Grubrich-Simitis, I. (1981). Extreme traumatization as cumulative trauma: Psycho-analytic investigations of the effects of concentration camp experiences on survivors and their children. *Psychoanalytic Study of the Child* 36: 415–50.

Grubrich-Simitis, I. (1984). From concretism to metaphor: Thoughts on some theoretical and technical aspects of the psychoanalytic work with children of holocaust survivors. *Psychoanalytic Study of the Child* 39: 301–19.

Hegel, G. (1835/1920). *Philosophy of Fine Art*, Vol. 1 (translated by F. P. B. Osmaston). London: Bell.

Hemley, R. (1998). *Nola: A Memoir of Faith, Art, and Madness*. Saint Paul, MI: Graywolf Press.

Hornstein, G. (2000). *To Redeem One Person is to Redeem the World: The Life of Frieda Fromm-Reichmann*. New York: The Free Press.

Jones, E. (1931). The problem of Paul Morphy: A contribution to the psychoanalysis of chess. *International Journal of Psycho-Analysis* 12: 1–23.

Karon, B. (2003). The tragedy of schizophrenia without psychotherapy: Washington School of Psychiatry 2001 Frieda Fromm-Reichmann Lecture. *Journal of the American Academy of Psychoanalysis and Dynamic Psychiatry* [special issue: The schizophrenic person and the benefits of the psychotherapies – Seeking a PORT in the storm] 31: 89–118.

Karon, B. and Vandenbos, G. (1981). *Psychotherapy of Schizophrenia: The Treatment of Choice*. New York: Jason Aronson.

Lamb, W. (1998). *I Know This Much is True*. New York: HarperCollins.

LaVia, D., Goldberg, L., McAfee, L., Roberts, V. and Silver, A.-L. (1986, October). *Chronicity and Change in the Therapist*. Presented to the 32nd Annual Chestnut Lodge Symposium, 'Aspects of Chronicity.'

McGlashan, T. (1984). The Chestnut Lodge follow-up study: I & II. *Archives of General Psychiatry* 41: 573–601.

McGlashan, T. (1986a). The Chestnut Lodge follow-up study, III & IV. *Archives of General Psychiatry* 43: 20–30, 167–76.

McGlashan, T. (1986b). Predictors of shorter-, medium-, and longer-term outcome in schizophrenia. *American Journal of Psychiatry* 143: 50–55.

Neugeboren, J. (1997). *Imagining Robert: My Brother, Madness, and Survival – A Memoir*. New York: William Morrow and Co.

Sandin, B. (1993). When being is not to be. In G. Benedetti and P. Furlan (eds) *The Psychotherapy of Schizophrenia: Effective Clinical Approaches – Controversies, Critiques and Recommendations*. Seattle: Hogrefe and Huber Publishers.

Schafer, R. (1970). The psychoanalytic vision of reality. *International Journal of Psycho-analysis* 51: 279–97.

Searles, H. F. (1961). Phases of patient–therapist interaction in the psychotherapy of chronic schizophrenia. In *Collected Papers on Schizophrenia and Related Subjects*. New York: International Universities Press.

Silver, A.-L. (ed) (1989). *Psychoanalysis and Psychosis*. Madison, CT: International Universities Press.

Silver, A.-L. (1993). Countertransference, Ferenczi, and Washington, DC. *Journal of the American Academy of Psychoanalysis* 21: 637–54.

Silver, A.-L. (1996). William James and Gertrude Stein: Psychology affecting literature. *Journal of the American Academy of Psychoanalysis* 24: 321–39.

Silver, A.-L. (1997). Chestnut Lodge, then and now: Work with a patient with schizophrenia and obsessive compulsive disorder. *Contemporary Psychoanalysis* 33: 227–49.

Silver, A.-L. and Feuer, P. (1989). Fromm-Reichmann's contributions at staff conferences. In *Psychoanalysis and Psychosis*. Madison, CT: International Universities Press.

Spiegelman, A. (1986). *Maus: A Survivor's Tale*. New York: Pantheon.

Stein, G. (1934). *The Making of Americans: The Hersland Family*. New York: Harcourt, Brace and World.

Chapter 16

Can very bad childhoods drive us crazy?

Science, ideology and taboo

John Read and Paul Hammersley

INTRODUCTION

This chapter discusses the political and ideological factors influencing research into the relationship between adverse childhood experiences and psychosis in adulthood. These factors are used, along with a critique of methodology, to understand the very different findings, and conclusions, of two recent large studies in this field.

The chapter summarises international studies of public opinion and concludes that the majority of ordinary people understand the causes of psychosis as lying in the psycho-social domain rather than the bio-genetic. We then examine who is more correct: the public or one wing of one profession (biological psychiatry) and the pharmaceutical industry? A review of the fast-growing body of relevant research literature concludes that a strong relationship between childhood trauma and adulthood psychosis has now been demonstrated beyond contention, and that the relationship appears to be a causal one, with or without a genetic predisposition. This relationship is particularly marked in relation to hallucinations, and to the content of psychotic symptoms in general.

The research and clinical implications are discussed. These include an urgent need for clinicians to assess all clients properly for trauma histories and, where abuse is identified, to offer appropriate trauma-focussed counselling. The oft-neglected implications for the prevention of psychosis are highlighted.

CONTRADICTORY FINDINGS

In 2004 two distinguished research teams each published a study examining childhood abuse and psychosis. The findings of one 'gave no support to child sexual abuse being associated with schizophrenic disorders later in life' (Spataro *et al.* 2004: 420). The authors also announced that 'the findings to date do not support an association between child sexual abuse and schizophrenia' (ibid.: 419). The other study found that adults abused as children (sexually, physically, emotionally or psychologically) were 2.5, 7.3 and 9.3 times more likely to be psychotic on the three different measures of psychosis used (Janssen *et al.* 2004). These researchers concluded: 'The results suggest that early childhood trauma increases the risk of positive psychotic symptoms. This finding fits well with recent models that suggest that early adversities may lead to psychological and biological changes that increase psychosis vulnerability' (ibid.: 38).

How can we make sense of such different outcomes and contradictory conclusions? Before examining the methodology of these two studies and the previous research literature, we will first discuss some powerful factors, sometimes ignored by researchers, that can influence what researchers find, the questions they ask in the first place and how they and subsequent reviewers interpret their findings. The same forces also influence which findings are acted upon by practitioners, professional training programmes, service funders and policymakers.

HOW OBJECTIVE IS SCIENTIFIC RESEARCH?

Contradictory findings and conclusions about 'schizophrenia' do not only occur in relation to the role of child abuse. The causes of, and solutions to, madness remain hotly contested (Bentall 2003; Geekie 2004). The debate began before the invention of schizophrenia (Read 2004a) and no resolution is on the horizon. For instance:

'Schizophrenia is a chronic, severe, and disabling brain disease.' In June 2003 this was the opening statement of the U.S. government agency, the National Institute for Mental Health, in their public information website about the topic of our book. Such an opinion can be found in most 'educational' material, from psychiatric textbooks to drug-company sponsored pamphlets. We disagree. The heightened sensitivity, unusual experiences, distress, despair, confusion and disorganisation that are currently labelled 'schizophrenic' are *not* symptoms of a medical illness. The notion that 'mental illness is an illness like any other', promulgated by biological psychiatry and the pharmaceutical industry, is not supported by research and is extremely damaging to those with this most stigmatising of psychiatric labels. . . . It is responsible for unwarranted and destructive pessimism about the chances of 'recovery', and has ignored – or even actively discouraged discussion of – what is actually going on in these people's lives, in their families, and in the societies in which they live.

(Read *et al.* 2004a: 3)

Is the 'nature–nurture' debate still important?

Some might argue that it is now so obvious that human behaviour is determined by interactions between social environment and genetic constitution that the 'nature–nurture' debate is of historical interest only. However, the relative emphasis we place on each of these essential ingredients continues to have significant consequences. The growing tendency to highlight genetic predispositions to social problems, such as criminal behaviour, alcoholism, violence and gambling, provides governments with an excuse not to fund primary prevention programmes targeted at the social causes of such problems (Davies and Burdett 2004).

Where important decisions hinge on whether problems have social causes, it remains important that research does inform the nature–nurture debate. Scientists, however, can sometimes be overly optimistic about the extent to which research actually influences the debate. There are powerful forces at work that determine not only which findings are acted upon, but also what sorts of research questions are asked and which studies are funded (Kuhn 1996).

We can also be naïve at times about the degree to which we, as researchers, are truly objective. Surrounded by ideologies and powerful economic and political interests, can any of us really claim to have reached the lofty heights of total intellectual detachment? Do some of us confuse being free from ideology with conforming to a dominant paradigm?

An extreme example

It is hard to find a more powerful example of the political motivations and consequences of the nature–nurture debate, and of the extent to which we can delude ourselves that we are following value-free scientific processes when informing that debate, than events in America and Europe just 60 years ago. On the basis of scientific psychiatric theories that many conditions and behaviours are genetically based, over half a million people were sterilised in Finland, Norway, Sweden, Denmark, Germany and the USA (Read and Masson 2004). In California there were 10,000 eugenic sterilisations by 1932, mostly for 'insanity'. Among the first to recommend these eugenic sterilisations was Eugen Bleuler, the inventor of schizophrenia (Bleuler 1911/1950; Read 2004a). The ensuing murder of several hundred thousand 'mental patients' in Europe was described by the eminent psychiatrists directly responsible (for the science and the killings) as 'mercy killing' for people they diagnosed as having lives 'of negative value'.

Attempts to narrow the gene pool in order to eliminate 'mental illnesses' are still with us, in the form of 'genetic counselling', to discourage people diagnosed as 'schizophrenic' from having children (Read and Masson 2004). The genetic theories themselves have many other consequences beyond genetic counselling. A particularly grotesque illustration of the continuing power of the 'medical model' of madness to distort reality in general, particularly in terms of ignoring trauma, is the recent discovery that about two thirds of Israel's psychiatric inpatients are Holocaust survivors and that many or most have been, for fifty years, diagnosed as having the genetically-based illness 'schizophrenia' and treated accordingly (Read and Masson 2004).

Indeed, the latter part of the 20th century saw a major tipping of the balance in the nature–nurture debate about the causes of human distress towards genetic and other biological explanations. More and more problems of living, from being very worried or very sad to drinking too much or eating too little, were redefined as 'mental illnesses' (Mosher *et al.* 2004). It has become almost impossible to discuss the issues without using the term 'mental illness'.

The last 50 years have 'witnessed the relentless pursuit of biological explanations for psychosis' (Martindale 2004: ii). What caused this dramatic increase in emphasis on biology? One factor is the political convenience of not having to pay attention to, or spend money on, the social causes of human distress. Furthermore, as individuals we are all sometimes tempted to avoid facing painful life events and to accept, instead, a medical-sounding label which explains everything away. Tremendous advances in our technological ability to study chromosomes and brains have also played a huge role. We must not forget, however, the entry of a brand new player into the nature–nurture debate. The pharmaceutical industry has much to gain from emphasising biological causes. It has done so brilliantly and ruthlessly, particularly in the field of psychosis. The first 'massive public relations foray by a pharmaceutical company into a previously small market – institutional psychiatry' was the aggressive sales campaign developed to promote the 'anti-psychotics' in the 1950s, which was then 'used time and again to sell new drugs to the psychiatric market' (Mosher *et al.* 2004: 115).

Public opinion

While some experts were lurching towards the nature end of the spectrum, the majority of the species plodded on with the same old belief that bad things happen and can drive us crazy. The public places far more emphasis on adverse life events than on biology or genetics. This has been found by studies in Australia, Austria, England, India, Ireland, Germany (east and west), New Zealand, Turkey and the USA (Read and Haslam 2004) and, most recently, in Russia and Mongolia (Dietrich *et al.* 2004). The same is true of the 1% of the public unfortunate enough to be diagnosed 'schizophrenic' (Holzinger *et al.* 2002). A London study found that the public's most endorsed causal model of schizophrenia was: 'Unusual or traumatic experiences or the failure to negotiate some critical stage of emotional development'. This was followed by: 'Social, economic, and family pressures . . . Subjects agreed that schizophrenic behaviour had some meaning and was neither random nor simply a symptom of an illness' (Furnham and Bower 1992: 206).

The public also prefers psycho-social solutions to medical interventions (Read and Haslam 2004). Reasons for rejecting anti-psychotic drugs include 'lack efficacy because they do not deal with the roots of the problem,' and 'prescribed for the wrong reasons (e.g., to avoid talking about problems, to make people believe things are better than they are, as a straitjacket)' (Jorm et al. 2000: 404). In Canada 90% or more endorse work/recreation opportunities, involvement of family/friends and group homes. Only 49% endorse drug treatment and 42% (only 18% of relatives) endorse psychiatric hospitals (Thompson et al. 2002). When Austrians are asked what they would do if a relative became psychotic the most common response is: 'Talk to them' (Jorm et al. 2000: 403).

Some experts genuinely think that the atypical position on the nature–nurture dimension adopted by biological psychiatry and the drug companies has been arrived at entirely by value-free scientific research, while the position adopted by everyone else in the world is just an ill-informed opinion. (When patients adopt the same view as the rest of the public this is evidence of their 'lack of insight'.) The term 'mental health literacy' (Jorm 2000), describing level of agreement with bio-genetic ideology, has been coined to bemoan the public's ignorance. 'What is most surprising is that psychological interventions are seen by the public as highly effective for psychotic disorders' (ibid.: 397). 'If the public's mental health literacy is not improved, this may hinder public acceptance of evidence-based mental health care' (ibid.: 396), meaning drugs.

One of the first research papers emanating from the World Psychiatric Association's campaign to improve attitudes about schizophrenia portrays as 'sophisticated' and 'knowledgeable' the belief that schizophrenia is a 'debilitating disease' caused by a biochemical imbalance (Thompson et al. 2002). The study was funded by drug company Eli Lilly.

Such destigmatisation programmes are another example of the implications, in the real world, of academic debates about nature and nurture. They also illustrate the ability of scientists and vested interests to ignore the relevant research. Those responsible, for decades, for trying unsuccessfully to persuade us all that 'mental illness is an illness like any other' ignore findings from a raft of studies showing that the more we do accept this 'medical model' ideology the more frightened, prejudiced and distancing we become (Dietrich et al. 2004; Read and Haslam 2004; Walker and Read 2002).

Researching two taboos

So the two studies with which we began this chapter did not occur within some magical bubble protecting the scientists involved from professional or political forces and personal preconceptions. In fact an ideologically-based bubble, originating with the preconception that 'schizophrenia' is a genetic-ally-based brain disease, for decades protected the topic of these studies from being researched at all (Read 1997). The many factors involved in keeping the possibility of a relationship between child abuse and psychosis virtually taboo included:

- the difficulty brain researchers have understanding that the environment can alter the neurology and biochemistry of the brain – especially in childhood (Read *et al.* 2001a) – leading to the faulty assumption that brain dysfunction is automatically evidence of a bio-genetic illness
- the illusion that the bio-psycho-social/vulnerability-stress model is a genuine integration of paradigms, when it is actually a relegation of psycho-social factors to the peripheral role of trigger or exacerbator (Read *et al.* 2004b, Read *et al.* 2001a)
- ignoring the fact that the original vulnerability-stress model clearly included 'acquired vulnerability' which included trauma and family experiences (Zubin and Spring 1977: 109)
- the distorting influence of the dependence of the psychiatric profession's journals, conferences and research institutions on drug company money (Mosher *et al.* 2004)
- drug company promulgation of the 'fact' that schizophrenia is a genetically-based brain disease with little or nothing to do with life events (Mosher *et al.* 2004; Read *et al.* 2004a)
- psychosis researchers excluding trauma as a causal variable (Read 1997)
- trauma researchers excluding psychosis as an outcome variable (ibid.)
- reviewers not paying attention to research that didn't match their preconceptions (ibid.)
- the reinterpretation of psychotic symptoms, if trauma is identified, as non-psychotic, and subsequent re-diagnosis (eg to PTSD; ibid.)
- the positing of spurious intervening variables, such as suggesting that being abused as a child has a genetic predisposition similar to that posited for 'schizophrenia' (ibid.)
- fear of being accused of 'family-blaming' (Aderhold and Gottwalz 2004; Read *et al.* 2004b)
- the failure of mental health staff to ask about abuse (Hammersley *et al.* 2004; Muenzenmaier *et al.* 1993; Read in press; Wurr and Partridge 1996), particularly if the client is diagnosed 'schizophrenic' (Read and Fraser 1998a) or the clinician has a strong bio-genetic orientation (Young *et al.* 2001)
- the failure to respond appropriately when clients do disclose abuse (Agar and Read 2002; Read in press), thereby preventing any learning about whether clients improve with abuse-focussed psychotherapy rather than just medication, especially if the client has a diagnosis indicative of psychosis (Read and Fraser 1998b) or the clinician is either a psychiatrist

(Lab *et al.* 2000) or has a strongly bio-genetic understanding of schizo-phrenia (Cavanagh *et al.* 2004)
• minimising of the prevalence and effects of child abuse in general (Herman 1992).

The last reason in the list represents a second, equally powerful, taboo that operates in tandem with the 'thou shalt not research the psychosocial causes of a known genetic illness' imperative. This ability to minimise the prevalence and effects of child abuse has manifested itself in many forms (Herman 1992). The archetypal distortion was committed by Freud (1896/1962: 203). After having observed that 'at the bottom of every case of hysteria there are one or more occurrences of premature sexual experience', Freud, under pressure from his profession, retracted and blamed instead children's fantasies about sex with their parents (Masson 2003). Just thirty years ago the leading psychiatric textbook in the USA reported the incidence of incest as one per million (Henderson 1975). When research in the 1980s corrected this psychiatric silliness some people, understandably, could not accept the distressing statistics that emerged. We witnessed a backlash in the form of an organised international movement claiming, wrongly, that it is easy to plant abuse memories and that mental health staff frequently do so, exaggerating the frequency with which inaccurate allegations are made and vilifying everyone involved in what they like to denigrate with the term 'the sexual abuse industry'.

Contrary to the notion that many of us are busy trying to 'plant' abuse memories in our clients, study after study shows that the majority of child abuse cases go undetected by mental health services (Read in press; Read and Fraser 1998a).

All in all, then, this is an unsafe battleground on which to try to demonstrate the role of nurture (or, more accurately, the lack thereof) in the aetiology of madness. There are so many reasons why the experts do not want to see what so many of our clients have told us, and what so many people tell the slowly increasing number of researchers who ask.

It's not just child abuse

Before returning to our two contradictory studies and the rest of the research findings, we should note that child abuse is just one of many psycho-social issues that have been clearly demonstrated to play a causal role in psychosis. Poverty (Harrison *et al.* 2001; Read 2004b), racism (Janssen *et al.* 2003; Read 2004b) and hostility or communication difficulties within families (Read *et al.* 2004b) are among the proven causal factors which, in our current obsession with neurons, chromosomes and drugs, are frequently ignored, minimised or obfuscated.

MAKING SENSE OF THE RESEARCH

Spataro et *al.*

The first of our two 2004 studies examined 1612 documented cases of child sexual abuse and recorded subsequent rates of treatment for various diagnoses, and compared these to treatment rates among the general population (Spataro *et al.* 2004). The abused males were 1.3 times more likely, and the abused females 1.5 times more likely, to have been treated for a 'schizophrenic disorder' than the general population. However these differences 'did not reach significance' (419). Therefore the conclusion that the study 'gave no support to child sexual abuse being associated with schizophrenic disorders later in life' (420) seems, at first glance, reasonable.

Professor Paul Mullen, one of Spataro's co-researchers, has done more than most researchers to demonstrate and publicise the prevalence and effects of child sexual abuse (CSA) and other adversities in childhood. He responds firmly to colleagues who minimise these effects. He recently wrote the following about a paper arguing that CSA is unrelated to depression and anxiety disorders:

> There are still those who would obscure and obfuscate the dreadful consequences of childhood abuse in general, and child sexual abuse in particular, and it would be shameful if such people were encouraged, however inadvertently, by this study. . . . If in science in general, and epidemiology in particular, you keep asking the same question over and over again eventually you will, purely from the play of chance, obtain an answer at variance with the previous answers. . . . The question that needs addressing is why this study failed to go where so many have gone before. The answer is almost certainly to be found in the methodology.
>
> (Mullen 2003: 340–1)

Might these statements also apply to the study which found no relationship between child sexual abuse and schizophrenia? Spataro, Mullen and colleagues list numerous limitations to their methodology, all of which, they acknowledge, 'reduce the probability of finding a positive association between CSA and mental disorders' (Spataro *et al.* 2004: 419). These limitations included: the presence of people in the general population sample who had suffered CSA, and the inclusion of only severe forms of CSA. Of crucial relevance to the topic at hand was the fact that 'the average age of our subjects was in their early 20s thus many have yet to pass the peak years for developing schizophrenic and related disorders' (419). In fact the general population sample was significantly older than the subjects and had, therefore, a significantly greater chance of developing schizophrenia.

A further serious problem with the study was not mentioned. All the abuse cases had come to the attention of the police or child protection services and, after examination by forensic doctors, the individuals had been 'ascertained as having been sexually abused' (416). The researchers understood that 'those whose sexual abuse comes to official notice at the time are a minority' (418). Indeed, in a recent study of 191 women who had suffered CSA the average time taken to tell anyone at all, let alone legal authorities, was 16 years (McGregor 2003). What Spataro *et al.* missed is that, after coming to the attention of the authorities, the majority would have been removed from the abusive situation. Many would have received some form of early therapeutic intervention. Early identification of, and appropriate response to, child abuse are significant predictors of better long-term outcomes, partly via the resultant impact on attributions of blame for the abuse (Barker-Collo and Read 2003). Therefore, this major sample bias will have further significantly reduced the strength of the relationship between CSA and subsequent treatment for schizophrenia found in this particular study (Read and Hammersley 2005).

We therefore agree with the authors when they point out, specifically in relation to their schizophrenia finding: 'Care must be taken in interpreting this and other negative findings' (419). Nevertheless they categorically stated that their study 'gave no support to child sexual abuse being associated with schizophrenic disorders later in life' (420). How many times will we see this sentence cited by 'those who would obscure and obfuscate the dreadful consequences of childhood abuse' in the coming years? Will obfuscators also cite all the study's limitations and remind readers that despite them all, the men who had been sexually abused as children were 1.3 times more likely, and the abused females 1.5 times more likely, to have been treated for a 'schizophrenic disorder' than the general population?

Now let's address the question of whether this was, like the study about anxiety and depression that Mullen quite rightly found so worrying, an aberrant finding flying in the face of previous research. Spataro *et al.* are adamant it was not. They bluntly assert, without even feeling the need to try to support the statement in any way: 'The findings to date do not support an association between child sexual abuse and schizophrenia.' They add that this hypothesis 'has claimed considerable public, if not professional, attention' (Spataro *et al.* 2004: 419). This raises the question of whether professional attention may have been somewhat selective.

Spataro and colleagues also failed to find, in their own study, the repeatedly documented relationship between child abuse and alcohol- and drug-related disorders. In this instance, however, they were quick to see this finding as aberrant, pointing out that it 'runs counter to much of the existing literature' (ibid.), to which they obviously have paid attention.

With just a modicum of attention one can find a host of studies documenting a relationship between child abuse and psychosis in general, and the symptoms of schizophrenia in particular. At least two reviews of these studies were available for Spataro *et al.* to consult (Morrison *et al.* 2003; Read, 1997). They cited neither.

Prevalence of child abuse in psychiatric populations

The first type of evidence, albeit indirect, is the extraordinarily high percentage of child abuse cases found in samples of adult and adolescent users of mental health services. A recent review of the prevalence of child abuse among psychiatric patients found no less than 40 studies on which to draw – even when limiting the review, in order to focus on samples with high proportions of psychosis, to inpatient samples and samples of outpatients in which at least 50% had diagnoses of psychosis. In these 40 studies the majority – 69% of the women and 60% of the men – had suffered either CSA or child physical abuse (CPA; Read *et al.* 2004c).

These are probably underestimates because patients under-report child abuse to mental health staff (Dill *et al.* 1991; Read in press). When researchers surveyed female inpatients after they returned to the community 85% disclosed CSA (Mullen *et al.* 1993). Furthermore the 69% and 60% findings do not include neglect or psychological/emotional abuse (Thompson and Kaplan, 1999). The review found rates of childhood neglect for adult inpatients ranging from 22% to 62% (Read *et al.* 2004c). In a community survey, women emotionally abused as children were five times more likely to have had a psychiatric admission (Mullen *et al.* 1996). In a study of adult outpatient 'schizophrenics' 35% had suffered emotional abuse as children, 42% physical neglect and 73% emotional neglect (Holowka *et al.* 2003).

Child abuse and severity of disturbance

Of course not all service users, even in inpatient samples, are diagnosed psychotic. It would be surprising, however, if the relationship of child abuse to specific diagnoses in the 40 samples was weaker for the more severe diagnoses like 'schizophrenia' than for the other diagnoses, because child abuse is related to severity of disturbance no matter how you measure it. Psychiatric patients subjected to CSA or CPA have earlier first admissions, longer and more frequent hospitalisations, spend longer in seclusion, receive more medication, are more likely to try to kill themselves and to self-mutilate, and have higher global symptom severity (Beck and van der Kolk 1987; Briere *et al.* 1997; Lipschitz *et al.* 1999; Mullen *et al.* 1993; Pettigrew and Burcham 1997; Read 1998; Read *et al.* 2001b; Sansonnet-Hayden *et al.* 1987).

While some studies find that psychosis, including schizophrenia, is no more or less related to child abuse than other diagnoses (e.g. Ritsher *et al.* 1997; Wurr and Partridge 1996), we document below some of the many studies showing that psychosis and schizophrenia are more strongly related than other diagnoses to child abuse.

Research measures of psychosis and schizophrenia

The 2004 review mentioned above identified nine studies showing that abuse survivors score higher than non-abused people on the schizophrenia and paranoia scales of the Minnesota Multiphasic Personality Inventory (MMPI) or the psychosis scale of the Symptom Checklist 90-Revised (SCL-R). In five of the nine these scales were more strongly related to abuse than the other clinical scales (Read *et al.* 2004c).

Clinical diagnoses

If one is paying attention one can find a large number of studies, using actual clinical diagnoses, producing similar findings to the MMPI and SCL-R studies (Read *et al.* 2004c). Here are some of them.

In a sample of adult outpatients diagnosed 'schizophrenic' 85% had suffered some form of childhood abuse or neglect (73% emotional neglect, 50% sexual abuse; Holowka *et al.* 2003). In a study of over 500 child guidance clinic attenders, 35% of those who became 'schizophrenic' as adults had been removed from home because of neglect – double the rate of any other diagnosis (Robins 1996). A study of over 1000 people found that those whose mother–child interactions when they were three were characterised by 'harshness towards the child; no effort to help the child' were, at age 26, significantly more likely to be diagnosed with 'schizophreniform disorder' but not mania, anxiety or depression (Cannon *et al.* 2002). Among 139 female outpatients 78% of those diagnosed 'schizophrenic' had suffered CSA; the percentages for other diagnoses were: panic disorder 26%, anxiety disorders 30% and major depressive disorder 42% (Friedman *et al.* 2002). In a study of 426 inpatients diagnosed psychotic (Neria *et al.* 2002), the CPA rate for the women was 29%, compared to 5% in the general population using identical methods (Kessler *et al.* 1995). Among children admitted to a psychiatric hospital, 77% of those who had been sexually abused were diagnosed psychotic, compared to 10% of the other children (Livingston 1987).

Hallucinations and delusions

Since its invention, it has been repeatedly demonstrated that 'schizophrenia' has none of the attributes of a meaningful construct required by scientific disciplines other than psychiatry (Bentall 2003). After decades of psychiatry and psychology ignoring its disjunctive nature (whereby different people can be diagnosed without having anything at all in common), and its poor reliability and validity (Read 2004c), some researchers have put aside the concept and, instead, study less heterogeneous and better-defined constructs, such as hallucinations and delusions (Bentall 2004). Bentall (2003) prefers to call these 'complaints' rather than use the paradigm-driven term 'symptoms'.

Several studies have now shown that the complaints of people diagnosed 'schizophrenic' are more common in those who suffered CSA or CPA, both in clinical samples (Muenzenmaier *et al.* 1993; Read and Argyle 1999; Read *et al.* 2003; Ross *et al.* 1994) and in the general population (Berenbaum 1999; Janssen *et al.* 2004; Ross and Joshi 1992).

In a landmark study inpatients diagnosed 'schizophrenic' that had suffered CSA or CPA had significantly more 'positive symptoms' of schizophrenia (but slightly fewer 'negative symptoms') than those not abused. The complaints significantly related to abuse were, in order of the strength of the relationship: voices commenting, ideas of reference, thought insertion, paranoid ideation, reading others' minds and visual hallucinations (Ross *et al.* 1994).

Recent reviews have confirmed the particularly strong relationship with auditory hallucinations, particularly voices commenting and command hallucinations (Read *et al.* 2004c; Read *et al.* 2005). A study of 200 outpatients found that those subjected to CSA were significantly more likely than non-abused patients to hear voices commenting and commands to harm self or others, and to have visual, tactile or olfactory hallucinations. The same held true for CPA (Read *et al.* 2003). The relationship between CSA and psychotic 'symptoms' holds across diagnostic boundaries. A study of adult bipolar affective disorder patients found that those subjected to CSA were twice as likely to have auditory hallucinations and six times as likely to hear voices commenting (Hammersley *et al.* 2003).

These findings that adults abused as children are more likely to hallucinate have been replicated with adolescent and child inpatients (Famularo *et al.* 1992; Sansonnet-Hayden *et al.* 1987). Hallucinations are particularly common in incest survivors (Ellenson 1985; Ensink 1992; Heins *et al.* 1990; Read and Argyle 1999).

A large prospective general population study found that adults abused as children are four times more likely than non-abused people to experience psychotic hallucinations and 3.9 times more likely to experience psychotic delusions (Janssen *et al.* 2004). However, after controlling for other diagnoses the relationship with hallucinations (but not the relationship with delusions) became 'statistically imprecise' – falling to 2.5 times more likely. This may reflect the frequency with which hallucinations are also present in other diagnoses, including dissociative disorders (Moskowitz *et al.* in press; Ross 2004; Ross and Joshi 1992) and PTSD (Morrison *et al.* 2003).

The recent reviews confirm this study's finding that child abuse is related to delusions, but suggest this is more the case for paranoid delusions than for grandiose delusions. The reviews find little evidence of a relationship with thought disorder. There is no data yet about catatonia. A consistent finding is that there appears to be no relationship with the 'negative symptoms' of 'schizophrenia' (Read *et al.* 2004c; Read *et al.* 2005).

The content and meaning of the complaints

One of the saddest consequences of the dominance of bio-genetic ideology is that many clinicians have been taught that it is not necessary to listen to what people are actually saying about their experiences. Once they have identified the 'symptoms of schizophrenia' they automatically feel they know what the problem, and the solution, is. This ignoring of the content and meaning of people's complaints is paralleled in researchers, who are under the additional pressure to produce numbers that can be tested for statistical significance. The human significance is lost.

In severely maltreated children 'the content of the reported visual and/or auditory hallucinations or illusions tended to be strongly reminiscent of concrete details of episodes of traumatic victimization' (Famularo *et al.* 1992: 866). The same has been found in adolescents (Sansonnet-Hayden *et al.* 1987) and adults (Heins *et al.* 1990). Ensink found that the hallucinations of adult CSA survivors contain both 'flash-back elements and more symbolic representations' of traumatic experiences (1992: 126). High rates of sexual delusions have been found in incest survivors diagnosed psychotic (Beck and van der Kolk 1987). In a New Zealand study of 200 outpatients there was a significant relationship between child abuse and content pertaining to evil or the devil (Read *et al.* 2003).

In a smaller New Zealand study the content of half (54%) of the hallucinations and delusions of abused inpatients were obviously abuse-related. For example, a woman who had been sexually abused by her father from the age of five heard 'male voices outside her head and screaming children's voices inside her head' (Read and Argyle 1999). Other studies have also presented numerous examples of the content of hallucinations and delusions in abuse survivors being clearly abuse-related (Beck and van der Kolk 1987; Ensink 1992; Heins *et al.* 1990; Read *et al.* 2003).

Controlling for mediating variables

Many of the studies discussed thus far are correlational. While these studies have been instrumental in breaking the silence about the fact that there clearly is a relationship between child abuse and 'schizophrenia', they can't tell us whether the relationship is a causal one. To address causality researchers must control for other factors that might account for the relationship, such as other adverse events or circumstances in childhood, and subsequent re-victimisation.

After controlling for other childhood disruptions and disadvantages, women whose CSA involved intercourse were 12 times more likely than non-abused females to have had psychiatric admissions and 26 times more likely to have tried to kill themselves (Mullen *et al.* 1993). In a study of female psychiatric patients (Briere *et al.* 1997), 53% of those who had suffered

CSA had 'nonmanic psychotic disorders (e.g., schizophrenia, psychosis not otherwise specified)' compared to 25% of those who were not victims of CSA. After controlling for 'the potential effects of demographic variables, most of which also predict victimisation and/or psychiatric outcome' (Read and Argyle 1999: 1469) CSA was still related to psychotic disorders ($p = .001$).

Another study controlled for subsequent re-traumatisation in the form of rapes or attempted rapes (ASA) and serious physical assaults (APA) after age 16. In a regression analysis, childhood abuse (CSA or CPA) remained a significant predictor of hallucinations even after taking into account (i.e. without) APA and ASA. This was the case for auditory hallucinations in general and voices commenting in particular, and also for tactile hallucinations (Read *et al.* 2003).

However, the study that has thus far controlled for the largest range of confounding variables is the second of the two with which we began this chapter (Janssen *et al.* 2004).

Janssen et *al.*

In a prospective study of a general population sample, 4045 adults assessed as psychosis-free were interviewed again three years later. Those abused as children (sexually, physically, emotionally or psychologically) were 13 times more likely to have developed Brief Psychiatric Rating Scale pathology-level psychosis. After controlling for age, sex, level of education, unemployment, urbanicity, ethnicity, discrimination, marital status, presence of any psychiatric diagnosis, life-time drug use, and positive psychotic symptoms or mental health care in first-degree relatives, those who had been abused as children were still 9.3 times more likely than non-abused participants to have developed pathology level psychosis.

Dose response

Yet another source of evidence for the relationship between child abuse and 'schizophrenia', and the complaints associated with this diagnosis, are studies showing that the more severe the abuse the stronger the relationship (as is the case for other diagnoses). For example, incest (compared to extra-familial CSA) or being subjected to both CSA and CPA (compared to just one) are related to significantly higher rates of hallucinations (Read and Argyle 1999; Read *et al.* 2003). In a study of incest survivors, cumulative trauma score (multiple types of abuse and multiple abusers) was significantly higher in those who later experienced auditory or visual hallucinations (Ensink 1992). Among non-patients predisposition to auditory, but not visual, hallucinations was significantly higher in those who reported multiple trauma (Morrison and Petersen 2003). The 'dose response' becomes even more evident when re-traumatisation is included. In one study outpatients who had experienced both CSA and ASA had particularly high rates of the following complaints: hallucinations – non-abused 18.5%, CSA + ASA 86%; delusions – non-abused 27%, CSA + ASA 71%; thought disorder – non-abused 13%, CSA + ASA 71% (Read *et al.* 2003).

Janssen *et al.*'s findings dramatically confirm the dose response. Those who had experienced child abuse of mild severity were 2.0 times more likely than non-abuse participants to have pathology-level psychosis, compared to 10.6 for those who had suffered moderate-severity abuse. Those who had suffered high-severity abuse were 48.4 times more likely to have pathology-level psychosis.

Genetic predisposition?

By controlling for psychotic symptoms in first-degree relatives, and still finding that abused people are nine times more likely to become psychotic, Janssen *et al.* provide data contrary to the view that only people with a genetic predisposition go mad. The same findings emerge from research demonstrating the relationship between urban living and schizophrenia (Lewis *et al.* 1992; Mortensen *et al.* 1999). Children growing up in deprived economic conditions with no family history of psychosis are seven times more likely to develop schizophrenia than non-deprived children (Harrison *et al.* 2001). One of the rare studies of the genetics of schizophrenia that evaluated the families adopting the offspring of parents diagnosed 'schizophrenic' found that only 4% of those children raised by 'healthy adoptive' families were assessed as 'severe + psychotic', compared to 34% of the children raised by 'disturbed' adoptive families (e.g. 'expelling relation to offspring'), leading to the conclusion that 'in healthy rearing families the adoptees have little serious mental illness, whether or not their biological mothers were schizophrenic' (Tienari 1991: 463).

The century-old assumption that 'schizophrenia' is a predominantly bio-genetically based phenomenon seems to have a blinding effect on the amount of attention schizophrenia researchers give to studies about child abuse and neglect. It is a dangerously weak premise on which to base such important presuppositions. When all the methodological flaws in the studies sustaining this notion of a genetic predisposition are taken into account, there is no robust evidence of its existence (Joseph 2004). It seems that combinations of bad things happening early enough, often enough, or sufficiently severely, can – as the public have always believed – drive us crazy, with or without a genetic predisposition.

CONCLUSIONS

It will be interesting to see which of the two large prospective studies published in 2004 receives more attention. Will it be the one showing that severely abused children are 48 times more likely to develop psychosis than non-abused children, or the one that claims there is no evidence of such a relationship?

The theoretical implications of what we pay attention to are profound. They have been outlined repeatedly elsewhere (e.g. Bentall 2003; Morrison *et al.* 2003; Read and Ross 2003). One recent review identified 39 research topics now awaiting investigation as a result of having broken the taboo that there is nothing to research here (Read *et al.* 2004c).

The clinical implications are obvious. A range of effective, evidence-based, psycho-social treatments for psychosis are available (Aderhold and Gottwalz 2004; Gottdiener 2004; Johannessen 2004; Martindale *et al.* 2000; Morrison 2002, 2004; Mosher 2004; Silver *et al.* 2004) and must be made available to everyone, including those who have been traumatised as children (Read and Ross 2003). We saw earlier that the public prefers such treatments to anti-psychotic drugs, which are neither as effective nor as safe as the drug companies would have us believe (Mosher *et al.* 2004; Ross and Read 2004). People diagnosed psychotic must be offered real choices about treatment approaches. First, however, we must move beyond ideologically-based pre-suppositions and learn to ask people with psychotic complaints about trauma (Hammersley *et al.* 2004; Read in press; Thompson and Kaplan 1999; Young *et al.* 2001).

The final words of the study that we hope, despite the forces aligned against it, will receive the attention it merits, are:

> The importance of identifying patients who have abuse histories is undeniably important in accurately diagnosing and treating symptoms and in intervening effectively with maladaptive interpersonal patterns. Many researchers and clinicians have called for routine abuse inquiry in all mental health settings. The results of this study lend credence to this suggestion.
>
> (Janssen *et al.* 2004: 43)

Less obvious, perhaps, are the political implications of continuing to attend selectively only to those research findings that appear to give credibility to our current over-emphasis on 'nature' at the expense of 'nurture'. Not least among these is the probability of increased funding for programmes designed to improve the quality of lives of children and their families and thereby reduce rates of psychosis in future generations (Davies and Burdett 2004). Indeed, it is entirely possible to conclude that the data gathered by Spataro, Mullen and their colleagues, rather than showing no significant relationship between child abuse and psychosis, actually demonstrate that removing children from abusive situations offers a high degree of protection from subsequent adult psychosis.

Things *are* changing. The relationship between child abuse and the complaints of people diagnosed 'schizophrenic' is finally, after decades of being ignored, firmly on the research agenda. British cognitive psychologists have been among the first to understand the issues and include them in their research and reviews (e.g. Bentall 2003; Freeman and Garety 2002; Morrison *et al.* 2003). An entire book has just been devoted to *Understanding Trauma and Psychosis* (Larkin and Morrison in press). Another new book, positing a trauma-based dissociative sub-type of schizophrenia, concludes that there is a large body of supporting data for a trauma model of psychosis (Ross 2004). Efforts are underway to see that *DSM-V* reflects the fact that psychotic symptoms can be traumatic in origin and dissociative in kind (Moskowtiz *et al.* in press). Some brain researchers are beginning to see the significance of the fact that the biochemical and neurological deficits found in adults diagnosed 'schizophrenic' are very similar to those found in traumatised children (Read *et al.* 2001a).

Indeed things have changed so much that studies are appearing at a rapidly accelerating pace. Many were published between the original writing of this chapter and publication of this book (e.g. Whitfield 2005). These recent studies are reviewed by Read *et al.* (2005). One of them found that, among 8580 British adults, those with a psychotic disorder were 15 times more likely than people with no psychiatric disorder to have suffered sexual abuse. As in many previous studies the relationship of sexual abuse to psychosis was stronger than its relationship to other disorders. Other victimisation experiences in childhood were also strongly related to psychosis in adulthood. Time in a children's institution was 12 times more common in those with psychosis than in those with no disorder; running away from home was 11 times more likely; violence in the home nine times more likely; and bullying four times more likely. Even after controlling for the interrelationships between these and other adverse events sexual abuse remained significantly related to psychosis ($p = .001$), and was the most strongly related to psychosis of all the events. The authors cautiously concluded: 'This is suggestive of a social contribution to aetiology' (Bebbington *et al.* 2004: 220).

We end with the statements of five users of mental health services. They are taken from a New Zealand survey, in which 45% of the respondents had been diagnosed as having schizophrenia and 40% with bipolar disorder (Lothian and Read 2002). Consistent with the studies mentioned earlier, two thirds reported sexual, physical or emotional abuse, but only 20% had been asked about abuse when assessed by mental health staff. The majority (69%) of those who reported abuse thought the abuse was connected to their mental health problems. Only 17% thought their primary clinician saw the connection. They were also significantly less likely than the non-abused participants to believe that their diagnosis accurately described their problems.

The stress involved in being physically and sexually abused and surviving into adulthood burdened with all the shame and memories caused massive distress and crisis.

The multiple abuse that followed went on and on whilst I was going in and out of hospital.

I think there was an assumption that I had a mental illness and, you know, because I wasn't saying anything about my abuse I'd suffered no-one knew.

There were so many doctors and registrars and nurses and social workers in your life asking you about the same thing, mental, mental, mental, but not asking you why.

I just wish they would have said what happened to you, what happened, but they didn't.

REFERENCES

Aderhold, V. and Gottwalz, E. (2004). Family therapy and schizophrenia: Replacing ideology with openness. In J. Read *et al.* (eds) *Models of Madness.* Hove, UK: Brunner-Routledge.

Agar, K. and Read, J. (2002). What happens when people disclose sexual or physical abuse to staff at a community mental health centre? *International Journal of Mental Health Nursing* 11: 70–9.

Barker-Collo, S. and Read, J. (2003). Models of response to childhood sexual abuse: Their implications for treatment. *Trauma, Violence and Abuse* 4: 95–111.

Bebbington P. *et al.* (2004) Psychosis, victimization and childhood disadvantage: Evidence from the second British National Survey of Psychiatric Morbidity. *British Journal of Psychiatry* 185: 220–26.

Beck, J. and van der Kolk, B. (1987). Reports of childhood incest and current behavior of chronically hospitalized psychotic women. *American Journal of Psychiatry* 144: 1474–6.

Bentall, R. (2003). *Madness Explained: Psychosis and Human Nature.* London: Penguin.

Bentall, R. (2004). Abandoning the concept of schizophrenia: The cognitive psychology of hallucinations and delusions. In J. Read *et al.* (eds) *Models of Madness.* Hove, UK: Brunner-Routledge.

Berenbaum, H. (1999). Peculiarity and reported child maltreatment. *Psychiatry* 62: 21–35.

Bleuler, E. (1911/1950). *Dementia Praecox or the Group of Schizophrenias* (translated by J. Zinkin). New York: International Universities.

Briere, J. *et al.* (1997). Lifetime victimization history, demographics and clinical status in female psychiatric emergency room patients. *Journal of Nervous and Mental Disease* 185: 95–101.

Cannon, M. *et al.* (2002). Evidence for early-childhood, pan-developmental impairment specific to schizophreniform disorder. *Archives of General Psychiatry* 59: 449–56.

Cavanagh, M. *et al.* (2004). Childhood abuse inquiry and response: A New Zealand training programme. *New Zealand Journal of Psychology* 33: 137–44.

Davies, E. and Burdett, J. (2004). Preventing 'schizophrenia': Creating the conditions for saner societies. In J. Read *et al.* (eds) *Models of Madness*. Hove, UK: Brunner-Routledge.

Dietrich, S. *et al.* (2004). The relationships between public causal beliefs and social distance toward mentally ill people. *Australian and New Zealand Journal of Psychiatry* 38: 348–54.

Dill, D. *et al.* (1991). The reliability of abuse history reports: A comparison of two inquiry formats. *Comprehensive Psychiatry* 32: 166–9.

Ellenson. G. (1985). Detecting a history of incest. *Social Casework*, November, 525–32.

Ensink, B. (1992). *Confusing Realities*. Amsterdam: Vu University.

Famularo, R. *et al.* (1992). Psychiatric diagnoses of maltreated children: Preliminary findings. *Journal of the American Academy of Child and Adolescent Psychiatry* 31: 863–7.

Freeman, D. and Garety, P. A. (2002). Cognitive therapy for an individual with a long-standing persecutory delusion: Incorporating emotional processes into a multi-factorial perspective on delusional beliefs. In A. P. Morrison (ed.) *A Casebook of Cognitive Therapy for Psychosis*. New York: Brunner-Routledge.

Friedman, S. *et al.* (2002). The incidence and influence of early traumatic life events in patients with panic disorder: A comparison with other psychiatric outpatients. *Anxiety Disorders* 16: 259–72.

Freud, S. (1896/1962). The aetiology of hysteria. In *The Standard Edition of the Complete Psychological Works of Sigmund Freud Vol. 3* (edited and translated by J. Strachey). London: Hogarth Press.

Furnham, A. and Bower, P. (1992). A comparison of academic and lay theories of schizophrenia. *British Journal of Psychiatry* 62: 201–10.

Geekie, J. (2004). Listening to the voices we hear: Clients' understandings of psychotic experiences. In J. Read *et al.* (eds) *Models of Madness*. Hove, UK: Brunner-Routledge.

Gottdiener, W. (2004). Psychodynamic therapy for schizophrenia: Empirical support. In J. Read *et al.* (eds) *Models of Madness*. Hove, UK: Brunner-Routledge.

Hammersley, P. *et al.* (2003). Childhood traumas and hallucinations in bipolar affective disorder. *British Journal of Psychiatry* 182: 543–7.

Hammersley, P. *et al.* (2004). Learning to listen: Childhood trauma and adult psychosis. *Mental Health Practice* 7: 18–21.

Harrison, G. *et al.* (2001). Association between schizophrenia and social inequality at birth. *British Journal of Psychiatry* 179: 346–50.

Heins, T. *et al.* (1990). Persisting hallucinations following childhood sexual abuse. *Australian and New Zealand Journal of Psychiatry* 24: 561–5.

Henderson, D. (1975). Incest. In A. Freedman *et al.* (eds) *Comprehensive Textbook of Psychiatry* (2nd ed.). Baltimore: Williams and Wilkins.

Herman, J. (1992). *Trauma and Recovery*. New York: Basic Books.

Holowka, D. *et al.* (2003). Childhood abuse and dissociative symptoms in adult schizophrenia. *Schizophrenia Research* 60: 87–90.

Holzinger, A. *et al.* (2002). Subjective illness theory and antipsychotic medication compliance by patients with schizophrenia. *Journal of Nervous and Mental Disease* 190: 597–603.

Janssen, I. *et al.* (2003). Discrimination and delusional ideation. *British Journal of Psychiatry* 182: 71–6.

Janssen, I. *et al.* (2004). Childhood abuse as a risk factor for psychotic experiences. *Acta Psychiatrica Scandinavica* 109: 38–45.

Johannessen, J.-O. (2004). The development of early intervention services. In J. Read *et al.* (eds) *Models of Madness.* Hove, UK: Brunner-Routledge.

Jorm, A. (2000). Mental health literacy: Public knowledge and beliefs about mental disorders. *British Journal of Psychiatry* 177: 396–401.

Jorm, A. *et al.* (2000). Public knowledge of and attitudes to mental disorders. In G. Andrews and S. Henderson (eds) *Unmet Needs in Psychiatry.* Cambridge: Cambridge University Press.

Joseph, J. (2004). Schizophrenia and heredity: Why the emperor has no genes. In J. Read *et al.* (eds) *Models of Madness.* Hove, UK: Brunner-Routledge.

Kessler, R. *et al.* (1995). PTSD in the National Comorbidity Survey. *Archives of General Psychiatry* 52: 1048–60.

Kuhn, T. (1996). *The Structure of Scientific Revolutions* (3rd ed.). Chicago: University of Chicago Press.

Lab, D. *et al.* (2000). Mental health professionals' attitudes and practices towards male childhood sexual abuse. *Child Abuse and Neglect* 24: 391–409.

Larkin, W. and Morrison, A. (eds) (in press). *Understanding Trauma and Psychosis: New Horizons for Theory and Therapy.* Hove, UK: Brunner-Routledge.

Lewis, G. *et al.* (1992). Schizophrenia and city life. *Lancet* 340: 137–40.

Lipschitz, D. *et al.* (1999). Perceived abuse and neglect as risk factors for suicidal behavior in adolescent inpatients. *Journal of Nervous and Mental Disease* 187: 32–9.

Livingston, R. (1987). Sexually and physically abused children. *Journal of the American Academy of Child and Adolescent Psychiatry* 26: 413–5.

Lothian, J. and Read, J. (2002). Asking about abuse during mental health assessments: Clients' views and experiences. *New Zealand Journal of Psychology* 31: 98–103.

Martindale, B. (2004). The ISPS book series. In J. Read *et al.* (eds) *Models of Madness.* Hove, UK: Brunner-Routledge.

Martindale, B. *et al.* (eds) (2000). *Psychosis: Psychological Approaches and their Effectiveness.* London: Gaskell.

Masson, J. (2003). *The Assault on Truth: Freud's Suppression of the Seduction Theory.* New York: Ballantine Books.

McGregor, K. (2003). *It's a Two-Way Thing: Women Survivors of Child Sexual Abuse Describe their Therapy Experiences.* Unpublished doctoral dissertation, University of Auckland, New Zealand.

Morrison, A. (2002). *A Casebook of Cognitive Therapy for Psychosis.* London: Routledge.

Morrison, A. (2004). Cognitive therapy for people with psychosis. In J. Read *et al.* (eds) *Models of Madness.* Hove, UK: Brunner-Routledge.

Morrison, A. and Petersen, T. (2003). Trauma and metacognition as predictors of predisposition to hallucinations. *Behavioural and Cognitive Psychotherapy* 31: 235–46.

Morrison, A. *et al.* (2003). Relationships between trauma and psychosis: A review and integration. *British Journal of Clinical Psychology* 42: 331–53.

Mortensen, P. *et al.* (1999). Effects of family history and place of season of birth on the risk of schizophrenia. *New England Journal of Medicine* 340: 603–8.

Moskowitz, A. *et al.* (in press). Are psychotic symptoms traumatic in origin and dissociative in nature? In P. Dell (ed.) *Service Book for Dissociative Disorders Section of Fifth Edition of the Diagnostic and Statistical Manual.* New York: International Society for the Study of Dissociation.

Mosher, L. (2004). Non-hospital, non-drug, intervention with first-episode psychosis. In J. Read *et al.* (eds) *Models of Madness.* Hove, UK: Brunner-Routledge.

Mosher, L. *et al.* (2004). Drug companies and schizophrenia: Unbridled capitalism meets madness. In J. Read *et al.* (eds) *Models of Madness.* Hove, UK: Brunner-Routledge.

Muenzenmaier, K. *et al.* (1993). Childhood abuse and neglect among women outpatients with chronic mental illness. *Hospital and Community Psychiatry* 44: 666–70.

Mullen, P. (2003). Invited commentary: Abusive experiences and psychiatric morbidity in women primary care attenders. *British Journal of Psychiatry* 183: 340–1.

Mullen, P. *et al.* (1993). Childhood sexual abuse and mental health in adult life. *British Journal of Psychiatry* 163: 721–32.

Mullen, P. *et al.* (1996). The long-term impact of the physical, emotional, and sexual abuse of children: A community study. *Child Abuse and Neglect* 20: 7–21.

Neria, Y. *et al.* (2002). Trauma exposure and PTSD in psychosis: Findings from a first-admission cohort. *Journal of Consulting and Clinical Psychology* 70: 246–51.

Pettigrew, J. and Burcham, J. (1997). Effects of childhood sexual abuse in adult female psychiatric patients. *Australian and New Zealand Journal of Psychiatry* 31: 208–13.

Read, J. (1997). Child abuse and psychosis: A literature review and implications for professional practice. *Professional Psychology: Research and Practice* 28: 448–56.

Read, J. (1998). Child abuse and severity of disturbance among adult psychiatric inpatients. *Child Abuse and Neglect* 22: 359–68.

Read, J. (2004a). The invention of 'schizophrenia'. In J. Read *et al.* (eds) *Models of Madness.* Hove, UK: Brunner-Routledge.

Read, J. (2004b). Poverty, ethnicity and gender. In J. Read *et al.* (eds), *Models of Madness.* Hove, UK: Brunner-Routledge.

Read, J. (2004c). Does 'schizophrenia' exist? Reliability and validity. In J. Read *et al.* (eds) *Models of Madness.* Hove, UK: Brunner-Routledge.

Read, J. (in press). Breaking the silence: Learning why, when and how to ask about trauma, and how to respond to disclosures. In W. Larkin and A. Morrison (eds) *Understanding Trauma and Psychosis: New Horizons for Theory and Therapy.* Hove, UK: Brunner-Routledge.

Read, J. and Argyle, N. (1999). Hallucinations, delusions and thought disorders among adult psychiatric inpatients with a history of child abuse. *Psychiatric Services* 50: 1467–72.

Read, J. and Fraser, A. (1998a). Abuse histories of psychiatric inpatients: To ask or not to ask? *Psychiatric Services* 49: 355–9.

Read, J. and Fraser, A. (1998b). Staff response to abuse histories of psychiatric inpatients. *Australian and New Zealand Journal of Psychiatry* 32: 206–13.

Read, J. and Haslam, N. (2004). Public opinion. Bad things happen and can drive you crazy. In J. Read *et al.* (eds) *Models of Madness.* Hove, UK: Brunner-Routledge.

Read, J. and Hammersley, P. (2005). Child sexual abuse and schizophrenia (Correspondence). *British Journal of Psychiatry* 186: 76.

Read, J. and Masson, J. (2004). Genetics, eugenics and mass murder. In J. Read *et al.* (eds) *Models of Madness.* Hove, UK: Brunner-Routledge.

Read, J. and Ross, C. (2003). Psychological trauma and psychosis: Another reason why people diagnosed schizophrenic must be offered psychological therapies. *Journal of the American Academy of Psychoanalysis and Dynamic Psychiatry* 31: 247–67.

Read, J. *et al.* (2001a). The contribution of early traumatic events to schizophrenia in some patients: A traumagenic neurodevelopmental model. *Psychiatry: Interpersonal and Biological Processes* 64: 319–45.

Read, J. *et al.* (2001b). Assessing suicidality in adults: Integrating childhood trauma as a major risk factor. *Professional Psychology: Research and Practice* 32: 367–72.

Read, J. *et al.* (2003). Sexual and physical assault during childhood and adulthood as predictors of hallucinations, delusions and thought disorder. *Psychology and Psychotherapy: Theory, Research and Practice* 76: 1–22.

Read, J. *et al.* (2004a). 'Schizophrenia' is not an illness. In J. Read *et al.* (eds) *Models of Madness.* Hove, UK: Brunner-Routledge.

Read, J. *et al.* (2004b). Unhappy families. In J. Read *et al.* (eds) *Models of Madness.* Hove, UK: Brunner-Routledge.

Read, J. *et al.* (2004c). Childhood trauma, loss and stress. In J. Read *et al.* (eds) *Models of Madness.* Hove, UK: Brunner-Routledge.

Read, J. *et al.* (in press). The relationship between child abuse and psychosis: Public opinion, evidence, pathways and implications. In W. Larkin and A. Morrison (eds) *Understanding Trauma and Psychosis: New Horizons for Theory and Therapy.* Hove, UK: Brunner-Routledge.

Read, J. *et al.* (2005). Childhood trauma, psychosis and schizophrenia: A literature review with theoretical and clinical implications. *Acta Psychiatrica Scandinavica* 112: 330–50.

Ritsher, J. *et al.* (1997). A survey on issues in the lives of women with severe mental illness. *Psychiatric Services* 48: 1273–82.

Robins, L. (1996). *Deviant Children Growing Up.* London: Williams and Wilkins.

Ross, C. (2004). *Schizophrenia: Innovations in Diagnosis and Treatment.* Binghampton, NY: Haworth Press.

Ross, C. and Joshi, S. (1992). Schneiderian symptoms and childhood trauma in the general population. *Comprehensive Psychiatry* 33: 269–73.

Ross, C. and Read, J. (2004) Antipsychotic medication: Myths and facts. In J. Read *et al.* (eds) *Models of Madness: Psychological. Social and Biological Approaches to Schizophrenia.* London: Brunner-Routledge.

Ross, C. *et al.* (1994). Childhood abuse and positive symptoms of schizophrenia. *Hospital and Community Psychiatry* 45: 489–91.

Sansonnet-Hayden, H. *et al.* (1987). Sexual abuse and psychopathology in hospitalized adolescents. *Journal of the American Academy of Child and Adolescent Psychiatry* 26: 753–7.

Silver, A. *et al.* (2004). Psychodynamic psychotherapy of schizophrenia: Its history and development. In J. Read *et al.* (eds), *Models of Madness.* Hove, UK: Brunner-Routledge.

Spataro, J. *et al.* (2004). Impact of child sexual abuse on mental health: Prospective study in males and females. *British Journal of Psychiatry* 184: 416–21.

Thompson, A. *et al.* (2002). Attitudes about schizophrenia from the pilot site of the WPA worldwide campaign against the stigma of schizophrenia. *Social Psychiatry and Psychiatric Epidemiology* 37: 475–82.

Thompson, A. and Kaplan, C. (1999). Emotionally abused children presenting to child psychiatry clinics. *Child Abuse and Neglect* 23: 191–6.

Tienari, P. (1991). Interaction between genetic vulnerability and family environment. *Acta Psychiatrica Scandinavica* 84: 460–5.

Walker, I. and Read, J. (2002). The differential effectiveness of psycho-social and bio-genetic causal explanations in reducing negative attitudes towards 'mental illness'. *Psychiatry: Interpersonal and Biological Processes* 65: 313–25.

Whitfield, C. (2005). Adverse childhood experiences and hallucinations. *Child Abuse and Neglect* 29: 797–810.

Wurr, C. and Partridge, I. (1996). The prevalence of a history of childhood sexual abuse in an acute adult inpatient population. *Child Abuse and Neglect* 20: 867–72.

Young, M. *et al.* (2001). Evaluating and overcoming barriers to taking abuse histories. *Professional Psychology: Research and Practice* 32: 407–14.

Zubin, J. and Spring, B. (1977). Vulnerability: A new view of schizophrenia. *Journal of Abnormal Psychology* 86: 103–26.

Index